Berthoud Library

Fitness Information for Teens

Second Edition

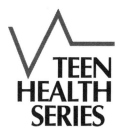

TEEN HEALTH SERIES

Second Edition

Fitness Information for Teens

Health Tips about Exercise, Physical Well-Being, and Health Maintenance

Including Facts about Conditioning, Stretching, Strength Training, Body Shape and Body Image, Sports Nutrition, and Specific Activities for Athletes and Non-Athletes

Edited by Lisa Bakewell

Omnigraphics

P.O. Box 31-1640, Detroit, MI 48231

Bibliographic Note

Because this page cannot legibly accommodate all the copyright notices, the Bibliographic Note portion of the Preface constitutes an extension of the copyright notice.

Edited by Lisa Bakewell

Teen Health Series

Karen Bellenir, *Managing Editor*
David A. Cooke, M.D., *Medical Consultant*
Elizabeth Collins, *Research and Permissions Coordinator*
Cherry Stockdale, *Permissions Assistant*
EdIndex, Services for Publishers, *Indexers*

* * *

Omnigraphics, Inc.
Matthew P. Barbour, *Senior Vice President*
Kevin M. Hayes, *Operations Manager*

* * *

Peter E. Ruffner, *Publisher*

Copyright © 2009 Omnigraphics, Inc.
ISBN 978-0-7808-1045-7

Library of Congress Cataloging-in-Publication Data

Fitness information for teens : health tips about exercise, physical well-being, and health maintenance including facts about conditioning, stretching, strength training, body shape and body image, sports nutrition, and specific activities for athletes and non-athletes / edited by Lisa Bakewell. -- 2nd ed.
    p. cm.
  Includes bibliographical references and index.
  Summary: "Provides basic consumer health information for teens on maintaining health through physical activity. Includes index, resource information and recommendations for further reading"--Provided by publisher.
   ISBN 978-0-7808-1045-7 (hard cover : alk. paper) 1. Physical fitness for youth. I. Bakewell, Lisa.
  RJ133.F58 2008
  613.7'043--dc22
                                                                2008031334

Table Of Contents

Part Three: Activities To Try

Part Four: Maintaining Health And Fitness

Part Five: Avoiding Fitness Busters

Part Six: If You Need More Information

Preface

About This Book

According to the U.S. Department of Health and Human Services, physical inactivity contributes to obesity, one of the most serious chronic health conditions threatening the nation today. The President's Council on Physical Fitness and Sports (PCPFS) says that adolescence itself is a risk factor for physical inactivity because, during the teen years, opportunities to participate in organized sports decrease and fewer hours are spent in physical education classes. Additionally, teens walk less once they start driving, and activities like watching television, listening to music, playing video games, and online computing can lead to the development of a sedentary lifestyle.

Fitness can impact a teen's schoolwork, job opportunities, and social activities because teens who are fit tend to feel better, physically and mentally, and perform daily activities with less fatigue. Fitness also helps prevent or delay the development of disorders such as diabetes, high blood pressure, heart disease, osteoporosis, stroke, and some forms of cancer. Furthermore, fitness habits adopted during adolescence can help an individual maintain an active, healthy lifestyle throughout the adult years.

Fitness Information For Teens, Second Edition provides updated facts about the importance of being physically fit. It describes how to make healthy lifestyle decisions, how to develop a successful exercise program, and how to make better food choices. It explains exercise fundamentals and describes common types of exercise equipment. Activities for athletes and non-athletes are outlined, and a special section about how to avoid fitness barriers is included. Mental wellness, proper sleep habits, body image, self-esteem, and drug issues (including the use of steroids) are discussed, and the use of physical activity to alleviate stress, depression, and anxiety is explained. The book concludes with a directory of resources and suggestions for additional reading.

How To Use This Book

This book is divided into parts and chapters. Parts focus on broad areas of interest; chapters are devoted to single topics within a part.

Part One: Before You Get Started begins with information on the steps to building a healthy lifestyle through fitness. It explains what fitness is, and answers the question: "Why should I be active?" Information on body image, self-esteem, and the importance of sports physicals is also included.

Part Two: Fitness Fundamentals talks about the body's skeletal muscles, including what they are, where they are, what they do, how to exercise them, and why stretching is important. Facts about measuring physical activity intensity and making an exercise plan are included along with a discussion about how to use common types of exercise equipment. Suggestions are also provided for choosing the correct shoes and exercise apparel.

Part Three: Activities To Try features a wide variety of fitness activities for athletes and non-athletes, including individual hobbies, team sports, and recreational pursuits. Individual chapters for each activity offer basic information, including how to participate, the needed equipment, safety tips, and how the activity fits into an active lifestyle. The part concludes with information about fitness activities for teens with physical challenges.

Part Four: Maintaining Health And Fitness provides facts about staying healthy by paying attention to other essential components of overall fitness. These include nutrition and weight control, hydration, dietary supplements, mental wellness, sleep needs, and locker room hygiene.

Part Five: Avoiding Fitness Busters describes some of the most common physical and mental barriers to achieving fitness goals, including lack of motivation, boredom, health issues, weather, sports injuries, and substance abuse. Negative consequences associated compulsive exercise and the female athlete triad, a life-threatening combination of amenorrhea, osteoporosis, and disordered eating, are also discussed

Part Six: If You Need More Information includes information about the President's Challenge, a directory of fitness organizations, and suggestions for additional reading.

Bibliographic Note

This volume contains documents and excerpts from publications issued by the following government agencies: Centers for Disease Control and Prevention (CDC); National Institute of Arthritis and Musculoskeletal and Skin Diseases (NIAMS); National Institute of Child Health and Human Development (NICHD); National Women's Health Information Center (NWHIC); President's Council on Physical Fitness and Sports; and Weight-Control Information Network (WIN).

In addition, this volume contains copyrighted documents and articles produced by the following organizations: A.D.A.M., Inc.; American Academy of Orthopaedic Surgeons; American Academy of Family Physicians; American College of Sports Medicine (ACSM); American Council on Exercise (ACE); American Heart Association, Inc.; American Orthopaedic Foot and Ankle Society; Aquatic Exercise Association; DrMirken.com; iEmily.com; *IMPACT Magazine*, IMPACT Productions; Iowa State University Extension Service; Kidnetic/International Food Information Council; National Center for Drug Free Sport; National Sleep Foundation; Nemours Foundation; President's Challenge; Racquetball Manufacturers Council; and *Sunset Magazine*, Sunset Publishing Company.

Full citation information is provided on the first page of each chapter. Every effort has been made to secure all necessary rights to reprint the copyrighted material. If any omissions have been made, please contact Omnigraphics to make corrections for future editions.

The photograph on the front cover is from Sue McDonald/iStock photo.

Acknowledgements

In addition to the organizations listed above, special thanks are due to the *Teen Health Series* research and permissions coordinator, Elizabeth Collins, and to its managing editor, Karen Bellenir.

About The *Teen Health Series*

At the request of librarians serving today's young adults, the *Teen Health Series* was developed as a specially focused set of volumes within Omnigraphics' *Health Reference Series*. Each volume deals comprehensively with a topic selected according to the needs and interests of people in middle school and high school.

Teens seeking preventive guidance, information about disease warning signs, medical statistics, and risk factors for health problems will find answers to their questions in the *Teen Health Series*. The *Series*, however, is not intended to serve as a tool for diagnosing illness, in prescribing treatments, or as a substitute for the physician/patient relationship. All people concerned about medical symptoms or the possibility of disease are encouraged to seek professional care from an appropriate health care provider.

If there is a topic you would like to see addressed in a future volume of the *Teen Health Series*, please write to:

Editor
Teen Health Series
Omnigraphics, Inc.
P.O. Box 31-1640
Detroit, MI 48231

A Note About Spelling And Style

Teen Health Series editors use *Stedman's Medical Dictionary* as an authority for questions related to the spelling of medical terms and the *Chicago Manual of Style* for questions related to grammatical structures, punctuation, and other editorial concerns. Consistent adherence is not always possible, however, because the individual volumes within the *Series* include many documents from a wide variety of different producers and copyright holders, and the editor's primary goal is to present material from each source as accurately as is possible following the terms specified by each document's producer. This sometimes means that information in different chapters or sections may follow other guidelines and alternate spelling authorities. For example, occasionally a copyright holder may require that eponymous terms be shown in possessive forms (Crohn's disease *vs.* Crohn disease) or that British spelling norms be retained (leukaemia *vs.* leukemia).

Locating Information Within The *Teen Health Series*

The *Teen Health Series* contains a wealth of information about a wide variety of medical topics. As the *Series* continues to grow in size and scope, locating the precise information needed by a specific student may become more challenging. To address this concern, information about books within the *Teen Health Series* is included in *A Contents Guide to the Health Reference Series*. The *Contents Guide* presents an extensive list of more than 14,000 diseases, treatments, and other topics of general interest compiled from the Tables of Contents and major index headings from the books of the *Teen Health Series* and *Health Reference Series*. To access *A Contents Guide to the Health Reference Series*, visit www.healthreferenceseries.com.

Our Advisory Board

We would like to thank the following advisory board members for providing guidance to the development of this *Series*:

Dr. Lynda Baker, Associate Professor of Library and Information Science, Wayne State University, Detroit, MI

Nancy Bulgarelli, William Beaumont Hospital Library, Royal Oak, MI

Karen Imarisio, Bloomfield Township Public Library, Bloomfield Township, MI

Karen Morgan, Mardigian Library, University of Michigan-Dearborn, Dearborn, MI

Rosemary Orlando, St. Clair Shores Public Library,
St. Clair Shores, MI

Medical Consultant

Medical consultation services are provided to the *Teen Health Series* editors by David A. Cooke, M.D. Dr. Cooke is a graduate of Brandeis University, and he received his M.D. degree from the University of Michigan. He completed residency training at the University of Wisconsin Hospital and Clinics. He is board-certified in internal medicine. Dr. Cooke currently works as part of the University of Michigan Health System and practices in Ann Arbor, MI. In his free time, he enjoys writing, science fiction, and spending time with his family.

Part One

Before You Get Started

Chapter 1

Fitness: Steps To A Healthy Life

Why Get Fit?

Exercise is an important part of a lifetime of good health. Exercising is also fun and is something you can do with friends. It also can help you accomplish the following:

- Feel less stressed

- Boost your self-esteem

- Feel more ready to learn in school

- Keep a healthy weight

- Build and keep healthy bones, muscles, and joints

There are many ways exercise can help you, both today and in the future.

Short-Term, Long-Term Benefits

Short-term benefits of exercise are the body's responses right after starting. The long-term benefits are improvements that occur over weeks, months, and years from regular exercising or training.

About This Chapter: This chapter includes text from "Why Get Fit?" "Exercise: How Much And What Kind?" "How Do I Get Started?" and "How To Know If You Are Getting A Good Workout," National Women's Health Information Center, Office on Women's Health (www.girlshealth.gov), August 2007.

Some short-term benefits include the following:

- Helps you feel good about yourself
- Relaxes and refreshes your body
- Gives you a break from daily routines and worries

Here are some examples of long-term benefits:

- Lowers high blood pressure
- Helps you lose weight and gain strength the healthy way by lowering body fat and increasing muscle
- Lowers risk of cancer, diabetes, heart disease, and osteoporosis (bone loss)

Most people can benefit from exercise. In fact, making physical activity a regular part of your life early on is one of the most important things you can do to improve your health. If you have an injury or think there is a health reason why you may not be able to exercise safely, talk with your doctor before starting a new exercise program or sport. You should also talk with a doctor first if you have and of these conditions:

- Asthma
- High blood pressure
- Heart trouble
- Dizzy spells
- Extreme breathlessness after physical activity
- Arthritis or bone problems
- Severe muscle, ligament, or tendon problems
- Fatigue or feel tired most of the time

Exercise: How Much And What Kind?

No matter what your shape—apple, pear, ruler, or hourglass—there's an exercise for you. To make physical activity a regular part of your life, you should use these tips:

> ### 🖙 Remember!!
>
> The more time you spend in front of the television or playing video games, the less time you have to be active. Not being active is called sedentary. Leading a sedentary lifestyle can cause weight gain and even obesity (dangerously high weight), which can lead to type 2 diabetes, high cholesterol levels, and high blood pressure. These three health issues can hurt your heart and make it easier for you to get certain diseases. Make physical activity a regular part of your life. It can help you protect your health.
>
> Source: National Women's Health Information Center, Office on Women's Health, August 2007.

- Pick exercises you like to do, and choose a few different exercise options so you don't get bored.

- Aim to exercise most days of the week. If you're not very active right now, start slowly and work your way up to being active every day.

There are three levels of physical activity:

- **Light:** Not sweating; not breathing hard (slow walking, dancing)

- **Moderate:** Breaking a sweat; can talk but can't sing (walking fast, dancing)

- **Vigorous:** Sweating, breathing hard; can't talk or sing (running, swimming laps)

No matter what fitness level you are at, your activity can include these two types of exercise:

- **Resistance Exercise:** Weight-training exercise using weight machines, resistance bands, or doing push-ups is called resistance exercise. This activity, done two or more days per week, increases strength and builds muscle.

- **Weight-Bearing Exercise:** Walking, running, hiking, dancing, gymnastics, soccer, and other activities that work bones and muscles against gravity is called weight-bearing exercise. This activity makes bones stronger.

✔ Quick Tip

You need to exercise for about 60 minutes every day. Setting aside 60 minutes all at once each day is one way to get in enough exercise, but if you wait until the end of the day to squeeze it in, you probably won't exercise enough or at all.

Try this instead: If you're not active for 60 minutes straight, it's okay to exercise for 10 or 20 minutes at a time throughout the day.

Source: National Women's Health Information Center, Office on Women's Health, August 2007.

What Kind Of Exercise Does Your Body Need?

Exercise should increase your heart rate and move the muscles in your body. Swimming, dancing, skating, playing soccer, or riding a bike are all examples of exercise that do these things. A well-rounded fitness program would include something from each of these four basic fitness areas:

- **Cardio-Respiratory Endurance:** The ability to exercise your heart and lungs nonstop over certain time periods is called cardio-respiratory endurance and is the same thing as aerobic endurance. When you exercise your heart beats faster and sends more oxygen to your body. If you are not fit, your heart and lungs have to work harder during exercise. Long runs and swims are examples of activities that can help your heart and lungs work better.

- **Muscular Strength:** The ability to move a muscle against resistance is called muscular strength. To become stronger, you need to push or pull against resistance, such as your own weight (like in push-ups), using free weights (note: talk to an instructor before using weights), or even pushing the vacuum cleaner. Regular exercise keeps all of your muscles strong and makes it easier to do daily physical tasks.

- **Muscular Endurance:** The ability of a muscle, or a group of muscles, to keep pushing against resistance for a period of time is called muscular endurance. Push-ups are often used to test endurance of arm and shoulder muscles. Aerobic exercise also helps to improve your muscular endurance. Activities such as running increase your heart rate and make your heart muscle stronger.

- **Flexibility:** The ability to move joints and use muscles as much as they can possibly be used is called flexibility. Sitting on the floor and reaching for your toes is a good measure of the level of flexibility in your lower back and the backs of your upper legs. When you are flexible, you are able to bend and reach with ease. Being flexible can help prevent injuries like pulled muscles. This is why warming up and stretching are so important. If you force your body to move in a way that you aren't used to, you risk tearing muscles, as well as ligaments and tendons.

Table 1.1. Exercises And The Muscles They Work

Exercise	Muscles Worked
Push-ups	Chest, shoulders, arms, abdominals
Sit-ups	Abdominals
Jumping jacks	Calves (lower leg), inner/outer thigh, butt
Running	Calves, front/back thigh
Jumping rope	Calves, thighs, abdominals, shoulders, arms
Swimming	Nearly all major muscles
Dancing	Nearly all major muscles (depending on type of dance)
Walking	Arms, calves, front/back thigh, abdominals
Squats	Calves, front/back thigh, butt
Inline skating	Inner/outer thigh, butt
Hula hoop	Lower back, abdominals

Source: American Council on Exercise.

How Do I Get Started?

There are lots of things that might get in the way of regular exercise. Many people find it hard to get started for many different reasons. For each challenge, though, there is a solution, and you don't have to be an athlete or be involved in an organized sport to be fit. You just have to sit less and move more. Check out these exercise challenges and possible solutions:

- **I am too busy.** Try exercising after school, or pick a time that works best for you each day. It's up to you to make the time and effort.

- **Exercise bores me.** Try out different activities. Sick of jogging? Try inline skating. Not interested in lifting weights? Try Pilates.

- **It's hard to stick with it.** Try exercising with a friend or a family member to give one another support.

- **I don't have equipment or access to a health club.** Choose activities that don't require special equipment, such as jogging or walking. Find resources within your community that are either low-cost or free, such as park and recreation programs.

- **I don't know how.** Start with activities that you don't have to learn new skills for such as walking, climbing stairs, or jogging. Exercise with friends who are either beginners like you or who are more experienced and can teach you what they know. Take a class to learn new things, such as a Pilates class, at your community center or health club.

Once you get past these challenges, decide when you are going to exercise and which activities you would like to do to get a good workout.

How To Know If You Are Getting A Good Workout

To know if you are exercising hard enough and at a safe level, you will need to figure out your target heart rate. Your target heart rate can depend on the type of exercise you are doing.

- **Moderate exercise** includes activities like fast walking, swimming, dancing, or water aerobics.

- **Vigorous exercise** includes activities like jogging, aerobics, basketball, fast swimming, or fast dancing. This level of exercise is more intense.

✔ Quick Tip

For moderate-intensity physical activity, a person's target heart rate should be 50 to 70 percent of his or her maximum heart rate. This maximum rate is based on the person's age. An estimate of a person's maximum age-related heart rate can be obtained by subtracting the person's age from 220. For example, the estimated maximum age-related heart rate for a 14-year-old would be calculated as 220 - 14 = 206 beats per minute (bpm). The 50% and 70% levels would be:

- **50% Level:** 206 x 0.50 = 103 bpm

- **70% Level:** 206 x 0.70 = 144 bpm

Thus, moderate-intensity physical activity for a 14-year-old person will require that the heart rate remain between 103 and 144 bpm during physical activity.

For vigorous-intensity physical activity, a person's target heart rate should be 70 to 85 percent of his or her maximum heart rate. To calculate this range, follow the same formula except change "50% and 70%" to "70% and 85%". For example, the estimated maximum age-related heart rate for a 14-year-old would be calculated as 220 - 14 years = 206 beats per minute (bpm). The 70% and 85% levels would be:

- **70% level:** 206 x 0.70 = 144 bpm

- **85% level:** 206 x 0.85 = 175 bpm

Thus, vigorous-intensity physical activity for a 14-year-old person will require that the heart rate remains between 144 and 175 bpm during physical activity.

Source: Adapted from "Target Heart Rate and Estimated Maximum Heart Rate," Centers for Disease Control and Prevention (CDC) at www.cdc.gov/nccdphp/dnpa/physical/measuring/target_heart_rate.htm, May 2007.

To figure out your target heart rate:

- Stop exercising briefly to take your heart rate (pulse). Take it within five seconds of when you stop exercising. It is recommended that you take your pulse at the wrist. Place the tips of the index and middle fingers over the artery (on the inside of your wrist) and press lightly. Do not use your thumb since it has a pulse of its own. Take a full 60-second count of the heartbeats, or take your pulse for 30 seconds and multiply by two. Start the count on a beat, which is counted as "zero."

- Use the formula in the "Quick Tip" box to figure out your target heart rate, or later, when you're back on your computer, use the calculator at http://www.girlshealth.gov/fitness/THR_Calc.cfm. The calculator will give your maximum and minimum heart rate. This is called your target zone. See if the number you remembered as your pulse falls within this zone. Try to exercise in this zone.

You can also try using the talk/sing test to make sure you are working out at the right level using these three steps:

- If you can talk while you are doing a physical activity, you are probably moving at a pace that is good for you.

- If you are too breathless to talk, you should slow down.

- If you can sing while you are doing a physical activity, you may not be working hard enough; so, you should pick up the pace.

You may also be looking to measure your exercise success in pounds or by how much weight you lose. If so, it is important to know that muscle weighs more than fat, so weighing yourself won't tell you if you are fit. Being able to exercise in your target heart rate zone is a better sign of your fitness level.

Chapter 2

Defining Fitness

Fitness Fundamentals: Guidelines for Personal Exercise Programs

What Is Fitness?

Physical fitness is to the human body what fine tuning is to an engine. It enables you to perform up to your potential. Fitness can be described as a condition that helps you look, feel, and do your best and gives you the ability to perform daily tasks vigorously and alertly with energy left over. Physical fitness is the ability to endure, to bear up, to withstand stress, and to carry on in circumstances where an unfit person could not continue. It is a major basis for good health and well-being.

Physical fitness involves the performance of the heart, lungs, and the muscles of the body. And, since what we do with our bodies also affects what we can do with our minds, fitness influences to some degree qualities such as mental alertness and emotional stability.

As you undertake your fitness program, it's important to remember that fitness is an individual quality that varies from person to person. It is

About This Chapter: This chapter includes excerpts from "Fitness Fundamentals: Guidelines For Personal Exercise Programs," The President's Council on Physical Fitness and Sports, October 2004. Additional text from Nemours Foundation is cited separately within the chapter.

influenced by age, sex, heredity, personal habits, exercise, and eating practices. You can't do anything about the first three factors. However, it is within your power to change and improve the others where needed.

Knowing The Basics

Body composition is often considered a component of fitness. It refers to the makeup of the body in terms of lean mass (muscle, bone, vital tissue, and organs) and fat mass. An optimal ratio of fat to lean mass is an indication of fitness. The right types of exercises will help you decrease body fat and increase (or maintain) muscle mass.

> ### ✎ What's It Mean?
>
> Physical Fitness: A condition or state of being that helps you look, feel, and do your best. It is the ability to do tasks full of energy and still be able to do other things with your time such as schoolwork and activities with family and friends. It is a basis for good health and well-being. Fitness involves performance of the heart and lungs and the muscles of the body. Fitness can also influence how alert you are and how you feel emotionally.
>
> Source: "Why Get Fit," National Women's Health Information Center, Office on Women's Health, August 2007.

A Workout Schedule

How often, how long, how hard you exercise—and what kinds of exercises you do—should be determined by what you are trying to accomplish. Your goals, your present fitness level, age, health, skills, interests, and convenience are among the factors you should consider. For example, an athlete training for high-level competition would follow a different program than a person whose goals are good health and the ability to meet work and recreational needs.

Your exercise program should include something from each of the four basic fitness components described in Chapter One. Each workout should begin with a warm-up and end with a cool down. As a general rule, space your workouts throughout the week and avoid consecutive days of hard exercise.

Here are the amounts of activity necessary for the average healthy person to maintain a minimum level of overall fitness, including some of the popular exercises for each category:

- **Warm-Up:** Five to 10 minutes of exercise such as walking, slow jogging, knee lifts, arm circles or trunk rotations. Low-intensity movements that simulate movements to be used in the activity can also be included in the warm-up.

- **Muscular Strength:** A minimum of two 20-minute sessions per week that include exercises for all the major muscle groups. Lifting weights is the most effective way to increase strength.

- **Muscular Endurance:** At least three 30-minute sessions each week that include exercises such as calisthenics, pushups, sit-ups, pull-ups, and weight training for all the major muscle groups.

- **Cardiorespiratory Endurance:** At least three 20-minute bouts of continuous aerobic (activity requiring oxygen) rhythmic exercise each week. Popular aerobic conditioning activities include brisk walking, jogging, swimming, cycling, rope jumping, rowing, cross-country skiing, and some continuous action games like racquetball and handball.

- **Flexibility:** Ten to 12 minutes of daily stretching exercises performed slowly and without a bouncing motion. This can be included after a warm-up or during a cool down.

- **Cool Down:** A minimum of five to 10 minutes of slow walking or some type of low-level exercise, combined with stretching.

A Matter Of Principle

The keys to selecting the right kinds of exercises for developing and maintaining each of the basic components of fitness are found in these principles:

- **Specificity:** Pick the right kind of activities to affect each component. Strength training results in specific strength changes. Also, train for the specific activity you're interested in. For example, optimal swimming performance is best achieved when the muscles involved in swimming are trained for the movements required. It does not necessarily follow that a good runner is a good swimmer.

- **Overload:** Work hard enough at levels that are vigorous and long enough to overload your body above its resting level and bring about improvement.

- **Regularity:** You can't hoard physical fitness. At least three balanced workouts a week are necessary to maintain a desirable level of fitness.

- **Progression:** Increase the intensity, frequency, and/or duration of activity over periods of time in order to improve.

Some activities can be used to fulfill more than one of your basic exercise requirements. For example, in addition to increasing cardiorespiratory endurance, running builds muscular endurance in the legs, while swimming develops the arm, shoulder, and chest muscles. If you select the proper activities, it is possible to fit parts of your muscular endurance workout into your cardiorespiratory workout and save time.

What's The Right Weight For My Height?

Reprinted with permission from www.kidshealth.org. Copyright © 2007 The Nemours Foundation. This information was provided by KidsHealth, one of the largest resources online for medically reviewed health information written for parents, kids, and teens. For more articles like this one, visit www.KidsHealth.org, or www.TeensHealth.org.

"What's the right weight for my height?" is one of the most common questions girls and guys have. It seems like a simple question. But, for teens, it's not always an easy one to answer. Why not? People have different body types, so there's no single number that's the right weight for everyone. Even among people who are the same height and age, some are more muscular or more developed than others. That's because not all teens have the same body type or develop at the same time.

It is possible to find out if you are in a healthy weight range for your height, though—it just takes a little effort. Read on to discover how this works. You'll also be able to put your measurements into our calculator and get an idea of how you're doing.

Growth And Puberty

Not everyone grows and develops on the same schedule, but teens do go through a period of faster growth. During puberty, the body begins making hormones that spark physical changes like faster muscle growth (particularly in guys) and spurts in height and weight gain in both guys and girls. Once these changes start, they continue for several years. The average person can expect to grow as much as 10 inches (25 centimeters) during puberty before he or she reaches full adult height.

Remember!!
Some teens, especially those who go through puberty on a later time schedule, may feel too skinny. The good news is that their growth, development, and weight gain almost always catch up to the other people their age later on.

Source: Copyright © 2007 The Nemours Foundation.

Most guys and girls gain weight more rapidly during this time as the amounts of muscle, fat, and bone in their bodies changes. All that new weight gain can be perfectly fine—as long as body fat, muscle, and bone are in the right proportion. Because some kids start developing as early as age eight and some not until age 14 or so, it can be normal for two people who are the same height and age to have very different weights.

It can feel quite strange adjusting to suddenly feeling heavier or taller. So it's perfectly normal to feel self-conscious about weight during adolescence—a lot of people do.

Figuring Out Fat Using BMI

Experts have developed a way to help figure out if a person is in the healthy weight range for his or her height. It's called the body mass index, or BMI. BMI is a formula that doctors use to estimate how much body fat a person has based on his or her weight and height.

The BMI formula uses height and weight measurements to calculate a BMI number. This number is then plotted on a chart, which tells a person whether he or she is underweight, average weight, at risk of becoming overweight, or overweight.

Figuring out the body mass index is a little more complicated for teens than it is for adults (that puberty thing again). BMI charts for teens use percentile lines to help individuals compare their BMIs with those of a very large group of people the same age and gender. There are different BMI charts for guys and girls under the age of 20.

A person's BMI number is plotted on the chart for their age and gender. A teen whose BMI is at the 50th percentile is close to the average of the age group. A teen whose weight falls between the 85th and 95th percentile is considered overweight because 85% to 95% of the age group has a lower BMI. A teen above the 95th percentile is considered obese. A teen below the fifth percentile is considered underweight because 95% of the age group has a higher BMI.

✔ **Quick Tip**

To figure out your BMI, use the BMI Calculator Tool at Nemours Foundation's Teen Health site. The internet address is http://www.kidshealth.org/teen/food_fitness/dieting/weight_height.html.

Before you start, you'll need an accurate height and weight measurement. Bathroom scales and tape measures aren't always precise, so the best way to get accurate measurements is by being weighed and measured at your doctor's office or school.

Source: Copyright © 2007 The Nemours Foundation.

What Does BMI Tell Us?

Although you can calculate BMI on your own, it's a good idea to ask your doctor, school nurse, or fitness counselor to help you figure out what it means. That's because a doctor can do more than just use BMI to assess a person's current weight. He or she can take into account where a girl or guy is during puberty and use BMI results from past years to track whether that person may be at risk for becoming overweight. Spotting this risk early on can be helpful because the person can then make changes in diet and exercise to help avert developing a weight problem.

People don't like looking overweight, but weight problems can be more serious than someone's appearance. People who are overweight as teens increase their risk of developing health problems, such as diabetes and high blood pressure. Being overweight as a teen also makes a person more likely to be overweight as an adult. And adults who are overweight may develop other serious health conditions, such as heart disease.

Although BMI can be a good indicator of a person's body fat, it doesn't always tell the full story. People can have a high BMI because they have a large frame or a lot of muscle (like a bodybuilder or athlete) instead of excess fat. Likewise, a small person with a small frame may have a normal BMI but could still have too much body fat. These are other good reasons to talk about your BMI with your doctor.

How Can I Be Sure I'm Not Overweight or Underweight?

If you think you've gained too much weight or are too skinny, a doctor should help you decide whether it's normal for you or whether you really have a weight problem. Your doctor has measured your height and weight over time and knows whether you're growing normally.

If concerned about your height, weight, or BMI, your doctor may ask questions about your health, physical activity, and eating habits. Your doctor may also ask about your family background to find out if you've inherited traits that might make you taller, shorter, or a late bloomer (someone who develops later than other people the same age). The doctor can then put all this information together to decide whether you might have a weight or growth problem.

If your doctor thinks your weight isn't in a healthy range, you will probably get specific dietary and exercise recommendations based on your individual needs. Following a doctor's or dietitian's plan that's designed especially for you will work way better than following fad diets. For teens, fad diets or starvation plans can actually slow down growth and sexual development, and the weight loss usually doesn't last.

What if you're worried about being too skinny? Most teens who weigh less than other teens their age are just fine. They may be going through puberty on

♣ It's A Fact!!
Why You Need More Than A Scale

People overweight for their height can have major differences in body composition (the amounts of muscle, fat, and bone they have). An athlete might be considered overweight because of extra muscle, while a less fit person of the same height and weight might have less muscle but be overweight because of too much body fat.

Source: Copyright © 2007 The Nemours Foundation.

a different schedule than some of their peers, and their bodies may be growing and changing at a different rate. Most underweight teens catch up in weight as they finish puberty during their later teen years and there's rarely a need to try to gain weight.

In a few cases, teens can be underweight because of a health problem that needs treatment. If you feel tired or ill a lot, or if you have symptoms like a cough, stomachache, diarrhea, or other problems that have lasted for more than a week or two, be sure to let your parents or your doctor know. Some teens are underweight because of eating disorders, like anorexia or bulimia, that require attention.

Getting Into Your Genes

Heredity plays a role in body shape and what a person weighs. People from different races, ethnic groups, and nationalities tend to have different body fat distribution (meaning they accumulate fat in different parts of their bodies) or body composition (amounts of bone and muscle versus fat). But genes are not destiny. (That may be a relief if you're looking at Aunt Mildred and wondering if you'll end up with her physique!) No matter whose genes you inherit, you can have a healthy body and keep your weight at a level that's normal for you by eating right and being active.

Genes aren't the only things that family members may share. It's also true that unhealthy eating habits can be passed down, too. The eating and exercise habits of people in the same household probably have an even greater effect than genes on a person's risk of becoming overweight. If your family eats a lot of high-fat foods or snacks or doesn't get much exercise, you may tend to do the same. The good news is these habits can be changed for the better. Even simple forms of exercise, such as walking, have huge benefits on a person's health.

It can be tough dealing with the physical changes our bodies go through during puberty. But at this time, more than any other, it's not a specific number on the scale that's important. It's keeping your body healthy—inside and out.

Chapter 3

Why Should I Be Active?

Physical Activity And Health

The Benefits Of Physical Activity

Physical activity can bring you many health benefits. People who enjoy participating in moderate-intensity or vigorous-intensity physical activity on a regular basis benefit by lowering their risk of developing coronary heart disease, stroke, non-insulin-dependent (type 2) diabetes mellitus, high blood pressure, and colon cancer by 30–50%. Additionally, active people have lower premature death rates than people who are the least active.

Regular physical activity can improve health and reduce the risk of premature death.

- Reduces the risk of developing coronary heart disease (CHD) and the risk of dying from CHD

- Reduces the risk of stroke

- Reduces the risk of having a second heart attack in people who have already had one heart attack

About This Chapter: This chapter includes excerpts from "Physical Activity and Health," the Department of Health and Human Services, Centers for Disease Control and Prevention (CDC), May 2007; and excerpts from "Physical Activity and the Stages of Motivational Readiness for Change Model," *Research Digest*, Series 4, Number 1, President's Council on Physical Fitness and Sports, March 2003.

- Lowers both total blood cholesterol and triglycerides and increases high-density lipoproteins (HDL or the "good" cholesterol)

- Lowers the risk of developing high blood pressure

- Helps reduce blood pressure in people who already have hypertension

- Lowers the risk of developing non-insulin-dependent (type 2) diabetes mellitus

- Reduces the risk of developing colon cancer

- Helps people achieve and maintain a healthy body weight

- Reduces feelings of depression and anxiety

- Promotes psychological well-being and reduces feelings of stress

- Helps build and maintain healthy bones, muscles, and joints

- Helps older adults become stronger and better able to move about without falling or becoming excessively fatigued

> ♣ **It's A Fact!!**
>
> *Can A Lack Of Physical Activity Hurt Your Health?*
>
> Evidence shows that those who are not physically active are definitely not helping their health, and may likely be hurting it. The closer we look at the health risks associated with a lack of physical activity, the more convincing it is that Americans who are not yet regularly physically active should become active.
>
> Source: "The Benefits of Physical Activity," Department of Health and Human Services, Center for Disease Control and Prevention (CDC), March 2008.

Physical Activity And The Stages Of Motivational Readiness For Change Model

[Editor's Note: Now that you know the benefits of becoming active, it's important to understand the Stages of Motivational Readiness For Change Model and what its stages mean to you as you strive to become more active. Each of the steps (precontemplation, contemplation, preparation, action, and maintenance) is discussed and ideas for goal setting at each stage are listed.]

Precontemplation

Individuals in the Precontemplation Stage are currently not active and are not thinking about becoming active. The goal for individuals in this stage is to begin thinking about becoming physically active and the role physical activity could have in their lives.

At this stage, it is important to assess your perception of the pros and cons of becoming physically active. You should thing about the benefits of physical activity including the health benefits such as reduced risk of cardiovascular disease (CVD) and improved cholesterol levels, blood pressure, osteoporosis, mood, stress, and energy levels.

It is equally important to think about the cons of physical activity, given that the negative aspects of being physically active may interfere with you starting a physical activity program. One example of a con is the belief that less time will be available for spending with family and friends if one becomes physically active. In this case, you might want to think about how to make physical activity a family activity or an activity that you can do with friends.

Related to the cons of physical activity, it is also important to think about specific barriers to physical activity. For example, one commonly reported barrier is lack of enjoyment of physical activity. You may have previously engaged in exercise and associate physical activity with sweating and other unpleasant physiological sensations. You should know, though, that research indicates that physical activity does not have to be at the vigorous level for you to experience the benefits of physical activity. Research studies have shown that the popular phrase "No pain, no gain" is untrue.

Another commonly reported barrier to physical activity is not having enough time and/or a lack of energy to be physically active. If time is a barrier, you can divide the physical activity over the course of the day. Additionally, you should remember that physical activity can actually lead to an increase in energy levels.

Environmental constraints, such as a lack of access to physical activity facilities and parks, are commonly reported barriers to physical activity. For example, joining a health club or purchasing physical activity equipment is expensive and many individuals perceive this as a barrier. However, health

♣ It's A Fact!!
Exercise Ups Brain Power

The next time you go for a run or take an indoor cycling class, think about this: You may be getting smarter. Or at the very least, stimulating the development of new cells in the learning centers of your brain.

Researchers at The Salk Institute for Biological Studies in La Jolla, California, examined the newly formed brain cells in mice.

They discovered that "voluntary exercise in a running wheel increased cell proliferation."

It is important to note that these mice were fully developed and yet still experienced brain cell regeneration, a function once believed to be limited to developing mammals.

But it wasn't just the exercise that helped increase cell development. A second, related study published in the same journal reports that cell development in this part of the brain also increased when the mice were placed in interesting, varied environments with plenty of stimuli.

So what makes for a good workout—a stimulating environment and challenging exercises—is also good for the brain.

Source: "Exercise Ups Brain Power," © American Council on Exercise (www.acefitness.org). All rights reserved. Reprinted with permission. Information was accessed May 2008.

clubs and special equipment are not necessary for physical activity participation. Simply purchasing a good pair of walking shoes is all that is needed to become an active person.

Another barrier that you may have is the fear of injury. Most injuries can be avoided by using appropriate techniques such as engaging in stretching and light activities before and after physical activity.

Goal setting is another behavioral strategy that is important for changing physical activity behavior. Goals should be implemented in every stage and your goals should vary depending on your stage of change. An example of a goal for a Precontemplater is reading an article about the benefits of physical activity. Ideally, you will begin thinking about becoming physically active and advance to the next stage, which is Contemplation.

Contemplation

Individuals in the Contemplation Stage are not currently physically activity but are thinking about becoming active. The goal of this stage is to increase the likelihood that you will take steps to become physically active. Similar to the Precontemplation Stage, you should consider the pros and cons of physical activity.

In taking steps towards becoming physically active, you should decide on what activities are best suited for your health and lifestyle. If you have been active in the past, you should consider the activities that you found enjoyable. Next, you can determine what activity that you can realistically fit into your daily schedule. It is important to increase your awareness of small changes that could be made to increase physical activity such as parking further away from a particular destination or taking the stairs instead of the escalator or elevator.

Specific physical activity goals can now be created. It is important that your goals be realistic given that unrealistic goals can lead to disappointment and frustration. You're likely to discontinue a physical activity program if your goals are set too high. It is important to start slowly and gradually increase physical activity over time.

Research indicates that individuals will be more likely to repeat a behavior if the behavior is rewarded. Therefore, it is important for you to reward yourself for meeting your goals. Research also indicates that individuals who have social support are more likely to maintain a physical activity program.

Regarding goal setting in the Contemplation Stage, you should set specific goals that involve taking specific steps toward becoming physically active. For example, one weekly goal may be to buy a good pair of walking shoes and talk to a family member about their plan to become physically active.

Preparation

Individuals in the Preparation Stage are engaging in physical activity but not at the recommended levels. The goal for you in this stage is to increase your physical activity participation to the recommended levels. You should develop a physical activity plan in which you engage in physical activity at the recommended levels (such as, 30 minutes or more of activity, at a moderate level of activity, on most days of the week).

Many of the same strategies described in the Contemplation Stage can also be applied in this stage, while carefully considering the goal differences between the two stages (such as, starting physical activity versus increasing activity to recommended levels). Similar to the Contemplation Stage, you should determine when and what type of activity works best with your lifestyle. Since you are already doing some activity, information obtained from your current activity can be used to devise your physical activity plan (for example, time of day for activity that works best with their schedule and the type of activity that is most enjoyable). Also, similar to the Contemplation Stage, social support, setting realistic goals, and reinforcing physical activity participation at the recommended levels are also important in this stage.

The key to the Preparation Stage is overcoming the barriers that prevent you from progressing from some activity to physical activity participation at the recommended levels. For example, you may discover that inclement weather interferes with your physical activity program. You may find that you participate in physical activity sporadically due to changes in weather conditions. This barrier can be overcome by developing a list of activities for when the weather prohibits physical activity outdoors (for example, walking in the mall, exercise videos, walking stairs).

Another factor that may influence regular physical activity is fatigue. You may be less likely to engage in physical activity on days you feel fatigued, but you might be surprised to know that physical activity may actually improve fatigue by increasing energy levels and improving quality of sleep.

Similarly, mood variations may lead to irregular activity patterns. Research indicates that physical activity can improve mood and it is important that you consider this when thinking about skipping a physical activity session.

Similar to the previous stages, goal setting can play an instrumental role in progressing you to the next stage of change. You should set specific goals that are daily, weekly, and that gradually increase your physical activity to the recommended levels. For example, your initial goal may be to engage in 60 minutes of physical activity per week and then gradually increase the goal to 150 minutes per week.

In order to assess attainment of your goals, self-monitoring becomes very important during the Preparation Stage. It is important for you to monitor your physical activity using a daily log that can be designed depending on your preferences. The key is that you utilize a log that you will adhere to and one that will help in the achievement of your goals. Another self-monitoring option is using a pedometer, which is an objective monitor worn to record and display number of steps taken per day.

Action And Maintenance

Individuals in the Action Stage are physically active at the recommended levels but have been regularly active for less than six months. Individuals in the Maintenance Stage are physically active at the recommended levels and have been for six or more months. The goal for individuals in the Action and Maintenance Stages is to maintain their physical activity participation.

One important strategy in the Action or Maintenance Stage is to identify risk factors for future relapse. Vacations, illness, stressful life events, and boredom of the physical activity routine are common situations may cause you to discontinue physical activity participation.

Illness contributes to a relapse when individuals fail to return to their physical activity program after recovering from an illness. It is important for you to recognize illness as a barrier and gradually return to your physical activity program once your physician agrees it is safe.

Because stressful life events can contribute to a relapse, it is important to remember that physical activity may be especially important during stressful times given that is can help alleviate stress and increase energy.

Finally, your types of physical activities should be varied to decrease the likelihood of boredom. If you prefer one type of activity such as walking, it is important to keep this activity interesting by varying the route, inviting friends, and/or walking indoors.

Similar to the Preparation Stage, it is important to set goals and monitor physical activity in the Action and Maintenance Stages. Both short and long-term goals should be made, and reinforcement should continue for achieving these goals. Goal setting is important because it decreases the likelihood of becoming bored with a particular physical activity program.

♣ It's A Fact!!
Everyone Can Benefit From Physical Activity

- **Teenagers:** Regular physical activity improves strength, builds lean muscle, and decreases body fat. Activity can build stronger bones to last a lifetime.

- **People trying to manage their weight:** Regular physical activity burns calories while preserving lean muscle mass. Regular physical activity is a key component of any weight-loss or weight-management effort.

- **People with high blood pressure:** Regular physical activity helps lower blood pressure.

- **People with physical disabilities, including arthritis:** Regular physical activity can help people with chronic, disabling conditions improve their stamina and muscle strength. It also can improve psychological well-being and quality of life.

- **Everyone under stress, including persons experiencing anxiety or depression:** Regular physical activity improves one's mood, helps relieve depression, and increases feelings of well-being.

- **Older adults:** Evidence indicates that muscle-strengthening exercises can reduce the risk of falling and fracturing bones and can improve the ability to live independently.

Source: From "Physical Activity And Health," Centers for Disease Control and Prevention (CDC), March 2008.

Chapter 4

Body Image And Self-Esteem

I'm fat. I'm too skinny. I'd be happy if I were taller, shorter, had curly hair, straight hair, a smaller nose, bigger muscles, longer legs.

Do any of these statements sound familiar? Are you used to putting yourself down? If so, you're not alone. As a teen, you're going through a ton of changes in your body. And as your body changes, so does your image of yourself. Lots of people have trouble adjusting, and this can affect their self-esteem.

Why Are Self-Esteem And Body Image Important?

Self-esteem is all about how much people value themselves, the pride they feel in themselves, and how worthwhile they feel. Self-esteem is important because feeling good about yourself can affect how you act. A person who has high self-esteem will make friends easily, is more in control of his or her behavior, and will enjoy life more.

Body image is how a person feels about his or her own physical appearance. For many people, especially people in their early teens, body image can be closely linked to self-esteem. That's because as kids develop into teens, they care more about how others see them.

What Influences A Person's Self-Esteem?

Puberty: Some teens struggle with their self-esteem when they begin puberty because the body goes through many changes. These changes, combined with a natural desire to feel accepted, mean it can be tempting for people to compare themselves to others. They may compare themselves to the people around them or to actors and celebs they see on TV, in movies, or in magazines.

But it's impossible to compare ourselves to others because the changes that come with puberty are different for everyone. Some people start developing early; others are late bloomers. Some get a temporary layer of fat to prepare for a growth spurt, others fill out permanently, and others feel like they stay skinny no matter how much they eat. It all depends on how our genes have programmed our bodies to act.

The changes that come with puberty can affect how both girls and guys feel about themselves. Some girls may feel uncomfortable or embarrassed about their maturing bodies. Others may wish that they were developing faster. Girls may feel pressure to be thin but guys may feel like they don't look big or muscular enough.

Outside Influences: It's not just development that affect self-esteem, though. Lots of other factors (like media images of skinny girls and bulked-up guys) can affect a person's body image too.

Family life can sometimes influence a person's self-esteem. Some parents spend more time criticizing their children and the way they look than praising them. This criticism may reduce a person's ability to develop good self-esteem.

People may also experience negative comments and hurtful teasing about the way they look from classmates and peers. Sometimes racial and ethnic prejudice is the source of such comments. Although these comments often come from ignorance on the part of the person who makes them, sometimes they can affect a person's body image and self-esteem.

Healthy Self-Esteem

If you have a positive body image, you probably like and accept yourself the way you are. This healthy attitude allows you to explore other aspects of growing up, such as developing good friendships, growing more independent from your parents, and challenging yourself physically and mentally. Developing these parts of yourself can help boost your self-esteem.

♣ It's A Fact!!

Resilience: People who believe in themselves are better able to recognize mistakes, learn from them, and bounce back from disappointment. This skill is called resilience.

Source: Copyright © 2006 The Nemours Foundation.

A positive, optimistic attitude can help people develop strong self-esteem. For example, saying, "Hey, I'm human," instead of "Wow, I'm such a loser," when you've made a mistake. Or not blaming others when things don't go as expected.

Knowing what makes you happy and how to meet your goals can help you feel capable, strong, and in control of your life. A positive attitude and a healthy lifestyle (such as exercising and eating right) are a great combination for building good self-esteem.

Tips For Improving Your Body Image

Some people think they need to change how they look or act to feel good about themselves. But actually all you need to do is change the way you see your body and how you think about yourself.

The first thing to do is recognize that your body is your own, no matter what shape, size, or color it comes in. If you are very worried about your weight or size, check with your doctor to verify that things are OK. But it is no one's business but your own what your body is like—ultimately, you have to be happy with yourself.

Next, identify which aspects of your appearance you can realistically change and which you can't. Everyone (even the most perfect-seeming celeb) has things about themselves that they can't change and need to accept—like their height, for example, or their shoe size.

If there are things about yourself that you want to change and can (such as how fit you are), do this by making goals for yourself. For example, if you want to get fit, make a plan to exercise every day and eat nutritious foods. Then keep track of your progress until you reach your goal. Meeting a challenge you set for yourself is a great way to boost self-esteem!

When you hear negative comments coming from within yourself, tell yourself to stop. Try building your self-esteem by giving yourself three compliments every day. While you're at it, every evening list three things in your day that really gave you pleasure. It can be anything from the way the sun felt on your face, the sound of your favorite band, or the way someone laughed at your jokes. By focusing on the good things you do and the positive aspects of your life, you can change how you feel about yourself.

Where Can I Go If I Need Help?

Sometimes low self-esteem and body image problems are too much to handle alone. A few teens may become depressed, lose interest in activities or friends—and even hurt themselves or resort to alcohol or drug abuse. If you're feeling this way, it can help to talk to a parent, coach, religious leader, guidance counselor, therapist, or an adult friend. A trusted adult—someone who supports you and doesn't bring you down—can help you put your body image in perspective and give you positive feedback about your body, your skills, and your abilities.

If you can't turn to anyone you know, call a teen crisis hotline (check the yellow pages under social services). The most important thing is to get help if you feel like your body image and self-esteem are affecting your life.

A Guy's Guide To Body Image

"A Guy's Guide to Body Image," November 2006, reprinted with permission from www.kidshealth.org. Copyright © 2006 The Nemours Foundation. This information was provided by KidsHealth, one of the largest resources online for medically reviewed health information written for parents, kids, and teens. For more articles like this one, visit www.KidsHealth.org, or www.TeensHealth.org.

Al's friend Rachel invited him to go to the lake for the day with her family. Rachel thought Al was fun to be around—plus he was cute. Rachel really hoped he'd say yes.

Al turned Rachel down. He liked Rachel, too, but was self-conscious about taking off his T-shirt. He worried that her family and others at the lake would see what he saw when he looked in the mirror—a scrawny excuse for a man. Al hadn't gone to the pool in more than a year because he was so self-conscious about his appearance.

The Truth About Guys

Many people think of guys as being carefree when it comes to their appearance. But the reality is that a lot of guys spend plenty of time in front of the mirror. It's a fact—some guys care just as much as girls do about their appearance.

You may hear a lot about being a tough guy, but how often do you hear that being a guy is tough? Guys might think that they shouldn't worry about how they look, but body image can be a real problem for them. Unlike girls, guys are less likely to talk to friends and relatives about their bodies and how they're developing. Without support from friends and family, they may develop a negative self-image. The good news is that self-image and body image can be changed.

Why Is Body Image Important?

Body image is a person's opinions, thoughts, and feelings about his or her own body and physical appearance. Having a positive body image means feeling pretty satisfied with the way you look, appreciating your body for its capabilities and accepting its imperfections. Body image is part of someone's total self-image. So how a guy feels about his body can affect how he feels about himself. If he gets too focused on not liking the way he looks, a guy's self-esteem can take a hit and his confidence can slide. (The same thing can happen to girls, too.)

How Puberty Affects Body Image

Although body image is just one part of our self-image, during the teen years, and especially during puberty, it can be easy for a guy's whole self-image to be based on how his body looks. That's because our bodies are changing so much during this time that they can become the main focus of our attention.

A change in your body can be tough to deal with emotionally—mainly because, well, your body is yours and you have become used to it.

Some guys don't feel comfortable in their changing bodies and can feel as if they don't know who they are anymore. Being the only guy whose voice is changing or who's growing body hair (or the only guy who isn't) can also make some guys feel self-conscious for a while.

Some guys go into puberty not feeling too satisfied with their body or appearance to begin with. They may have wrestled with body image even before puberty started (for example, battles with weight or dissatisfaction with height). For them, puberty may add to their insecurities.

♣ It's A Fact!!
When Body Worries Go Too Far

It's normal for a guy to have a few minor complaints about his looks, but a focus that's too intense can signal a problem. Body dysmorphic disorder is a mental health condition in which people are so preoccupied with what they believe are defects in the way they look that they spend hours of time and attention every day checking, fixing, or hiding appearance flaws. This body image disorder interferes with a person's ability to function or be happy, and requires a professional's help.

Source: Copyright © 2006 The Nemours Foundation.

It Could Be In Your Genes

It can be tough to balance what you expect to happen to your body with what actually does happen. Lots of guys can have high expectations for puberty, thinking they'll develop quickly or in a certain way.

The best way to approach your own growth and development is to not assume you'll be a certain way. Look at everyone in your family—uncles, grandfathers, and even female relatives—to get an idea of the kinds of options your genes may have in store for you.

When Everyone Else Seems Bigger

Not everyone's body changes at the same time or even at the same pace. It can be tough if all of your friends have already matured physically and are taller and more muscular. Most guys eventually catch up in terms of growth, although some will always be taller or more muscular than others—it's in their genes.

It's natural to observe friends and classmates and notice the different ways they're growing and developing. Guys often compare themselves with other guys in certain settings, and one of the most common is the locker room. Whether at a local gym or getting ready for a game at school, time in the locker room can be daunting for any guy.

Try to keep in mind in these situations that you aren't alone if you feel you don't "measure up." Many guys feel exactly the same way about their own bodies—even those whose physiques you envy. Just knowing that almost everyone else will go through the same thing can make all the difference.

You could try talking to a trusted male adult—maybe a coach, a doctor, a teacher, or your dad. Chances are they went through similar experiences and had some of the same feelings and apprehensions when their bodies were changing.

Picture Perfect?

Guys put enough pressure on themselves, but what about the pressure society puts on them to be perfect?

It used to be that only girls felt the pressure of picture-perfect images, but these days the media emphasis on men's looks creates a sense of pressure for guys, too. And sometimes (actually many times) that "as advertised" body is just not attainable. The men you see in those pictures may not even be real. Magazines and ad agencies often alter photographs of models, either by airbrushing the facial and muscular features, or by putting a good-looking face on someone else's buff body.

Building A Better Body Image

So in the face of all the pressure society places on guys—and guys place on themselves—what can you do to fuel a positive body image? Here are some ideas:

- **Recognize your strengths.** Different physical attributes and body types are good for different things—and sometimes the things you did well as a kid can change during puberty. What does your body do well? Maybe your speed, flexibility, strength, or coordination leads you to excel at a certain sport. Or perhaps you have non-sports skills, like drawing, painting, singing, playing a musical instrument, writing, or acting. Just exploring talents that you feel good about can help your self-esteem and how you think of yourself.

♣ It's A Fact!!

Big Bullies: Sometimes if people haven't caught up physically, bigger kids may tease them. Often, the guys who put others down do it because they aren't comfortable with their bodies. Putting someone else down makes them feel more powerful. A simple and effective way to deal with annoying guys like this is to be comfortable with who you are and get in touch with your strengths. Use humor and wit to combat a bully—he won't know what hit him.

Source: Copyright © 2006 The Nemours Foundation.

- **A good body doesn't always translate into athletic success.** Too often, the way guys see their body image is closely associated with their performance on a sports field or in the gym. The upside to this is that if you're good at a team sport, you might have a pretty good view of your body. But what if you don't like team sports or you got cut from a team you really wanted to make? In these cases, it helps to look at individual accomplishments.

If you don't like team sports, that's OK. Try finding another form of physical activity that really gets you going. Depending on your interests and where you live, that may be mountain biking, rock climbing, dancing, yoga, or even jogging. This will help you stay in shape and help you to appreciate skills may not have realized you had in a team environment.

If you like team sports but didn't make a particular team, don't let it get you down. Use this as an opportunity to discover what you're good at, not to lament what you aren't best at. Maybe try out for another team—so soccer wasn't for you, but maybe cross-country running will be.

♣ It's A Fact!!
Body Image And Eating Disorders

When you put yourself down about how you look, it can lead to negative feelings and can create a bad body image and poor self-esteem. Poor self-esteem and a bad body image can also lead to eating disorders that could put your health in danger.

If you start to have negative thoughts about your body and the way you look, think about all of the traits that make you special and unique. Look at your whole self—body and mind—in a positive way and write down what you see. Use these action steps everyday to boost your body image and self-esteem:

- Think positive thoughts about yourself.

- Focus on your strengths—not your weaknesses.

- Realize that you are better at some things than others.

- Set realistic goals. This means not setting goals too high or too low, but at a level you know you can reach. Then, you can always strive to do better than your goal.

- Give yourself credit when you reach a goal and praise yourself when you have done well.

- Learn to be assertive—express your thoughts, opinions, needs, and feelings openly—but without abusing others' rights.

- Don't compare yourself to others—remember, you're just fine the way you are.

- Practice positive body language. Walk tall, don't slump. When your body says, "I can" everyone will believe you can.

Important: If you are struggling with an eating disorder or just can't seem to feel better, talk to an adult you trust right away.

Source: Excerpts from "Mind-Emotion Commotion," National Women's Health Information Center, April 2007.

If none of these appeal to you, continue to practice the sport you were cut from and try again next year. The people around you probably won't remember that you didn't make the team—not being picked was a much bigger deal to you than it was to them.

- **Look into starting a strength training program.** Exercise can help you look good and feel good about yourself. Good physiques don't just happen—they take hard work, regular workouts, and a healthy diet. There's no need to work out obsessively. A healthy routine can be as simple as exercising 20 minutes to one hour three days a week. Another benefit to working out properly is that it can boost your mood—lifting weights can lift your spirits.

- **Don't trash your body, respect it!** To help improve your view of your body, take care of it. Smoking and other things you know to be harmful will take a toll after a while. Treating yourself well over time results in a healthier, stronger body—and that contributes to a better body image. Practicing good grooming habits—regular showering; taking care of your teeth, hair, and skin; wearing clean clothes, etc.—also can help you build a positive body image.

- **Be yourself.** Your body is just one part of who you are—along with your talent for comedy, a quick wit, or all the other things that make you unique. Your talents, skills, and beliefs are just as much a part of you as the casing they come in. So try not to let minor imperfections take over.

While it's important to have a positive body image, getting too focused on body image and appearance can cause a guy to overlook the other positive parts of himself. If you're like most guys who take care of their bodies and wear clothes that look good, you probably look great to others. You just might not be aware of that if you're too busy being self-critical.

Chapter 5

Sports Physicals

You already know that playing sports helps keep you fit. You also know that sports are a fun way to socialize and meet people. But you might not know why the physical you may have to take at the beginning of your sports season is so important.

In the sports medicine field, the sports physical exam is known as a preparticipation physical examination (PPE). The exam helps determine whether it's safe for you to participate in a particular sport. Most states actually require that kids and teens have a sports physical before they can start a new sport or begin a new competitive season. But even if a PPE isn't required, doctors still highly recommend them.

What is a sports physical?

There are two main parts to a sports physical: the medical history and the physical exam.

Medical History: This part of the exam includes questions about:

• serious illnesses among other family members;

- illnesses that you had when you were younger or may have now, such as asthma, diabetes, or epilepsy;

- previous hospitalizations or surgeries;

- allergies (to insect bites, for example);

- past injuries (including concussions, sprains, or bone fractures);

- whether you've ever passed out, felt dizzy, had chest pain, or had trouble breathing during exercise;

- any medications that you are on (including over-the-counter medications, herbal supplements, and prescription medications).

The medical history questions are usually on a form that you can bring home, so ask your parents to help you fill in the answers. If possible, ask both parents about family medical history.

Looking at patterns of illness in your family is a very good indicator of any potential conditions you may have. Most sports medicine doctors believe the medical history is the most important part of the sports physical exam, so take time to answer the questions carefully. It's unlikely that any health conditions you have will prevent you from playing sports completely.

Answer the questions as well as you can. Try not to guess the answers or give answers you think your doctor wants.

Physical Examination: During the physical part of the exam, the doctor will usually:

- record your height and weight;

- take a blood pressure and pulse (heart rate and rhythm) reading;

- test your vision;

- check your heart, lungs, abdomen, ears, nose, and throat;

- evaluate your posture, joints, strength, and flexibility.

Although most aspects of the exam will be the same for males and females, if a person has started or already gone through puberty, the doctor may ask girls and guys different questions. For example, if a girl is heavily involved in a lot of active sports, the doctor may ask her about her period and diet to make sure she doesn't have something like female athlete triad.

A doctor will also ask questions about use of drugs, alcohol, or dietary supplements, including steroids or other "performance enhancers" and weight-loss supplements, because these can affect a person's health.

Some schools may require that a PPE include an electrocardiogram, or EKG, for all athletes. An EKG, which takes about 10 minutes, measures the electrical activity of a person's heart. EKGs don't hurt—electrodes that measure heart rate and rhythm are placed on the chest, arms, and legs, and a specialist reads the results.

At the end of your exam, the doctor will either fill out and sign a form if everything checks out OK or, in some cases, recommend a follow-up exam, additional tests, or specific treatment for medical problems.

♣ It's A Fact!!
Why is a sports physical important?

A sports physical can help you find out about and deal with health problems that might interfere with your participation in a sport. For example, if you have frequent asthma attacks but are a starting forward in soccer, a doctor might be able to prescribe a different type of inhaler or adjust the dosage so that you can breathe more easily when you run.

Your doctor may even have some good training tips and be able to give you some ideas for avoiding injuries. For example, he or she may recommend specific exercises, like certain stretching or strengthening activities that help prevent injuries. A doctor can also identify risk factors that are linked to specific sports. Advice like this will make you a better, stronger athlete.

When and where should I go for a sports physical?

Some people go to their own doctor for a sports physical; others have one at school. During school physicals, you may go to half a dozen or so "stations" set up in the gym; each one is staffed by a medical professional who gives you a specific part of the physical exam.

If your school offers the exam, it's convenient to get the exam done there. But even if you have a PPE at school, it's a good idea to see your regular doctor for an exam as well. Your doctor knows you—and your health history—better than anyone you talk to briefly in a gym.

If your state requires sports physicals, you'll probably have to start getting them when you're in ninth grade. Even if PPEs aren't required by your school or state, it's still smart to get them if you participate in school sports. And if you compete regularly in a sport before ninth grade, you should begin getting these exams even earlier.

Getting a sports physical once a year is usually adequate. If you're healing from a major injury, like a broken wrist or ankle, however, get checked out after it's healed before you start practicing or playing again.

You should have your physical about six weeks before your sports season begins so there's enough time to follow up on something, if necessary. Neither you nor your doctor will be very happy if your PPE is the day before baseball practice starts and it turns out there's something that needs to be taken of care before you can suit up.

What if there's a problem?

What happens if you don't get the OK from your own doctor and have to see a specialist? Does that mean you won't ever be able to letter in softball or hockey? Don't worry if your doctor asks you to have other tests or go for a follow-up exam—it could be something as simple as rechecking your blood pressure a week or two after the physical.

Your doctor's referral to a specialist may help your athletic performance. For example, if you want to try out for your school's track team but get a slight pain in your knee every time you run, an orthopedist or sports medicine specialist can help you figure out what's going on. Perhaps the pain comes from previous overtraining or poor running technique. Maybe you injured the knee a long time ago and it never totally healed. Or perhaps the problem is as simple as running shoes that don't offer enough support. Chances are, a doctor will be able to help you run without the risk of further injury to the knee by giving you suggestions or treatment before the sports season begins.

It's very unlikely that you'll be disqualified from playing sports. The ultimate goal of the sports physical is to ensure safe participation in sports, not to disqualify the participants. Most of the time, a specialist won't find anything serious enough to prevent you from playing your sport. In fact, fewer than one percent of students have conditions that might limit sports participation, and most of these conditions are known before the PPE takes place.

Do I still have to get a regular physical?

In a word, yes. It may seem like overkill, but a sports physical is different from a standard physical.

The sports physical focuses on your well-being as it relates to playing a sport. It's more limited than a regular physical, but it's a lot more specific about athletic issues. During a regular physical, however, your doctor will address your overall well-being, which may include things that are unrelated to sports. You can ask your doctor to give you both types of exams during one visit; just be aware that you'll need to set aside more time.

Even if your sports physical exam doesn't reveal any problems, it's always a good idea to monitor yourself when you play sports. If you notice changes in your physical condition—even if you think they're small, such as muscle pain or shortness of breath—be sure to mention them to a parent or coach. You should also inform your physical education teacher or coach if your health needs have changed in any way or if you're taking a new medication.

☞ Remember!!
Just as professional sports stars need medical care to keep them playing their best, so do teenage athletes. You can give yourself the same edge as the pros by making sure you have your sports physical.

Part Two

Fitness Fundamentals

Chapter 6

Your Multitalented Muscles

Did you know you have more than 600 muscles in your body? They help you do almost everything—from pumping blood throughout your body to lifting your heavy backpack. You control some of your muscles and others, like your heart, do their jobs without you thinking about them at all.

Muscles are all made of the same material, a type of elastic tissue (sort of like the material in a rubber band). Thousands, or even tens of thousands, of small fibers make up each muscle. You have three different types of muscles in your body: smooth muscle, cardiac (say: kar-dee-ak) muscle, and skeletal (say: skel-uh-tul) muscle.

Smooth Muscles

Smooth muscles are sometimes also called involuntary muscles and they are usually in sheets, or layers, with one layer of muscle behind the other. You can't control this type of muscle. Your brain and body tell these muscles what to do without you even thinking about it. You can't use your smooth muscles to make a muscle in your arm or jump into the air.

But smooth muscles are at work all over your body. In your stomach and digestive system, they contract (tighten up) and relax to allow food to make its journey through the body. Your smooth muscles come in handy if you're sick and you need to throw up. The muscles push the food back out of the stomach so it comes up through the esophagus (say: ih-sah-fuh-gus) and out of the mouth.

Smooth muscles are also found in your bladder. When they're relaxed, they allow you to hold in urine (pee) until you can get to the bathroom. Then they contract so that you can push the urine out. These muscles are also in a woman's uterus, which is where a baby develops. There they help to push the baby out of the mother's body when it's time to be born.

You'll find smooth muscles at work behind the scenes in your eyes, too. These muscles keep the eyes focused.

A Hearty Muscle

The muscle that makes up the heart is called cardiac muscle. It is also known as the myocardium (say: my-uh-kar-dee-um). The thick muscles of the heart contract to pump blood out and then relax to let blood back in after

---

♣ It's A Fact!!
Exercise's Effects On Bones And Muscles

Exercise is critical for strong muscles and bones. Muscle strength declines as people age, but studies report that when people exercise they are stronger and leaner than others in their age group.

Exercise helps kids lower their risk of chronic pain in the future. Research has shown that it helps them prevent back and neck pain. The more flexible men are as teenagers, the lower their risk of neck tension in the future, according to a study published in the February 2006 *British Journal of Sports Medicine*. The same report found that women who had the greatest endurance strength as teenagers had a lower risk of tension neck than those with lower teenager endurance strength. However, men with the greatest endurance strength had higher rates of knee injuries later on.

Source: Excerpted from "Exercise (In Depth Report)," © 2008 A.D.A.M., Inc. Reprinted with permission.

it's circulated through the body. Just like smooth muscle, cardiac muscle works all by itself with no help from you. A special group of cells within the heart are known as the pacemaker of the heart because it controls the heartbeat.

Skeletal Muscle

Now, let's talk about the kind of muscle you think of when we say "muscle"—the ones that show how strong you are and let you boot a soccer ball into the goal. These are your skeletal muscles—sometimes called striated (say: stry-ay-tud) muscle because the light and dark parts of the muscle fibers make them look striped (striated is a fancy word meaning striped).

Skeletal muscles are voluntary muscles, which means you can control what they do. Your leg won't bend to kick the soccer ball unless you want it to. These muscles help to make up the musculoskeletal (say: mus-kyuh-low-skel-uh-tul) system—the combination of your muscles and your skeleton, or bones.

Together, the skeletal muscles work with your bones to give your body power and strength. In most cases, a skeletal muscle is attached to one end of a bone. It stretches all the way across a joint (the place where two bones meet) and then attaches again to another bone.

Skeletal muscles are held to the bones with the help of tendons (say: ten-dunz). Tendons are cords made of tough tissue, and they work as special connector pieces between bone and muscle. The tendons are attached so well that when you contract one of your muscles, the tendon and bone move along with it.

Skeletal muscles come in many different sizes and shapes to allow them to do many types of jobs. Some of your biggest and most powerful muscles are in your back, near your spine. These muscles help keep you upright and standing tall.

They also give your body the power it needs to lift and push things. Muscles in your neck and the top part of your back aren't as large, but they are capable of some pretty amazing things: Try rotating your head around, back and forth, and up and down to feel the power of the muscles in your neck. These muscles also hold your head high.

Face Muscles

You may not think of it as a muscular body part, but your face has plenty of muscles. You can check them out next time you look in the mirror. Facial muscles don't all attach directly to bone like they do in the rest of the body. Instead, many of them attach under the skin. This allows you to contract your facial muscles just a tiny bit and make dozens of different kinds of faces. Even the smallest movement can turn a smile into a frown. You can raise your eyebrow to look surprised or wiggle your nose.

And while you're looking at your face, don't pass over your tongue—a muscle that's attached only at one end. Your tongue is actually made of a group of muscles that work together to allow you to talk and help you chew food. Stick out your tongue and wiggle it around to see those muscles at work.

Major Muscles

Because there are so many skeletal muscles in your body, we can't list them all here. But here are a few of the major ones:

- In each of your shoulders is a deltoid (say: del-toyd) muscle. Your deltoid muscles help you move your shoulders every which way—from swinging a softball bat to shrugging your shoulders when you're not sure of an answer.

- The pectoralis (say: pek-tuh-rah-lus) muscles are found on each side of your upper chest. These are usually called pectorals (say: pek-tuh-rulz), or pecs, for short. When many boys hit puberty, their pectoral muscles become larger. Many athletes and bodybuilders have large pecs, too.

- Below these pectorals, down under your rib cage, are your rectus abdominus (say: rek-tus ab-dahm-uh-nus) muscles, or abdominals (say: ab-dahm-uh-nulz). They are also sometimes called abs for short.

- When you make a muscle in your arm, you tense your biceps (say: bye-seps) muscle. When you contract your biceps muscle, you can actually see it push up under your skin.

- Your quadriceps (say: kwad-ruh-seps), or quads, are the muscles on the front of your thighs. Many people who run, bike, or play sports develop large, strong quads.

- And when it's time for you to take a seat? You'll be sitting on your gluteus maximus (say: gloot-ee-us mak-suh-mus), the muscle that's under the skin and fat in your behind.

Chapter 7

Working Your Muscles

Flex Appeal: Biceps

Strong biceps don't just look good, they can make your life a lot easier too. Your bicep muscles come in handy for everyday tasks like brushing your teeth and buttoning your shirt. Sure, these jobs don't take much muscle strength, but your biceps are essential for other jobs that do take strength. Working with your triceps and shoulder muscles, your biceps lift an armload of schoolbooks or help haul groceries.

Don't worry, strength training won't make you turn out looking like some freaky guy. It's physically impossible for women (especially young women) to develop oversized muscles unless they take health-damaging supplements like steroids. You want to be healthy and strong, not a candidate for those theatrical world wrestling championships.

Where are my biceps?

Your biceps are the two muscles on the front of your upper arm between your shoulder and elbow. You can see your biceps when you flex your arms out to your sides like a bodybuilder. The size of your biceps doesn't determine how strong they are. A girl with small biceps could be stronger than another girl who has big biceps. What's important is that your biceps be able to do their job for you.

What do biceps do?

Biceps are very busy muscles. They're responsible for everything from helping you bend your elbows (how many times a day do you do that?) to turning the pages of a book. Your biceps also help your back muscles when you pull on things like a door or a dog's leash. If you like playing sports, biceps help you do things like throw a ball, swing a tennis racket, shoot baskets, or row.

How do I get strong biceps?

Your biceps get exercise throughout the day because they're used for so many different tasks. But this doesn't mean that they're as strong as they should be. You tone your biceps by challenging them with resistance training, like weight lifting. Any exercise that bends and straightens your arm will do the trick. Try these resistance training exercises designed specifically to strengthen your biceps: standing curls and concentration curls. [Visit iemily.com if you need instructions for performing these exercises.] Or you can always use your own body weight to do push-ups.

Whether you work your biceps while standing or sitting, the goal is to isolate this muscle, so that it's the one doing the work. You'll get the best results if you use resistance, such as dumbbells, a body bar, or stretchy rubber bands. Start with a light weight—one pound is plenty for most girls getting started—and gradually increase the weight or resistance as you get stronger.

When is the best time to work my biceps?

It's best to save exercises that work the smaller muscles, such as biceps and triceps, until the end of your workout. That way, these muscles are fresh to help out with more challenging exercises that require more muscle strength, such as push-ups and pull-ups. And don't forget to work the opposite muscle group. In this case, that's the triceps.

Weak Triceps Tripping You Up? Get Toned!

Where are my triceps?

Have you heard of batwings? Well, that's what some people call those flabby flaps that hang off untoned arms when you wave good-bye. And that's where you'll find your tricep muscles—at the back of the upper arm. Strong triceps keep your arms looking good and they can make your life a lot easier, too.

What do triceps do?

The triceps work opposite your biceps. Together, they are in charge of straightening your arm. They help you do everything from picking up your keys to reaching up to catch a Frisbee. If you like playing sports, triceps help you do things like throw a ball, swing a tennis racket, shoot baskets, or row.

How do I get strong triceps?

Your tricep muscles are small and hard to isolate. That means you have to concentrate and use proper form to strengthen them. To keep your triceps toned, you'll need to include exercises that involve straightening and bending your arms.

Try these resistance training exercises for your triceps: dips and kickbacks. [Visit iemily.com if you need instructions for performing these exercises.] These tricep toners probably won't be your favorite part of the strength training routine because they're difficult, but they work.

> ### ✎ What's It Mean?
>
> Parallel: Extending in the same direction.
>
> Lactic Acid: An acid produced in the muscle tissues during strenuous exercise.
>
> Source: www.iEmily.com
> © 2006 iEmily.com.

How do I stretch my triceps?

After you finish your strength training routine, be sure to stretch your muscles. Stretching helps your muscles get rid of the lactic acid that builds up and makes you feel sore a day or two after your workout. [Visit iemily.com if you need instructions for a tricep stretch that feels great after a challenging workout.]

♣ It's A Fact!!
What causes muscle soreness?

Your muscles should feel sore on some days after you exercise. If you go out and jog the same two miles at the same pace, day after day, you will never become faster, stronger or have greater endurance. If you stop lifting weights when your muscles start to burn, you won't feel sore on the next day and you will not become stronger. All improvement in any muscle function comes from stressing and recovering. On one day, you go out and exercise hard enough to make your muscles burn during exercise. The burning is a sign that you are damaging your muscles. On the next day, your muscles feel sore because they are damaged and need time to recover. Scientist call this DOMS, delayed onset muscle soreness.

It takes at least eight hours to feel this type of soreness. You finish a workout and feel great; then you get up the next morning and your exercised muscles feel sore. We used to think that next-day muscle soreness is caused by a buildup of lactic acid in muscles, but now we know that lactic acid has nothing to do with it. Next-day muscle soreness is caused by damage to the muscle fibers themselves. Muscle biopsies taken on the day after hard exercise show bleeding and disruption of the z-band filaments that hold muscle fibers together as they slide over each other during a contraction.

Scientists can tell how much muscle damage has occurred by measuring blood levels of a muscle enzyme called serum creatine phosphokinase (CPK). CPK is normally found in muscles and is released into the bloodstream when muscles are damaged. Those exercisers who have the highest post-exercise blood levels of CPK often have the most muscle soreness. Using blood CPK levels as a measure of muscle damage, researchers have shown that people who continue

Super Shoulders!

Tennis phenom Serena Williams gets that booming serve from strong delts. And gymnast Shannon Miller relies on her delts to pull herself up and around the uneven bars. When it comes to strength training, don't give your delts the cold shoulder.

Where are my delts?

Delts (short for deltoids) refers to a group of muscles around your shoulder joint. You have front, middle, and back deltoid muscles. They all work

to exercise when their muscles feel sore are the ones most likely to feel sore on the next day.

Many people think that cooling down by exercising at a very slow pace after exercising more vigorously, helps to prevent muscle soreness. It doesn't. Cooling down speeds up the removal of lactic acid from muscles, but a buildup of lactic acid does not cause muscle soreness, so cooling down will not help to prevent muscle soreness. Stretching does not prevent soreness either, since post-exercise soreness is not due to contracted muscle fibers.

Next-day muscle soreness should be used as a guide to training, whatever your sport. On one day, go out and exercise right up to the burn, back off when your muscles really start to burn, then pick up the pace again and exercise to the burn. Do this exercise-to-the-burn and recover until your muscles start to feel stiff, and then stop the workout. Depending on how sore your muscles feel, take the next day off or go at a very slow pace. Do not attempt to train for muscle burning again until the soreness has gone away completely. Most athletes take a very hard workout on one day, go easy for one to seven days afterward, and then take a hard workout again. World-class marathon runners run very fast only twice a week. The best weightlifters lift very heavy only once every two weeks. High jumpers jump for height only once a week. Shot putters throw for distance only once a week. Exercise training is done by stressing and recovering.

—by Gabe Mirkin, M.D.

Source: "What Causes Muscle Soreness?" By Gabe Mirkin, MD. © 2007 www.DrMirkin.com. Reprinted with permission.

together to support and move your shoulders and arms. Most people refer to the whole group of muscles as the delts.

What do my delts do?

Your shoulders come into play every time you move your arm. That's because the deltoid muscles help connect your arms to your upper body. Delts are essential for everyday stuff, too. Without them, you couldn't wave to your friends across the cafeteria or slam your locker shut before everything inside comes pouring out. If you like sports, your delts help you do everything from spiking a volleyball to swimming laps.

How do I get strong shoulders?

Most exercises that involve your arms will help strengthen your shoulders. Upper body exercises, such as push-ups and pull-ups, also work the shoulders. Here are a couple favorites that help you concentrate on strengthening your delts: standing lateral raise and overhead shoulder press. [Visit iemily.com if you need instructions for performing these exercises.]

How do I stretch my delts?

After you finish your strength training routine, be sure to stretch your muscles. Stretching helps your muscles get rid of the lactic acid that builds up and makes you feel sore a day or two after your workout. [You can find instructions for a great stretch that stretches out your delts and also helps with your back and arms on the iemily.com website.]

Fear Not the Strong Chest: Pectoral Muscles

Where are my pecs?

Your pectorals (called pecs) are the chest muscles under your breasts. The pecs run from your breastbone to the shoulder on each side. Maybe that's why so many marketing gimmicks promise you'll increase the size of your breasts if you buy their chest-toning gadgets. The truth is that working your pecs will only firm your pecs. Chest exercises won't make your breasts bigger or smaller.

What do my pecs do?

Strong pecs help you push and hug, as well as add oomph to any movements that involve your arms and shoulders. Powerful pecs help you maneuver your bike up a steep hill when your legs are giving out. They help you mow the lawn quickly and give your friend a hug when she finds the earring you lost when you slept over her house. Pecs give gymnasts the strength to perform those powerful vaults and bar routines and give cross-country skiers speed and control.

How do I get strong pecs?

Any movement that involves pushing or pressing a weight (or your own body weight) will strengthen your pectoral muscles. While you're working your pecs, you'll be strengthening your shoulder muscles and triceps too. What a bonus!

How do I stretch my pecs?

After you finish your strength training routine, be sure to stretch your muscles. Stretching helps your muscles get rid of the lactic acid that builds up and makes you feel sore a day or two after your workout. If you are on a bench, let your arms drop to the sides and hang out to stretch your chest muscles. Or try a butterfly chest stretch to get a good stretch for your pecs. [Visit iemily.com if you need instructions for performing this exercise.]

The Geometry Of Your Upper Back

Where are my rhomboids, traps, and lats?

Rhomboids, trapezius, and latissimus dorsi sound like shapes you study in geometry class. But, unlike geometric shapes, you can't see them. These upper back muscles are right behind you.

The latissimus dorsi muscles (called lats) run in a fan-shape fashion from your armpit to your spine. They help you lift your arms up overhead. You use your trapezius muscles (called traps) when you shrug your shoulder. These muscles cross your shoulders and run down along your spine in something like a diamond shape. The rhomboids, which pull your shoulder blades together, sit between your spine and those blades.

What do my upper back muscles do?

You may not give these muscles much thought, but every time you pull something—a tug of war rope, an oar, a car door—your upper back is working. Swimmers, who spend so much time pulling water out of their way, have well-developed upper backs and shoulders.

How do I get a strong upper back?

Any exercise that involves a pulling motion will strengthen your upper back muscles. Since there are a lot of muscles involved, there are a lot of exercises to choose from. Here are two to get you started: pull-ups and one-arm row. [Visit iemily.com if you need instructions for performing these exercises.]

How do I stretch my upper back?

After you finish your strength training routine, be sure to stretch your muscles. Stretching helps your muscles get rid of the lactic acid that builds up and makes you feel sore a day or two after your workout. An upper back stretch that feels great after a challenging workout is the folded bend or Child's Pose. [Visit iemily.com if you need instructions for performing this exercise.]

Get A Hard Core: Building Lower Back Muscles

Where are my lower back muscles?

You've heard at least one adult—your mother or father, a teacher, or friend—grumble about his or her aching back. Chances are the problem stemmed from the tailbone or lower back. You can avoid this misery by strengthening the muscles that run along both sides of your spine (formerly called erector spinae).

What do my lower back muscles do?

Together with your stomach muscles (abdominals, or "abs"), your lower back muscles act like a girdle supporting your torso. Strong lower back muscles give you the support you need to help a friend re-arrange her bedroom furniture. They also keep you comfortable when you're stuck at a desk doing homework for hours on end. Those lower back muscles are also the key to safety when you lift weights (or the kid you are babysitting). And gymnasts know a strong lower back puts the spring in back handsprings.

How do I get strong lower back muscles?

Some lower back exercises require no equipment. You can do them anywhere you have enough space to lie down. You can also strengthen your lower back—along with your abs and the rest of your torso—using a medicine ball, or weighted workout ball. Originally used by boxers in training, these balls are great tools for building a strong torso. And they're a fun way to work out with a friend. Try these resistance-training exercises for your lower back: back extension and ball pass. [Visit iemily.com if you need instructions for performing these exercises.]

How do I stretch my lower back muscles?

After you finish your strength training routine, be sure to stretch your muscles. Stretching helps your muscles get rid of the lactic acid that builds up and makes you feel sore a day or two after your workout.

Get Your Rear In Gear

Where are my glutes and quads?

The muscles that you sit on have an important sounding name, gluteus maximus (called glutes). Your glutes are one of the biggest muscles you've got, covering all of each cheek in your butt and extending down the back of your outer thigh. Four big muscles called the quadriceps (or quads) run down the front of your thigh.

What do my glutes and quads do?

Your glutes are in charge of straightening your leg from the hip. Every time you pedal a bike, climb stairs, or get up from a chair, you have your glutes to thank. Your quads straighten your leg from the knee. Strong glutes and quads boost your power, speed, and stamina for most activities and sports. Cyclists need them to crank up big hills. Speed skaters couldn't hold that low crouch without strong glutes and quads. Soccer players need them to sprint and boot the ball. Glutes and quads give figure skaters the lift they need to get airborne for double axels and triple toe loops. And kickboxers get their kick from strong glutes and quads.

Okay, so you don't want to be the next Bonnie Blair or Tara Lipinski and you're not into Tae-Bo. But it's still smart to work these big muscles. Strong glutes and quads help protect your hips and knees. And toning these muscles will help you walk those endless halls at school or dance until dawn.

How can I get strong glutes and quads?

It's tough to target the glutes alone, so butt strengthening exercises are often a package deal. You'll be working the quads and hamstrings (the muscles at the back of your thighs) at the same time. Try these resistance-training exercises designed specifically to strengthen your glutes and quads: squats, lunges, and step-ups. [Visit iemily.com if you need instructions for performing these exercises.]

How can I stretch my glutes and quads?

After you finish your strength training routine, be sure to stretch your muscles. Stretching helps your muscles get rid of the lactic acid that builds up and makes you feel sore a day or two after your workout. Stretches called the crossover stretch for your glutes and the lying quad stretch for the back of your legs great after a challenging workout. [Visit iemily.com if you need instructions for performing these exercises.]

Thigh Master

Where are my adductors and abductors?

In addition to the hamstrings on the back of your thighs and the quadriceps on the front of your thighs, you have outer and inner thigh muscles. The muscles that run down the outside of your thigh are called abductors. Your inner thigh muscles are called adductors.

What do my inner and outer thigh muscles do?

Your adductors and abductors help you move from side to side. Strong thigh muscles help you sidestep a brigade of charging snowballers and help you step aside just before your dog plows you over with an enthusiastic greeting. Basketball players need them to dodge a player on the way to the hoop. Kickboxers count on them for all those sidekicks. Tennis players need them to leap across the court for a wide ball. And girls who do aerobics use the inner and outer thigh muscles to do step patterns like the grapevine.

How do I get strong thighs?

Instead of doing boring leg lifts on the floor, try a standing exercise called the side lunge. [Visit iemily.com if you need instructions for performing this exercise.] While you stretch and strengthen your inner and outer thighs, you'll be working your quads and butt, as well as your hamstring muscles.

How do I stretch my inner and outer thighs?

After you finish your strength training routine, be sure to stretch your muscles. Stretching helps your muscles get rid of the lactic acid that builds up and makes you feel sore a day or two after your workout.

Tug Of War: Your Hamstring Muscles

Where are my hamstrings?

Your hamstrings are the muscles behind the thigh. This big muscle stretches all the way from your butt to the back of your knee.

What do my hamstrings do?

In a never-ending tug of war, the hamstrings straighten the knee, while the quadriceps (on the front of your thighs) bend it. You couldn't even walk if you didn't have hamstring muscles. Runners and other athletes tend to develop very strong hamstrings. But most of us forget about those muscles on the back of our thighs and end up with weak hamstrings. Strong quads and weak hams is a recipe for injury—that's why athletes spend a lot of time strengthening and stretching their hamstrings.

How do I get strong hamstrings?

The hamstrings, quads, and the muscles of your buttocks (glutes) work as a team. Quad and glute exercises such as lunges and squats also target the hamstrings. If you want to focus on the hamstrings alone, add an exercise that involves bending only the knee, not the hip and the knee. The most common one is called a hamstring curl. These can be done on a machine at the gym. Girls who don't have access to weight-training machines can get great results with elastic rubber tubing (sold at sporting goods stores). It doesn't take up any space and comes in cool, neon colors. Try a resistance training exercise for your hamstrings called the hamstring curl. [Visit iemily.com if you need instructions for performing this exercise.]

How do I stretch my hamstrings?

After you finish your strength training routine, be sure to stretch your muscles. Stretching helps your muscles get rid of the lactic acid that builds up and makes you feel sore a day or two after your workout. Hamstrings tend to be tight so it is especially important to include a hamstring stretch in your workout. [Visit iemily.com if you need instructions for performing this exercise.]

Give Those Legs A Lift: Building Strong Calf Muscles

Where are my calf muscles?

Their official names are gastrocnemius and soleus, but calf muscle is a lot easier to say. You'll find these muscles at the back of your lower leg. The gastrocnemius is the bulkier one, just below your knee. The soleus sits underneath the gastrocnemius and reaches down towards your ankle.

What do my calf muscles do?

The big gastrocnemius does the heavy lifting when you go up on tiptoes. That comes in handy for ballet but also when you're stuck in a crowd and you want to see over some guy's head. The smaller soleus gets in on the action whenever you bend your knees. In other words, your calf muscles are working almost all the time.

How do I get strong calves?

Any aerobic activity that involves pushing off with your toes works your calves. That includes pushing a skateboard uphill with one foot, walking, running, doing step aerobics, dancing, and kickboxing. [Visit iemily.com if you need instructions for performing calf strengthening exercises you can do while waiting for the bus or talking on the phone.]

How do I stretch my calves?

After you finish your strength training routine or after a run or aerobic workout, be sure to stretch your calf muscles. Stretching helps your muscles get rid of the lactic acid that builds up and makes you feel sore a day or two after your workout. [Visit iemily.com if you need instructions for performing a calf stretch that feels great after a challenging workout.]

Your Body: The Abdominal Muscles

Gut, stomach, tummy, belly. Whatever you call it, in medical-speak it's known as your abdomen and the muscles in it are called your abdominals, or "abs" for short.

What are abdominal muscles?

Abdominals are more than just the muscles that wrap around your middle. Strong abs provide the balance that keeps a ballerina on her toes. They protect a kickboxer's internal organs. Abs help yoginis do breathing exercises. And they support your lower back when you lift weights or lug books around in your backpack. Your abs are actually three different muscles with three different jobs. That means doing a variety of exercises will pay off in strong, healthy abs. Combine abdominal strength training with cardiorespiratory exercise (aerobics) to burn fat, and you'll soon have killer abs.

What do I use my abdominal muscles for?

The rectus abdominis muscles are found in the outermost part of your abdomen. They run down the front of your body from your rib cage to your pelvis. They help stabilize your body, support your spine, help you keep your balance and your back straight, and allow you to bend at the waist. You use them when you walk and run, and even when you breathe.

Your external and internal oblique muscles are found on the sides of your stomach. They define your waist. Your obliques are your "twister" muscles. They allow you to twist and turn at the waist. You use them when you pivot, play basketball, or swing a golf club.

How do I tone my abdominal muscles?

Basic crunches are the place to start, especially if you haven't been working out. Unless you already have very strong abs, you don't need to use weights. Lie down on the floor, and place your hands behind your head. Keep your focus on your abs and your gaze up toward the ceiling to avoid straining your neck. Also, because your abs are really three different muscles, doing a variety of exercises helps target them all. [Visit iemily.com if you need instructions for performing some additional crunches.] Do these on an exercise mat, a thick towel, or a carpet.

About iEmily

iEmily.com is a health website that provides teen girls with respectful, in-depth information about physical health and emotional well-being. The site includes articles reviewed by physicians, psychologists, and educators on nutrition, physical fitness, sexual health, emotional and psychological concerns, and other topics. iEmily.com also offers links to websites for additional information, as well as a list of hotlines for immediate help.

Chapter 8

Stretching: An Important Component Of Fitness

Flexible Benefits

We take part in aerobic activity to improve our cardiovascular endurance and burn fat. We weight-train to maintain lean muscle tissue and build strength. Those are the two most important elements of a fitness program, right?

Actually, there are three important elements. Often neglected is flexibility training. That neglect is regrettable, because flexibility training:

- Allows greater freedom of movement and improved posture;
- Increases physical and mental relaxation;
- Releases muscle tension and soreness;
- Reduces risk of injury.

Some people are naturally more flexible. Flexibility is primarily due to one's genetics, gender, age, and level of physical activity. As we grow older, we tend to lose flexibility, usually as a result of inactivity rather than the

About This Chapter: This chapter begins with "Flexible Benefits," reprinted with permission from the American Council on Exercise (www.acefitness.org), © 2001. All rights reserved. Additional information from the American Academy of Orthopaedic Surgeons is cited separately within the chapter.

aging process itself. The less active we are, the less flexible we are likely to be. As with cardiovascular endurance and muscle strength, flexibility will improve with regular training.

Stretch For Success

Before stretching, take a few minutes to warm up as stretching cold muscles can cause injury. Begin with a simple, low-intensity warm-up, such as easy walking while swinging the arms in a wide circle. Spend at least five to 10 minutes warming up prior to stretching.

Fitting Stretching Into A Compressed Schedule

Time constraints keep many people from stretching. Some complain they just don't have time to stretch; others hurry out of their fitness classes before the cool-down exercises are completed.

Ideally, at least 30 minutes, three times per week, should be spent on flexibility training. But even a mere five minutes of stretching at the end of an exercise session is better than nothing. And all aerobic activity should be followed by at least a few minutes of stretching.

Here are some tips for fitting stretching into an overstuffed schedule:

- If you don't have time to sufficiently warm up before stretching, try doing a few stretches immediately after a shower or while soaking in a hot tub. The hot water elevates muscle temperature enough to make them more pliable and receptive to stretching.

> **Remember!!**
>
> When performing any stretch:
>
> - Start each stretch slowly, exhaling as you gently stretch the muscle.
> - Try to hold each stretch for at least 10 to 30 seconds.
>
> Avoid these stretching mistakes:
>
> - Don't bounce a stretch. Holding a stretch is more effective and there is less risk of injury.
> - Don't stretch a muscle that is not warmed up.
> - Don't strain or push a muscle too far. If a stretch hurts, ease up.
> - Don't hold your breath.
>
> Source: © 2001 ACE.

- Try a few simple stretches before getting out of bed in the morning. Wake yourself up with a few full-body stretches by pointing the toes and reaching the arms above your head. This can clear your mind and help jump-start your morning.

- Take a stretching class such as yoga or Tai Chi. Scheduling a class will help you to stick with a regular stretching program.

Flexibility Exercises For Young Athletes

Source: "Flexibility Exercises For Young Athletes," reproduced with permission from Moseley C: *Your Orthopaedic Connection*. Rosemont, IL, American Academy of Orthopaedic Surgeons, © 2007. All rights reserved.

Staying injury-free throughout the sports season requires a proper pre-exercise stretching program. Here are some stretching exercises that members of the American Academy of Orthopaedic Surgeons believe to be a good general set of flexibility exercises for young athletes to perform before participating in any athletic activity.

Athletes must do each one of the exercises carefully, speed is not important. Once the exercise routine is learned, the entire program should take no longer than 10 minutes.

Be sure to warm up before doing any of these exercises. Good examples of warm up activities are slowly running in place and walking for a few minutes.

Seat Straddle Lotus

- Sit down, placing the soles of the feet together, and drop the knees toward floor. Place the forearms on the inside of the knees and push the knees toward the ground. Lean forward from the hips.

- Hold for five seconds.

- Repeat three to six times.

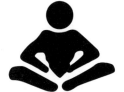

Figure 8.1. Seat Straddle Lotus

Seat Side Straddle

- Sit with legs spread, placing both hands on the same shin or ankle. Bring the chin toward the knee, keeping the leg straight.

- Hold for five seconds.

- Repeat three to six times.

- Repeat exercise on the opposite leg.

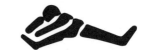

Figure 8.2. Seat Side Straddle

Seat Stretch

- Sit with the legs together, feet flexed, and hands on the shins or ankles. Bring the chin toward the knees.

- Hold for five seconds.

- Repeat three to six times.

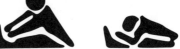

Figure 8.3. Seat Stretch

Knees To Chest

- Lie on the back with knees bent. Grasp the tops of knees and bring them out toward the armpits, rocking gently.

- Hold for five seconds.

- Repeat three to five times.

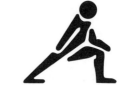

Figure 8.4. Knees To Chest

Forward Lunges

- Kneel on the left leg, placing the right leg forward at a right angle. Lunge forward, keeping the back straight. Stretch should be felt on the left groin.

- Hold for five seconds.

- Repeat three to six times.

- Repeat on opposite leg.

Figure 8.5. Forward Lunges

Side Lunges

- Stand with legs apart, bending the left knee while leaning toward the left. Keep the back straight and the right leg straight.

- Hold for five seconds.

- Repeat three to six times.

- Repeat on opposite leg.

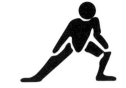

Figure 8.6. Side Lunges

Cross-Over

- Stand with legs crossed, keeping the feet close together and the legs straight. Try to touch the toes.

- Hold for five seconds.

- Repeat three to six times.

- Repeat with the opposite leg.

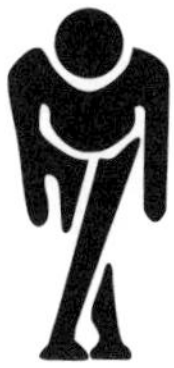

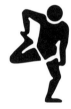

Figure 8.7. Cross-Over

Standing Quad Stretch

- Stand supported by holding onto a wall or chair. Pull the foot behind to the buttocks. Try to keep knees close together.

- Hold for five seconds.

- Repeat three to six times.

Figure 8.8. Standing Quad Stretch

Chapter 9

Exercise To Build Healthy Bones

Bone Up On Bone Loss, Exercise To Build Healthy Bones

Bone Health Is Important

Our bones give us the freedom to do the things we want to do. They help us to stand up straight, to run, to jump, and to play. That's why it is important for our bones to stay strong and healthy our whole lives long.

Unfortunately, many older people have bones that are weak and break easily. Osteoporosis is a condition in which bones are fragile, making them fracture or break much easier.

Osteoporosis usually doesn't show up in our bones until we are adults, but can start when we are young.

Between the ages 10 to 18 is when you make the bone that must last a lifetime. This bone is known as peak bone mass. To reach the best possible peak bone mass means getting enough exercise and calcium. Bones are like a bank account—if you deposit lots of exercise and calcium now, when you are young, you will have strong bones for later in life.

About This Chapter: This chapter includes information from "Bone Up On Bone Loss! Exercise To Build Healthy Bones!" U.S. Department of Health and Human Services, 2000; and excerpts from "What Girls Need To Know About Bone Health," National Women's Health Information Center, July 2007.

How Exercise Helps Bones

One important way to help keep your bones healthy for your entire life is through exercise. Exercise is the way you tell bones that they need to be strong. Just like exercising your muscles can make them grow bigger, exercising your bones makes them work harder, which helps them to build up bone mass. And building bone mass as a child or teenager is especially important because this is when our bones are growing the most.

Good Exercises For Healthy Bones

Weight-bearing exercise is one of the most important things kids can do right now to build bone mass and reduce the risk for osteoporosis later. Weight-bearing exercises make your bones and muscles work. For exercises, like jogging or jumping rope, your feet and legs are carrying your body weight. Regular weight-bearing exercise can help people reach the best possible peak bone mass when they are young and help keep that bone strength throughout life.

Some activities like swimming do not involve weight-bearing benefits. They do build strong muscles, though, which also helps to build strong bones.

The 1996 Surgeon General's Report on Physical Activity and Health recommends that everyone over age two should participate in at least 30 minutes of moderate physical activity, preferably, each day of the week. To keep your bones growing strong, gradually begin to exercise with more intensity and for longer periods of time.

Table 9.1. How Much Calcium Do Kids Need Each Day?

Age	Milligrams
1–3 years	500 mg
4–8 years	800 mg
9–18 years	1,300 mg

Source: U.S. Department of Health and Human Services, 2000.

♣ **It's A Fact!!**

Here Are Some Exercises For Strong Healthy Bones

- Walking
- Jogging
- Climbing stairs
- Hiking

- Aerobic dancing
- Racquet sports
- Dancing
- Cross country skiing

Jumping and running sports are also great exercises for bone health. Sports like basketball, volleyball, soccer, field hockey, and softball are other good ways to build strong bones too.

Source: U.S. Department of Health and Human Services, 2000.

Other Important Things For Healthy Bones

Our bodies continually remove and replace small amounts of calcium from our bones. If your body removes more calcium than it replaces, your bones will become weaker and have a greater chance of breaking.

In addition to proper exercise, other things like calcium are important for building strong and healthy bones. When we get enough calcium from the foods we eat and drink, our bodies don't have to take the calcium from our bones. Kids should start now to store plenty of calcium in their bones for later in life.

Milk and other dairy foods, such as cheese and yogurt, are excellent sources of calcium. One eight-ounce glass of milk has about 300 milligrams (mg) of calcium. Children and teens need about 1300 mg of calcium a day. Kids can also get calcium from alternative sources such as foods rich in calcium or supplements. Check the nutrition label on foods you buy to choose foods high in calcium and low in fat and calories.

Make A Commitment To Last A Lifetime

Healthy bones are important for a healthy body. Getting enough physical activity is the way to make your bones grow strong. Whether it's as part of a gym class, an after school sport, or just playing with friends, being active is a key to strong bones. Getting enough calcium when you are younger helps your bones to stay strong and healthy too. Don't forget, what you do for your bones now can have a big impact on what your bones do for you later in life.

What Girls Need To Know About Bone Health

What is osteoporosis?

Osteoporosis is a disease that thins and weakens bones to the point where they break easily. Hip, spine (backbone) and wrist bones are often involved. Osteoporosis is called a "silent disease" because bone loss happens without much notice. Having a bone break easily or getting a little shorter is often the first sign of this disease. While osteoporosis can strike at any age, over half of all women over age 65 have it.

There are certain factors that are linked to your chances of getting osteoporosis. These are called risk factors. Some risk factors cannot be changed, while others can be changed. Below are risk factors for osteoporosis that cannot be changed.

- **Sex:** Women are more likely to develop the disease than men.
- **Age:** The longer you live, the greater your chances are of getting the disease.
- **Family history:** This disease runs in families.
- **Body size:** Women who are small-boned and thin have a higher risk than women who are larger-boned and weigh more.
- **Ethnicity:** White and Asian women are at greater risk for this disease.

Below are risk factors for osteoporosis that can be changed.

- **Diet:** Getting enough calcium and vitamin D.
- **Physical activity:** Exercise helps keep bones strong and healthy.
- **Smoking:** Smoking can cause you to go through menopause earlier and boost your risk for osteoporosis.

Why should I be worried about bone health now?

Your peak bone-making years are your childhood and teen years. If you do not make enough bone as a kid, your risk for osteoporosis goes up. And, while not common, a young woman can get osteoporosis.

What is weight-bearing physical activity?

Weight-bearing physical activity is any activity in which your body works against gravity, so your feet and legs are supporting or carrying your weight. Examples of weight-bearing physical activities include walking, running, tennis, dancing, tae kwon do, hiking, hopscotch, and basketball.

Activities that are not weight-bearing include riding a bike, swimming, and skateboarding. These activities are good for overall health, though, and can be mixed in with weight-bearing activities.

How do calcium and physical activity make bones stronger?

To make bones strong and to keep them strong, the body needs both calcium and weight-bearing physical activity. One or the other is not enough to make bones strong—it takes both.

• **Calcium** helps bones to grow right. When the body makes new bone tissue, it first lays down a framework of a protein called collagen. Then, calcium from the blood spreads throughout the collagen framework. The hard crystals of calcium attach to the bone structure. Calcium and collagen work together to make bones both strong and flexible.

• **Physical activity** helps bones become stronger and thicker, just as a muscle gets stronger and bigger the more you use it. Bones are living tissue.

How much calcium do I need? Do I have to drink a lot of milk?

Girls ages nine to 18 should get 1300 milligrams of calcium per day. There are lots of ways to get calcium, including milk. Table 9.2 lists the amount of calcium that is found in different foods and drinks. As you can see, there are lots of good tasting foods and drinks you can choose to make sure you get enough calcium.

Table 9.2. Foods High In Calcium

Food	Portion Size	Calcium (mg)*
Plain, fat-free yogurt	1 cup	450
Grilled cheese sandwich**	1 sandwich	371
American cheese	2 ounces	350
Ricotta cheese, part skim	½ cup	340
Fruit yogurt	1 cup	315
Milk (fat-free, low-fat, or whole)	1 cup	300
Orange juice with added calcium	1 cup	300
Soy beverage with added calcium	1 cup	250–300
Cheese pizza	1 slice	220
Cheddar cheese	1 ounce	204
Tofu (made with calcium)	½ cup (about five one-inch cubes)	204
Macaroni and cheese	½ cup	180
Cottage Cheese	1 cup	138
Frozen yogurt (fat-free or low-fat)	½ cup	105
Broccoli, cooked or fresh	1 cup	90
Ice cream	½ cup	84
Bok choy, cooked or fresh	½ cup	80
Almonds, dry roasted	1 ounce(About 20–25 almonds)	71
White bread	2 slices	70

* Amount of calcium depends on the ingredients of many foods.

** Using 2 slices of white bread, 1½ ounces of cheese, and nonstick cooking spray.

Source: National Women's Health Information Center, July 2007.

Should I take a calcium supplement to make sure I get enough?

Girls who have allergies or other dietary limitations should ask their doctor about calcium supplements, but most girls can get enough calcium by eating the right types of foods.

Can I get too much calcium?

While it is possible to get too much calcium, it is not likely for most girls. Even with all the products that have added calcium, many girls take in far less calcium each day than the 1300 milligrams they need.

Can I get enough calcium if milk upsets my stomach?

Yes. Lactose intolerance means some girls get a stomachache or have gas after they have milk or other dairy products. The good news is that there are milk and other dairy products that are specially made for people with lactose intolerance. Look for milks, cheeses, cottage cheese, and other products that are made with the enzyme lactase, which helps people digest dairy. You can also buy Lactaid pills to chew or swallow with the first bite of dairy, which also have lactase. There are also other foods that have calcium like broccoli, almonds, and foods that have added calcium like orange juice and cereals. Remember to look for "calcium" on food labels.

Are dairy products fattening?

There are many low-fat or non-fat milk products available. Also, there is the same amount of calcium in non-fat and low-fat milk. Dairy products are a very important part of teen's diet. They provide calcium, vitamin D, and other nutrients that help prevent osteoporosis. There are good non-dairy sources of calcium, but dairy products offer the most calcium per serving. For example, one cup of fat-free or low-fat milk has about 300 milligrams of calcium. One cup of broccoli (cooked or fresh) has about 90 milligrams of calcium.

I've heard that soda is bad for my bones. Why?

Young girls often choose soft drinks over milk and other drinks high in calcium. If you drink sodas with caffeine and sugar, you will have less room for bone-healthy drinks like milk and other drinks that have extra calcium added to them.

What else can I do to improve my bone health?

Steer clear of alcohol and smoking, and make sure your diet is healthy overall. Smoking, drinking alcohol, and having eating disorders such as anorexia nervosa or bulimia can cause weaker bones. If you have any of these habits and would like to stop, ask an adult that you trust for help. It is best, though, to never start these dangerous behaviors.

My neighborhood is not very safe. How can I take part in weight-bearing activity while staying indoors?

There are plenty of indoor weight-bearing exercises that you can do to get strong, healthy bones. Dancing, lifting hand-held weights (or soup cans), jogging in-place, and push-ups can be done both indoors and outdoors.

What kinds of weight-bearing exercise can girls with physical disabilities do to keep their bones strong?

These are examples of weight-bearing exercises for girls with physical disabilities:

- **Wheelchair aerobics** combines upper body movements and stretches to improve flexibility. They are done in a seated position, often to music.

- **Arm cycling** (ergometry) is like bicycling, only it is done with the arms instead of the legs. A girl can use a stationary (non-moving) bike or arm-driven cycles made for outdoor use. Always wear a helmet when cycling outdoors.

- **Wheeling** involves moving a wheelchair forward, using the arms or legs, over an extended distance. This can be done inside or outside, using a regular wheelchair or a specialized sport wheelchair.

- **Resistance training** uses wide elastic bands. One end of a band is attached to a non-moving object such as a doorknob, leg of a bed, or a heavy table while the other end is held and stretched to exercise one part of the body at a time. Hand weights can also be used for this type of training.

- **Some sports** can be adapted for girls with physical disabilities, like wheelchair tennis and wheelchair basketball.

Chapter 10

Measuring Physical Activity Intensity

The intensity of physical activity, or how hard your body is working, is typically categorized as light, moderate, or vigorous based on the amount of energy or effort a person expends in performing the activity.

This chapter describes methods of estimating the relative intensity of any physical activity as it applies to your own level of health. Samples of exercises and their intensity levels are also provided.

Talk Test

Physical activity can add years to your life and life to your years. The talk test method of measuring intensity is simple. A person who is active at a light intensity level should be able to sing while doing the activity. One who is active at a moderate intensity level should be able to carry on a conversation comfortably while engaging in the activity. If a person becomes winded or too out of breath to carry on a conversation, the activity can be considered vigorous.

Target Heart Rate And Estimated Maximum Heart Rate

Measuring target heart rate and estimated maximum heart rate is another way of monitoring physical activity intensity. It is used to determine

About This Chapter: This chapter includes excerpts from "Measuring Physical Activity Intensity," Centers for Disease Control and Prevention (CDC), May 2007. Additional information from Kidnetic/International Food Information Council is cited separately within the chapter.

whether a person's pulse or heart rate is within the target zone during physical activity.

For moderate-intensity physical activity, a person's target heart rate should be 50 to 70 percent of his or her maximum heart rate. This maximum rate is based on the person's age. An estimate of a person's maximum age-related heart rate can be obtained by subtracting the person's age from 220. This answer is the estimated maximum age-related heart rate. Multiply this answer by 50 percent and 70 percent to find the target heart rate for moderate-intensity physical activity.

☞ Remember!!

The amount of time needed for exercise depends on the intensity of the exercise. Higher intensity activities require less time spent. Lower intensity activities require more time spent.

For vigorous-intensity physical activity, a person's target heart rate should be 70 to 85 percent of his or her maximum heart rate. To calculate this range, follow the same formula as used above, except change "50 and 70 percent" to "70 and 85 percent" to find the target heart rate for vigorous-intensity physical activity.

Taking Your Heart Rate

Generally, to determine whether you are exercising within the heart rate target zone, you must stop exercising briefly to take your pulse. You can take the pulse at the neck, the wrist, or the chest. We recommend the wrist. You can feel the radial pulse on the artery of the wrist in line with the thumb. Place the tips of the index and middle fingers over the artery and press lightly. Do not use the thumb. Take a full 60-second count of the heartbeats, or take for 30 seconds and multiply by 2. Start the count on a beat, which is counted as "zero."

Perceived Exertion (Borg Rating Of Perceived Exertion Scale)

Another method of determining physical activity intensity is the Borg Rating of Perceived Exertion (RPE). Perceived exertion is how hard you feel your body is working. It is based on the physical sensations you experience during physical activity including increased heart rate, increased respiration, breathing rate, increased sweating, and muscle fatigue. Although this is a subjective measure, experts have found a high correlation between a person's RPE and the actual heart rate during physical activity.

The numbers on the Borg Scale range from six to 20, where six means "no exertion at all" and 20 means "maximal exertion." Practitioners generally agree that RPE ratings between 12–14 (somewhat hard) on the Borg Scale suggests that your physical activity is being performed at a moderate level of intensity. If you describe your muscle fatigue and breathing as a level nine (very light), you would want to increase your intensity. On the other hand, if you feel your exertion is 19 (extremely hard), you would need to slow down your movements to achieve the moderate-intensity range.

Metabolic Equivalent (MET) Level

Another way of measuring physical activity intensity is by the metabolic equivalent, or MET, level. Although the intensity of certain activities is commonly characterized as light, moderate, or vigorous, many activities can be classified in any one or all three categories simply on the basis of the level of personal effort involved in carrying out the activity (like how hard one is working to do the activity). For example, one can bicycle at intensities ranging from very light to very vigorous.

✔ Quick Tip

The harder your body works, the higher the MET.

• One MET is the energy (oxygen) used by the body as you sit quietly, perhaps while talking on the phone or reading a book.

• Any activity that burns three to six METs is considered moderate-intensity physical activity.

• Any activity that burns more than six METs is considered vigorous-intensity physical activity.

Source: Centers for Disease Control and Prevention (CDC), May 2007.

✔ Quick Tip

Five Fun Ways To Get Physical

Who says you have to play sports to have fun and be fit? There are lots of great ways to put more action in your life. Being active helps you build strong bones and muscles. It also helps you look and feel your best. And it helps give you more energy to do other things.

Pick and choose some of these fun ways to get fit. Or think of your own ways to get moving. Your body will thank you.

1. **Use your feet.** Your feet were made for walking, so use them every chance you get. Walk to a friend's house, to the store, around the mall, or wherever it's safe to walk. While you're at it, walk your dog. Or offer to walk your neighbor's dog.

2. **Move to the beat.** Turn up the music and dance. Dance with your friends or on your own. And who says you can't do two things at once? Dance while you talk on the phone. Dance while you watch TV. You can even dance while you clean your room!

3. **Roll around town.** Make your muscles do the work on your bike, skates, or scooter as you enjoy the cool breeze. Don't forget to wear the gear: a helmet, and knee, wrist, and elbow pads for skating.

4. **Get your friends moving.** Gather a few friends to shoot hoops, kick around a soccer ball, play street hockey, or throw around a football or baseball. You don't need to be on a team to enjoy sports. Check out the rec center in your neighborhood for open gym times and other fun activities like tennis, swimming, or dance classes.

5. **Be a buddy.** Stuck babysitting or playing with younger brothers or sisters? Make it play time. Young kids love games like hopscotch, tag, hide-and-seek, Hula-Hoops, jump rope, squirt guns, T-ball, kickball, or flying a kite—especially when they're doing it with a "cool" older friend like you.

"Five Fun Ways To Get Physical," reprinted with permission from www.kidnetic.com, a website of the International Food Informational Council Foundation. © 2006 IFIC Foundation. All rights reserved.

The information below provides one method of characterizing physical activities at different levels of effort based on the standard of a metabolic equivalent (MET). This unit is used to estimate the amount of oxygen used by the body during physical activity.

General Physical Activities Defined By Level Of Intensity

The following is in accordance with Centers for Disease Control and Prevention (CDC) and American College of Sports Medicine (ACSM) guidelines.

Moderate Activity (3.0 to 6.0 METs; 3.5 to 5 kcal/min

- Walking at a moderate or brisk pace of 3 to 4.5 mph on a level surface.
- Using crutches
- Hiking
- Roller skating or in-line skating at a leisurely pace
- Bicycling 5 to 9 mph, level terrain, or with few hills
- Stationary bicycling—using moderate effort
- Water aerobics
- Calisthenics—light
- Yoga
- Gymnastics
- General home exercises, light or moderate effort, getting up and down from the floor
- Jumping on a trampoline
- Using a stair climber machine at a light-to-moderate pace
- Using a rowing machine—with moderate effort
- Weight training and body-building
- Boxing—punching bag
- Ballroom dancing
- Line dancing
- Square dancing
- Folk dancing
- Modern dancing, disco
- Ballet
- Table tennis—competitive
- Tennis—doubles
- Golf, wheeling, or carrying clubs
- Softball—fast pitch or slow pitch
- Basketball—shooting baskets
- Coaching children's or adults' sports

Vigorous Activity (Greater than 6.0 METs; more than 7 kcal/min)

- Racewalking and aerobic walking—5 mph or faster
- Jogging or running
- Wheeling your wheelchair
- Walking and climbing briskly up a hill
- Backpacking
- Mountain climbing, rock climbing, or rappelling
- Roller skating or in-line skating at a brisk pace
- Bicycling more than 10 mph or bicycling on steep uphill terrain
- Stationary bicycling—using vigorous effort
- Aerobic dancing—high impact
- Step aerobics
- Water jogging
- Teaching an aerobic dance class
- Calisthenics—vigorous effort
- Karate, judo, tae kwon do, jujitsu
- Jumping rope
- Performing jumping jacks
- Using a stair climber machine at a fast pace
- Using a rowing machine— with vigorous effort
- Using an arm cycling machine—with vigorous effort
- Circuit weight training
- Boxing—in the ring, sparring
- Wrestling—competitive
- Professional ballroom dancing—energetically
- Square dancing—energetically
- Folk dancing—energetically
- Clogging
- Tennis—singles
- Wheelchair tennis
- Most competitive sports
- Football game
- Basketball game
- Wheelchair basketball
- Soccer
- Rugby
- Kickball
- Field or in-line skate hockey
- Lacrosse

Chapter 11

Make An Exercise Plan

Physical fitness has many parts. When you are physically fit you have the energy and strength to perform daily activities without getting tired. Also, you have the energy to participate in leisure and recreation activities. When you are fit you have a strong heart, lungs, and muscles. Fitness benefits your daily activities, making it easier to meet daily demands. It also improves your mental health and your ability to cope with stressful events.

Why Do We Measure Physical Activity?

Physical Activity is a general term that encompasses most movements that are produced by skeletal muscles and result in an increase in energy expenditure. Being physically active leads to many lifestyle improvements, including physical and mental health benefits. Activities that would generally result in a change in energy expenditure include tumbling, walking to school, and playing games that require movement. You should try to be as active as possible at an early age. Building active habits now will help you keep these habits into adulthood.

The time for fitness is now. Children who are physically active and eat correctly grow into healthier and more active adults.

About This Chapter: This chapter includes excerpts from "Get Fit And Be Active," the President's Council on Physical Fitness and Sports, 2006.

✔ Quick Tip
Get In The Groove With The 10-Minute Move

Moving your body by running, jumping, walking, and playing gives you energy, makes your muscles stronger, and helps you feel good about yourself. Moving for 60 minutes every day is a great goal. But don't worry if that seems like too much to do at one time. Try doing your moves for just 10 minutes, but do them at least a few times each day.

See how many 10-minute moves you can do each day, like during a homework break or while you're watching TV. Do your favorite thing or try one of the ideas below. If you want to do more than 10 minutes at a time, you'll feel even better.

- Turn on your favorite music and dance.
- Walk to a friend's house that's a few blocks away.
- Go outside and rake leaves, pull weeds or sweep the sidewalk.
- Do inside chores like vacuuming, dusting or emptying the garbage.
- Do jumping jacks for one minute, march in place for one minute and step up and down a stair for one minute. Repeat until 10 minutes are up.
- Play tag with your younger brother or sister.
- Skip rope.
- Walk the dog.
- In-line skate.
- Do part of an exercise tape.
- Shoot baskets in the driveway or at the rec center.
- Practice the Hula-Hoop.
- Kick a soccer ball.
- Ride an exercise bike.
- Jog around the block.

Source: "Get In The Groove With The 10-Minute Move," reprinted with permission from www.kidnetic.com, a website of the International Food Informational Council Foundation. © IFIC Foundation. All rights reserved.

Measuring Physical Fitness

The five components of physical fitness are: aerobic capacity, muscular strength, muscular endurance, flexibility, and body composition. Each of these components of physical fitness is measurable.

- **Aerobic Capacity:** The ability of your heart and lungs to supply the muscles of your body with oxygen—an indicator of aerobic fitness. Exercises like cycling, running, swimming, and walking build this type of endurance. How quickly you can run a mile (or shorter distances for younger children) is a test of cardiorespiratory endurance.

- **Muscular Strength:** The amount of force you exert with a muscle. Your body has many muscles and all of them should be exercised to keep them strong. You can use your body weight, or additional weights, such as barbells. Weight-training machines are popular, too. Performing strength-training exercises can help you become strong and less likely to get injured when working or playing. Strength is good for your posture and creates strong bones.

- **Muscular Endurance:** The ability of your muscles to move for long periods of time, which is an indicator of a muscle's ability to do work. Exercises like curl-ups and push-ups are good for building muscular endurance. You need to build endurance so you have more energy and are able to play or work harder for longer periods of time. Good health conditions will help prevent the development of some diseases.

- **Flexibility:** The ability to move your muscles and joints through their full range of motion. It is beneficial in injury prevention and relaxation. Stretching increases flexibility. When stretching you should reach easily in a direction and hold the stretch, do not bounce.

- **Body Composition:** The amount of lean body mass, including bones, muscles, and tissues. Those items are compared to the amount of fat in your body. People who are physically fit generally will have much more lean body mass than fat body mass. Being active and exercising will give your body and muscles shape. People who exercise generally have less body fat than people who are inactive and aren't in shape. Adolescent boys and men tend to have less body fat than adolescent girls and women. If you want to know if your body mass composition is good, ask a physical education or health teacher to measure your percent body fat or to calculate your Body Mass Index (BMI).

F.I.T.T. Principles

To improve your fitness level and your chances of meeting the standards of the President's Challenge, you should follow these principles of exercise: Frequency, Intensity, Type, and Time (F.I.T.T.).

- **Frequency:** Set up a regular schedule for exercising. Try to accumulate at least one hour of activity daily with more vigorous workouts three to four days a week. You are likely to see improvements when you

---

♣ It's A Fact!!
American Council On Exercise (ACE)
Lists Most Common Fitness Myths

Consumers are constantly bombarded with fitness information and "expert" advice from questionable sources. The American Council on Exercise (ACE) recently conducted a survey of more than 1,500 ACE-certified fitness professionals to discover the exercise myths that they most commonly hear from their clients. The following are their top responses:

- **Women who lift weights will get bulky muscles:** Women usually do not have the genetic potential to develop large, bulky muscles because they don't have enough of the hormone, testosterone, needed for the development of muscle bulk. While steroids and other artificial means may cause some women to bulk up, strength training will not.

- **Spot reducing is possible:** Spot reducing is not possible. The concept is based on the flawed notion that it is possible to "burn off" fat from a specific part of the body by selectively exercising that area. However, numerous studies have refuted this claim. Only regular exercise training (aerobic and strength) and a sensible diet can eliminate excess body fat.

- **No pain, no gain:** Many incorrectly assume that exercise must hurt to be beneficial, when in fact exercising to the point of pain can do more harm than good. A sensible exercise program might be uncomfortable, but

exercise regularly and have a schedule for exercise. Also, you are more likely to continue those workouts when you have an exercise schedule.

- **Intensity:** For your muscles to get stronger or your body to get fit, you must work harder when exercising than when you are at rest. Your heart should beat faster and your breathing should increase when you are performing aerobic exercise and when you are lifting weights. Make sure you work harder when you are exercising, but don't overdo it. Lifting too much weight or working out too hard can cause injuries.

- **Type:** You need to exercise your body the same way that you are going to use it. For example, aerobic exercise will not build flexibility, and lifting weights will not increase your aerobic endurance. For flexibility,

---

should not be painful. It should put a reasonable demand on the cardio-respiratory and musculoskeletal systems to improve their function, without significantly increasing the risk of injury.

- **Exercise requires a hefty time commitment:** Any amount of regular exercise contributes to better overall health and well-being. ACE recommends a total of at least 30 minutes of physical activity a day to maintain health and reduce the risk of heart disease and cancer. Individuals desiring to lose weight and keep it off are advised to accumulate 60 minutes of physical activity each day.

- **If you exercise, you can eat whatever you want:** A sound nutrition program goes hand-in-hand with a sound exercise regimen. If the goal is to lose weight or maintain a healthy weight, consumers should add more fruits and vegetables to the diet, avoid processed high-sugar foods and control portion size.

- **There's a magic bullet or quick fix out there somewhere:** There is no quick fix. Many nutritional supplements are marketed using deceptive, misleading, or fraudulent advertising. A well-balanced diet coupled with regular exercise is still the safest and most effective way to achieve weight loss or performance goals.

you must stretch. For aerobic capacity, you must increase your heart rate. For strength, you must work your muscles.

- **Time:** Gradually increase the number of times you do an exercise, the length of time that perform an exercise, and how hard you exercise. It generally takes six to eight weeks to see physical improvements, but you will feel better shortly after starting to exercise.

Phases Of Exercise

There are four phases of exercise including a warm-up, stretching, exercise, and a cool-down.

- **Warm-Up:** Before you exercise, you should always warm up your body. When you warm up your body you increase your blood flow and get your muscles and joints ready to exercise. Most people are warmed up when they begin to sweat and breathe heavier. Warming up makes your muscles more limber and decreases your chance of being injured during exercise.

- **Stretching:** Once you have warmed up, you can complete stretching exercises that will prepare your whole body. You should specifically target the muscles that will be used while you are actively exercising.

- **Exercise:** Complete the exercise activities in which you choose to participate. Always make sure to take appropriate safety precautions (for example, wear protective gear) and to exercise for a duration and at an intensity that is appropriate for your fitness level.

- **Cooling Down:** Once you have completed exercising you are ready to cool down. It is just as important to cool down after exercise as it is to warm up before exercise. When you cool down you should let your breathing return to normal. It is best to walk around for a few minutes to make sure your breathing is normal and to let your heartbeat slow down. After you have walked around for a few minutes following vigorous exercise, you are ready to begin your cool down stretches. Stretching again after you have cooled down will help prevent injuries, help to increase your range of motion, and will prevent soreness. You should complete the stretches you did before the exercise and add more stretches for the specific muscles worked.

Chapter 12

Using Exercise Equipment

Heart Rate Monitors

Heart rate can be used to monitor how hard you are working during an activity (that is, exercise intensity), and to track changes in fitness level. The heart rate monitor (HRM) provides a convenient method for measuring and recording heart rate during exercise. The first HRM was introduced in the early 1980s, and many improvements have been made since then, such as:

- Coded transmission process (from chest strap to watch) to reduce interference with other HRMs.

- Ability to store heart rate data and to download stored data onto a computer and analyze with special software.

- Functions to aid in training.

About This Chapter: This chapter begins with "Heart Rate Monitors," by Scott Crouter, Ph.D.; "A Pedometer," by Patrick Schneider; "A Home Treadmill," by Michael Bracko, Ed.D., FACSM; "A Stationary Bicycle," by Allen Parcell, Ph.D., FACSM; "A Rowing Machine," by Timothy Hosea, M.D., FACSM; "A Stair Stepper/Climber," by Hank Williford, Ed.D., FACSM, and Michele Olson, Ph.D., FACSM; "An Elliptical Trainer," by Hank Williford, Ed.D., FACSM and Michelle Olson, Ph.D., FACSM; and "Selecting And Effectively Using Rubber Band Resistance Exercise," by William Kraemer, Ph.D., FACSM. Reprinted with permission from the American College of Sports Medicine. Copyright © 2005 American College of Sports Medicine. This text is a product of ACSM's Consumer Products Committee. Additional text from IMPACT Productions, and American Council on Exercise is cited separately within the chapter.

The use of a HRM to determine exercise intensity is based on the following physiological principal: as exercise intensity increases, oxygen consumption (VO2) and heart rate increase in a linear relationship. Heart rate is easier to measure than VO2 and the relationship between them has been established, as shown by the example in Figure 12.1.

Factors Affecting Heart Rate

Many factors can alter your heart rate:

- Stress

- Illness

- Overtraining and fatigue

- Medications

- Time of day

- Food and/or drink (i.e., caffeine); nutritional status

- Altitude

- Body temperature

- Hydration levels

- Weather conditions and/or ambient temperature

- Cardiac drift, which is the increase in heart rate seen over time while exercising at a constant

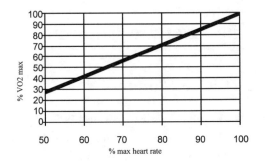

Figure 12.1. Percentages of VO2 Max And Max Heart Rate

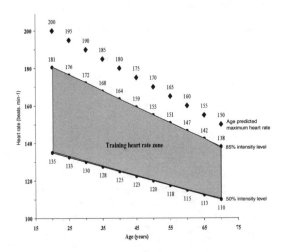

Figure 12.2. Training Heart Rate Zone

work load. Some studies have found that your heart rate can increase by as much as 5–20 beats per minute (bpm) during exercise lasting 20–60 minutes even when the intensity does not change.

Choosing Heart Rate Monitors

The following questions should be considered when selecting a heart rate monitor (HRM):

What does a HRM consist of? A HRM consists of a watch that is worn on your wrist, and a transmitter that you wear against your skin, around your chest. The electrodes in the transmitter pick up signals from your heart and send them wirelessly to the watch. These signals are continuously displayed.

What types of activities can I participate in while wearing a HRM? A HRM can be worn while participating in almost any physical activity, whether for work or recreation—yard work, indoor/outdoor walking and running, skating, biking (indoor/outdoor), rowing, etc. Most models are waterproof enough for swimming, though not for diving.

—by Scott Crouter, Ph.D.

A Pedometer

About Pedometers

The pedometer is a device about the size of a pager that typically attaches to the belt or waistband and is designed primarily to count steps. More recently, some pedometers are also capable of counting steps while placed in a shirt pocket or in a bag if it's held snug to the body.

Interestingly, Leonardo da Vinci is credited with the invention of the pedometer. Although the early mechanical pedometers were deemed unreliable, the electronic pedometer developed in the early 1990s is significantly more accurate and reliable.

Pedometers are capable of recording ambulatory activity such as walking, jogging, or running. They will not count steps during activities such as cycling, rowing, upper body exercise, etc.

☞ Remember!!
Staying Active Pays Off

Those who are physically active tend to live longer, healthier lives. Research shows that even moderate physical activity—such as 30 minutes a day of brisk walking—significantly contributes to longevity. A physically active person with such risk factors as high blood pressure, diabetes, or even a smoking habit can get real benefits from regular physical activity as part of daily life.

As many dieters have found, exercise can help you stay on a diet and lose weight. What's more, regular exercise can help lower blood pressure, control blood sugar, improve cholesterol levels, and build stronger, denser bones.

The First Step

Before you begin an exercise program, take a fitness test, or substantially increase your level of activity, make sure to answer the following questions. This physical activity readiness questionnaire (PAR-Q) will help determine your suitability for beginning an exercise routine or program.

- Has your doctor ever said that you have a heart condition or that you should participate in physical activity only as recommended by a doctor?

- Do you feel pain in your chest during physical activity?

How Do Pedometers Differ?

Pedometers can differ in the cost, internal mechanism and features.

- **Cost:** Pedometers typically range in cost from $10–$50 depending on the features.

- **Internal mechanism:** There are different mechanisms by which pedometers function. One common type consists of a spring-suspended lever arm that moves up and down in response to vertical acceleration of the hip. This movement opens and closes an electrical circuit and a

- In the past month, have you had chest pain when you were not doing physical activity?

- Do you lose your balance because of dizziness? Do you ever lose consciousness?

- Do you have a bone or joint problem that could be made worse by a change in your physical activity?

- Is your doctor currently prescribing drugs for your blood pressure or a heart condition?

- Do you know of any reason you should not participate in physical activity?

If you answered yes to one or more questions, if you are over 40 years of age and have been inactive, or if you are concerned about your health, consult a physician before taking a fitness test or substantially increasing your physical activity. If you answered no to each question, then it's likely that you can safely begin fitness testing and training.

Source: "Staying Active Pays Off," reprinted with permission from the American College of Sports Medicine. Copyright © 2005 American College of Sports Medicine. This text is a product of ACSM's Consumer Products Committee.

step is counted. Others use an accelerometer-type mechanism. Pedometers with this mechanism can distinguish between ambulatory activities of differing intensities (If you shake the pedometer up and down and it does not produce a clicking sound, it probably has an accelerometer-type mechanism).

- **Features:** While steps are the fundamental unit of the pedometer, some devices also calculate distance walked and estimate calories burned. In general, pedometers are most accurate in counting steps, less accurate in calculating distance walked, and even less accurate at estimating caloric expenditure. The calculation of distance walked requires the input of the user's stride length while the caloric expenditure feature requires the input of the user's body weight. Steps are the fundamental unit of the pedometer and all other features are dependent upon the device's step counting accuracy. Some of the newer devices also estimate the total time spent walking at a moderate intensity.

Choosing A Pedometer

The following questions should be considered when selecting a pedometer:

What feature(s) am I most interested in? Step counting is what most pedometers do best. Therefore, purchasing an accurate step counting pedometer should be a primary objective.

How can I test a pedometer's accuracy? One way to test a pedometer's accuracy is to perform a 20-step test. To do this, position the device on your belt or waistband in line with your knee on either side of the body and reset your pedometer to zero. Take 20 steps at your typical walking pace. Check to see if the pedometer reads between 18 and 22 steps. If it does, it is likely a reasonably accurate step counter. If not, try repositioning it on your belt or waistband and try the test again. If your pedometer repeatedly fails this test, look into purchasing a different type.

What factors can affect pedometer accuracy? Studies have shown that a variety of factors can potentially affect a pedometer's step counting accuracy, i.e., walking speed, waistband type, and abdominal size. In general, most pedometers are fairly accurate step counters at speeds of 2.5 mph and above. Even some of the more accurate pedometers miscount steps at slower speeds. With regard to waistband type, pedometers are generally more accurate step counters when attached to a firm waistband in an upright position (Loose waistbands typically result in a significant underestimation of steps). Abdominal size can also affect step-counting accuracy. Those with the horizontal lever arm mechanism appear to be more vulnerable to miscounting steps based on the tilt or angle at which the pedometer sits when fastened to the belt or waistband.

How do I use a pedometer to supplement my walking program? First, determine your baseline physical activity level. To do this, wear the pedometer for one full week without altering your typical routine. If you are routinely active, continue being so but, if you are not habitually active, do not start during this one-week period. You can use this step index to classify your activity level based on steps per day (Keep in mind that if you regularly participate in non-ambulatory activity, your steps per day value will not accurately represent your activity level).

For most healthy adults, 10,000 steps per day is a reasonable goal. If your baseline steps fall short of this value, try to increase your activity level by 1,000 steps per day every two weeks until you reach your goal. To put your step count into perspective, there are about 2,000 steps in a mile.

Children can also benefit from the use of pedometers. Typically active children should accumulate between 12,000 and 16,000 steps per day. Pedometers can be used to motivate children or youth to become more physically active.

To increase your daily step counts, look for opportunities to be more active. For example, take the stairs rather than the elevator, park at the far end of the parking lot (if it is safe to do so), go for walking breaks at work, etc. The instant feedback that a pedometer provides can serve as a motivator to accumulate more steps. Every step counts so even small increases added into your daily routine can make a difference.

—by Patrick Schneider

Table 12.1. Step Index

Steps Per Day	Activity Level
Less than 5,000	Sedentary
5,000–7,499	Low Active
7,500–9,999	Somewhat Active
10,000–12,500	Active
Greater than 12,500	Highly Active

Source: Developed by C. Tudor-Locke and D.R. Bassett Jr. (2004).

♣ It's A Fact!!

A Complete Physical Activity Program

A well rounded program of physical activity includes aerobic exercise and strength training exercise, but not necessarily in the same session. This blend helps to maintain or improve cardiorespiratory and muscular fitness and overall health and function. Regular physical activity will provide more health benefits than sporadic, high intensity workouts, so choose exercises you are likely to enjoy and that you can incorporate into your schedule.

American College of Sports Medicine (ACSM)'s physical activity recommendations for healthy adults, updated in 2007, recommend at least 30 minutes of moderate-intensity physical activity (working hard enough to break a sweat, but still able to carry on a conversation) five days per week, or 20 minutes of more vigorous activity three days per week. Combinations of moderate- and vigorous-intensity activity can be performed to meet this recommendation. Typical aerobic exercises include walking and running, stair climbing, cycling on a stationary or moving bike, rowing, cross-country skiing, and swimming.

In addition, strength training should be performed a minimum of two days each week, with 8–12 repetitions of 8–10 different exercises that target all major muscle groups. This type of training can be accomplished using body weight, resistance bands, free weights, medicine balls, or weight machines.

Source: "A Complete Physical Activity Program," reprinted with permission from the American College of Sports Medicine. Copyright © 2005 American College of Sports Medicine. This text is a product of ACSM's Consumer Products Committee.

A Home Treadmill

Selecting A Home Treadmill

Treadmills are a popular choice of equipment for those who want to engage in physical activity. Below are useful guidelines for you to consider before making a purchase. Be sure to try it out before you buy. Doing so will allow you to find a treadmill that meets your specific needs. A treadmill may be either motorized or human-powered. Manual treadmills are less expensive and safer because the running belt stops moving when you do. However, manual treadmills usually have smaller running belts, making it difficult to jog or run, let alone maintain a brisk walk. Often, the difficulty in getting the belt to move smoothly on a non-motorized treadmill increases the likelihood of holding on to the handrail in an effort to generate power, causing an inconsistent pace. This inconsistent pace may cause muscle strain or difficulty in elevating your heart rate. Additionally, the holding on may elevate blood pressure from breathholding. Exercise at home should be easy and something to look forward to. If it is difficult to get the machine to work, you are less likely to exercise. For these reasons, you may want to consider a motorized treadmill.

Safety

- Stability of platform when level and with elevation: feels solid, not wobbly.

- Doesn't have parts that hit you or cramp your movements in an unnatural fashion.

- Automatic emergency shut-off key, clip, or tether.

- Side rails or safety bars for balance: They should be reachable and sturdy, but out of the way of swinging arms.

Maintenance And Durability

- Is the company reliable and reputable?

- Can the treadmill be easily assembled and maintained?

- Cost of maintenance?

- Does the treadmill come with a warranty? What does the warranty cover and for how long?

- Are local technicians available for service?

Power And Performance

- **Treadmill motor:** Should have a minimum continuous duty rating of 1.5 h.p. motor (2.5 to 3.0 h.p. is preferred). To test the motor, plant your feet firmly on the belt while the machine is running at its lowest speed, checking for any hesitation, groaning or grinding.

- **Power supply:** Does the treadmill require 110 or 220v? 220v will probably require circuit alterations in the room where it will be used.

- **Belt size:** Should be at least 18 to 20 inches wide and 48 inches long. Narrow, short running belts make it more difficult and less enjoyable because the chances of tripping or falling off of the belt increase with a narrow belt. The platform should be low to the floor and have ample space to straddle the treadmill belt.

- **Speed range:** Speed range should be 0.1 to a minimum of 8 mph. This speed range should satisfy most walkers as well as runners. Low starting speed is an important issue. We recommend a safe starting speed of 0.1 mph with slow incremental increase in belt speed. The stop should be smooth stop (not sudden). The motor should be able to maintain speed regardless of treadmill elevation and weight of user.

- **Incline:** Should range from 0 percent to at least 10 percent. Incline mechanisms can be either electric or manual. Manual cranks are found generally on lower end treadmills to keep the price down. The treadmill should not wobble at high elevations.

Operation

- Is the control panel accessible and easy to read?

- Does the control panel have the capacity for manual use separate from software used for automated programming?

- Is the noise level acceptable?

- Is the belt heavy duty as to not stretch with extended use?

Other Considerations

- Weight of treadmill

- Space available and height of ceiling

- Aesthetics

- Storage potential

- How accurate is the calibration?

Using A Home Treadmill

Treadmills should be positioned away from walls to avoid injury due to falls. Be sure that the back of the treadmill has at least six to eight feet of clearance from a ledge, wall or window. The power supply and wiring should be located away from walking paths or taped to prevent tripping when stepping on or off of the running belt.

Make sure the running belt is properly adjusted before use. Belts that are too loose or too tight will cause wear and tear on the treadmill, which result in expensive repair or replacement costs. The deck beneath the belt should be laminated to protect it from friction wear and tear. This deck absorbs the hundreds of pounds of force from each step.

Make sure that you follow the directions included with purchase for maintaining the belt deck connection. Increased friction and heat will cause "amp draw," which pulls power away from the electrical components of your machine. Discuss appropriate lubrication and maintenance with the sales people at the store where you purchased you treadmill.

Your treadmill should come equipped with arm grips, siderails, or safety bars. These are excellent for defining the running/walking area for your exercise bout. They allow you to catch yourself it you trip or fall. When stepping off a treadmill while the belt is moving it is advisable to use these rails for safety.

The treadmill should come equipped with an emergency shut-off key, clip or tether. These are a safety must, especially with young children around. The tether feature is preferred, since an automatic stop button may not be in reach as you fall.

Many treadmills come with sophisticated electronic displays that allow you to design workouts to your needs. For some, this programming is basically a motivation and selling point. All you need is enough variety to keep your workouts motivating and interesting. The bare minimum display and programming features should include distance, speed, time, incline and possibly

> ## ♣ It's A Fact!!
> ## Free Weights Vs. Strength-Training Equipment
>
> Have you wondered which method of strength training is better, free weights or strength-training equipment? The truth is, each has its advantages and disadvantages.
>
> The choice depends on your level of experience and your exercise goals, and to some extent, your personal preference. An understanding of these factors will help you decide if free weights or machines—or a combination of both—will help you reach your goals.
>
> ### The Free-Weight Advantage
>
> - Free weights incorporate the stabilizing muscles that enable you to perform the movements you choose to make and may be more effective in producing overall muscular strength and power gains.
>
> - Free-weight exercises tend to more closely match the movement patterns you're likely to need for specific sports.
>
> - Free weights are more versatile—you can do a wide variety of exercises with a simple set of dumbbells. You can, for example, hold the weights with palms facing forward, facing your body, or facing the wall behind you. In doing so, you can do three different exercises that will work your muscles in different ways.
>
> - Free weights tend to be inexpensive, are portable and take up little space.

calories expended. It is important that you be able to use the treadmill in the manual mode.

Important Points To Remember

- **Before you get on:** Before you get on the treadmill, experiment with the controls. Speed it up, slow it down, increase and decrease the incline and test the emergency off button.

- **Posture when walking or running:** Shoulders back, head up and slightly forward, chin up and abdominals tight. Look forward, not down at your feet.

The Free-Weight Disadvantage

- You must learn to balance the weight while exerting force. This can be difficult—and potentially dangerous—if you are lifting weights overhead.

- The isolation of specific muscles can be difficult. To target the muscle you want, you must use very precise technique.

- Free weights can be swung for momentum rather than lifted slowly and steadily, which works the muscles better.

- Training alone can lead to injury if you don't use proper technique.

The Machine Advantage

- Machines are generally safer and easier to use, an advantage for beginners learning a specific movement.

- Some machines are more efficient than free weights at isolating a specific muscle or muscle group. This is important when you're strengthening a specific body part or rehabilitating an injury.

- Machines ensure correct movements for a lift, which helps prevent cheating when muscle fatigue sets in.

- Machine workouts can take less time because you can move easily from machine to machine. Changing the resistance is easy; you just insert a pin or enter a code.

- **Stride length:** Relax and maintain the normal stride you would use when walking on the ground. Don't chop your steps.

- **Where you are:** It is important to pay attention to where you are on the treadmill. Don't drift sideways or allow yourself to go to the back of the belt.

- **Make it a habit:** A treadmill is only as good for your health as the frequency with which you use it. Set a specific time of day, set a specific number of minutes and make it routine.

—by Michael Bracko, Ed.D., FACSM

♣ It's A Fact!!

The Machine Disadvantage

- Most machines involve moving a weight along a predetermined path, making it difficult to strengthen the stabilizer muscles.

- Machines are much more limited, with most devices allowing only one exercise.

- Most machines are geared to the average-sized person, so if you're shorter or taller than average, you may find it difficult to use some machines. However, some companies have developed equipment that is scaled down to suit many smaller men and women.

Generally speaking, if you are beginning a strength-training program for the first time, or have been away from your program for months or even years, then it's a good idea to try the resistance-training machines for the first 10 to 12 weeks of your program.

Doing so will give your body the time it requires to adjust without putting undue stress on your muscles and joints. Using machines may also be easier and less discouraging if you're a novice, because free weights require some coordination to use.

A Stationary Bicycle

Selecting A Stationary Bicycle

Stationary bicycles are a safe and effective means of exercise. They provide a means of low-impact cardiovascular exercise, are generally quiet in operation, and are efficient with their use of space.

There are two major characteristics to consider when selecting a stationary bicycle. First, the seating position on the bicycle, and second, the method of resistance. Exercisers may choose the standard upright bicycle or semi-recumbent (sitting) stationary bicycles, which may be more comfortable for some individuals. For resistance, stationary bicycles use friction belts or wheels, magnets, hydraulics, or fans. Additionally, many bicycles are equipped with computers that will report workout data and in some cases even direct exercise sessions. All these characteristics influence the cost of stationary bicycles.

Experienced exercisers may want to use free weights because of the additional training benefits they offer. That said, the combination of both free weights and machines can add variety to your workout.

If you are a health club member, be sure to ask the fitness instructor to show you how to use the free weights and machines properly. If you forget how, ask until you feel confident that you are using the proper technique to complete each exercise.

If you are exercising at home, be sure to purchase an exercise tape that outlines the proper technique to follow. Good technique is essential if you want to reach your strength training goals, while avoiding injury.

Source: "Free Weights vs. Strength Training Equipment," reprinted with permission from the American Council on Exercise (www.acefitness.org), © 2004. All rights reserved.

You must consider your needs and interests when purchasing a stationary bicycle. Position is important. Most upright bicycles come with a large, well-padded saddle, so comfort for most will not be an issue. However, for individuals with lower back pain, mobility, or balance concerns, a semi-recumbent stationary bicycle may offer a safer, more comfortable option. Computer, size, and resistance mechanism options will allow you to select the stationary bicycle to meet your fitness goals. Remember, more expensive models do not inherently make you more fit. An inexpensive model used regularly can adequately provide the necessary resistance to increase cardiovascular fitness.

Safety

- Stability; wide base for ergometer
- Protected or covered flywheel and/or fans

Maintenance And Durability

- Established, reputable company

- Assembly requirements

- Warranties and local maintenance

- Annual maintenance costs

- Availability of replacement parts

Power, Performance, And Operation

- Capable of providing adequate resistance

- Consider noise generated by fans

- Adequately adjusts for proper fit on the bicycle

- Comfortable seat, saddle, and handlebars

- Consider the size of the assembled unit

- Are the electrical requirements, if any, available in your exercise area?

- Guidelines for assembly and operation should be clear and complete.

Using A Stationary Bicycle

Stationary bicycles should be positioned so that all moving parts are allowed safe clearance. You should also have adequate room to safely mount and dismount the machine.

Position on a bicycle is critical to enjoyable and effective cycling. Handlebar and saddle height are the primary considerations. When you adjust your position on a bicycle, you are attempting to distribute your body weight evenly between your arms and your seat. First, adjust the saddle so that it is level with the floor. "Pointed up" will put pressure on the groin area. "Pointed down" will put too much weight on your arms and shoulders. Next, adjust the saddle height so there is a slight bend in the knee when the pedal is at the bottom of the stroke. An additional saddle height guideline is that your hips should not rock back and forth when you pedal. A saddle that is too high will result in too much pressure in the groin region and may cause soreness and/or numbness.

Finally, adjust the handlebars to allow for a comfortable forward-leaning position. Handlebars that are too high will put excessive pressure on your seat, while handlebars that are too low may result in lower back soreness and arm and shoulder fatigue. It will take several cycling sessions and some additional adjustments to find your perfect position. Be patient. One of the biggest reasons people stop cycling is because of discomfort. Proper positioning on a bicycle will provide for comfortable and enjoyable exercise.

Important Points To Remember

- **Spend time test-riding stationary bicycle models before you buy.** Adjustability, noise, and ease of operation should be considered in the store, not in your living room.

- **Proper position is imperative.** Be patient and complete in your positioning process.

- **Make it a habit.** A stationary bicycle is only good for your health if you use it. Set attainable goals for regular use of your home exercise equipment.

—by Allen Parcell, Ph.D., FACSM

A Rowing Machine

Selecting A Rowing Machine

Rowing is an efficient and effective low-impact exercise that utilizes the arms, abdomen, back and legs, providing a total-body workout. This activity offers the opportunity for a wide range of training from fat burning and aerobic conditioning to high-intensity anaerobic and interval VO2 max training. The rowing stroke is a smooth, continuous, non-impact movement. If you have a history of low back pain, special attention must be given to developing proper rowing technique to prevent injury.

The rowing machine should mimic the smooth motion of rowing on the water. The machine and platform must be of sturdy construction and able to easily support the weight of the person rowing. The seat should be comfortable, but not too soft. The seat must slide back and forth smoothly and allow for full extension and flexion of the knees. There should be plenty of room in front of the person rowing to allow for full extension of the shoulders and arms at the beginning of the rowing motion. The "oar" handle should be centered in front and enable a full range of motion in a straight horizontal plane. There should be a smooth, seamless uptake of the resistance throughout the rowing stroke. Avoid machines that feature a jerky sensation of resistance change, or sudden change in resistance. The rowing machine should allow for the easy adjustment of the resistance, even from one stroke to another.

Many rowing machines are equipped with a monitor that will indicate pace, distance, power output (watts), calories burned, and heart rate. Some may also be programmed for a workout including distance or time rowed and the rest period between intervals. More sophisticated monitors provide a visual display of the force of a stroke and/or continuous tracking against an imaginary "pace" boat for each interval in a workout. They may also keep a personal electronic log of your workout and results. One manufacturer even has an annual worldwide ranking online for various ages, body weights, and distance rowed and sponsors a world indoor rowing championship. Some machines provide detailed instruction on rowing technique and have Web sites for training tips, maintaining a personal workout log, and motivational competitions.

Rowing machines are manufactured with four different types of resistance: air, water, magnetic, and piston. The industry standard utilizes air resistance, and the less expensive machines are piston-driven. Magnetic machines are the quietest. Air and magnetic machines allow for the fastest change in resistance. Water and piston machines claim to provide the closest replication to the feeling of rowing on water. Water machines are the heaviest. The air machines should have a cover made of narrow mesh over the flywheel to prevent injury to the fingers. Some piston and air resistance machines can be folded for easy storage.

The rowing machine should mimic the smooth motion of rowing on the water. The following may be effective in developing a smooth and effective stroke.

- **The rowing stroke:** The rowing stroke is a continuous motion. The starting point is generally referred to as the catch. At this point, the knees are flexed or bent with the shins vertical and the shoulders and arms reaching forward. This is the position that mimics the oar being placed into the water prior to the drive phase of the stroke. The drive phase is initiated by the legs as they extend. The arms remain straight until the knees are mostly extended, and then the elbows flex bringing the oar handle into the upper stomach. The drive ends at the finish when the legs are fully extended, shoulders are back, elbows are flexed and the oar handle is against the upper stomach. The recovery phase is the phase of the rowing stroke where the rower returns to the catch position to initiate another drive phase. The recovery begins with the hands and arms moving away from the body and the elbows extending. The upper body moves forward over the hips as the hands move past the knees, the knees begin to flex and the seat moves up the slide to the catch position.

Proper Use Of A Rowing Machine

The rowing machine must be placed on a solid level surface. There must be open space around the machine to allow for the full arc of the rowing motion. Before purchasing a rowing machine, measure the space in which you intend to use it and store it to make sure it will fit. Some models allow for storage in a vertical position. The machine must be stable in this vertical position and not place in an area where it may be knocked over.

A common error when rowing on a machine is allowing the knees to flex prior to the hands passing over the knees during the recovery. This forces the rower to lift the oar handle over the knees before the catch and may lead to injury. Another common mistake is allowing the seat to slide out from under the rower prior to the handle moving back on the drive. This puts the back in a weaker position and may lead to a back injury if done with enough force.

The effort put into the rowing stroke is a combination of the stroke rate and resistance setting. Generally there is a greater stress put on the back with the slower stroke rate. The resistance setting should be lower for the long aerobic workouts. Aerobic training for the beginner can start at 15 minutes with a five-minute warm-up and five-minute cool-down. When a person rows regularly for several weeks or months, and their fitness level increases, the time of the workout can increase to 20 minutes, then 25, and 30 minutes. To increase the intensity of the workout, the resistance and stroke rate can be increased. However, any attempt to combine a slower stroke rate with high resistance may lead to back injury.

In addition the rower should not suddenly pull as hard as possible in an attempt to achieve maximal effort in a single stroke or two. This places a sudden large stress on the lower back and may result in injury. The pace of a workout should be reached over three to five strokes or more. A warm-up consisting of slow, easy rowing for four to five minutes will help reduce the risk of injury and improve the benefits of a workout.

Care Of A Rowing Machine

All rowing machines should be kept clean, with regular wiping of the handle with a disinfectant. The handle should fit comfortably in the hand and be covered with a non-slip rubber surface. Should a rower develop blisters and/or bleeding, the handle must be appropriately cleaned.

Special care must be taken to avoid twisting the chain or cord attached to the handle to avoid damage to the chain. When the rowing machine is not being used, the handle should be placed against the flywheel to avoid unnecessary stretching of the pull cord.

Regular maintenance and cleaning of the machine will help ensure the proper operation and safety. The manufacturer should clearly detail a maintenance program in the owner's manual and should provide a warranty.

—by Timothy Hosea, M.D., FACSM

A Stair Stepper/Climber

Selecting A Stair Stepper/Climber

Stair steppers, elliptical trainers, and climbers are often thought of as similar pieces of equipment, but they are very different. The stair stepper provides only lower body strength training and aerobic exercise. The elliptical trainer has an orbital motion that encompasses walking, running, climbing, and related cardiovascular workouts. Additionally, some elliptical trainer models incorporate upper-body workouts, providing a total-body workout.

☞ Remember!!

Safety Reminders:
Rowing Machine Operation

- Make sure the machine has been properly cleaned and maintained prior to use.

- Make sure that the proper rowing technique is always used.

- Avoid twisting or excessively stretching the cord.

- Always warm-up before a workout session and increase the length and intensity of training gradually over weeks and months.

- Never start a rowing interval with maximal effort in a single stroke.

Source: Hosea, ACSM, 2005.

The climber allows for upper body and lower body strength training as well as aerobic training. These machines provide the ability to tone thigh and gluteal muscles equally well when compared to other exercise programs or machines.

Spend some time analyzing your needs and interests to decide on the type of stepper or climber you want. For example, is this to be used as a basic daily exercise program, or are you training for a specific event? Many of these machines feature a console with programs that can range from basic to sophisticated. Training for a specific event may indicate a need for a wider range of options and programs, including the ability to customize programs to meet your specific needs. The more features, options, and programs, the more costly the stepper/climber.

Basic consoles should display calories burned, distance climbed, rate of speed, and intensity level. Intensity may be controlled manually, and some basic models may have a few programs from which to choose. The best way to select the right stair stepper is to try out a number of different models.

Safety

It is essential that your machine have solid construction and a stable frame. In steppers, the stepping action should be smooth and independent (pushing one step down should not push the other step up). Self-leveling pedals will allow the user to keep the step flat throughout the workout. It is important that these machines be ergonomically sound and that you position yourself to maximize the safety and effectiveness of your workout. This means that the handrails should be positioned so that your workout posture is upright with the knees behind the toes. Bending forward places a great amount of stress on the back. Using the handrails to support part of the body weight reduces the total caloric expenditure and may result in a posture that is biomechanically unsound. Last, but not least, read all of the manufacturer's instructions to get the most out of your machine.

Using A Stair Stepper/Climber

Steppers should be positioned so that there is easy access onto and off of the steps. The path immediately behind the steps should be free of power cords and other tripping hazards. The area immediately above the stepper should be open and allow plenty of room to stand tall, even when the steps are at the top of the stepping range.

Make sure the stepper responds according to the manufacturer's directions. Test all of the arrows or buttons that control the intensity, and make sure the display screen is working properly.

The stepper should have side rails, a rail in the front, and/or moving posts on the side. When using the stationary rails, your hands should rest lightly to assist with balance. Posture should be upright—make the legs do the work. If using the moving posts, again, use a light grip to assist with balance and to add upper body movement to the workout.

Unlike the treadmill, there is no emergency shut-off key. You simply need to stop the motion of the pedals by riding the pedals to the floor. Step off, one foot at a time, and release the pedals gently.

Make sure you understand all of the machine's characteristics before engaging in a workout. Thoroughly understanding the instructions will result in a safer and more effective workout for you.

Important Points To Remember

- Before you get on, read the instructions.

- Understand how to increase and decrease the intensity of the workout. Have your water bottle, reading material, and other necessary items prepared and safely stowed in an accessible place.

- Just because you are not running does not mean you should step with any old shoe. Wear athletic shoes that support the foot, heel, and ankle. Dress comfortably by avoiding restrictive clothing.

- Be sure your posture is upright. Stand tall and look forward. If you're looking down to read, rest your neck every few minutes by changing the head position.

- Stepping rate: Choose an initial stepping rate that slightly raises the pulse rate. Remember the faster the pedals move, the faster you must move to keep up. More pedal resistance allows you to slow your stepping rate. The height of each step should approximate the stepping action for climbing a normal step. The stepping height should feel comfortable on the knees and ankles.

Maintenance And Durability

- Is the manufacturing company reliable and reputable?

- Does the stepper require assembly? Can this be completed by the consumer?

- What costs are associated with lubrication and replacement of parts? Which parts are most likely to wear and where can those parts be purchased?

- Does the stepper come with a warranty? What does it cover and for how long?

- Are local technicians available for service?

Power And Performance

- Check on the weight limit of the machine. Is it safe for all users?

- Most home models require 110–220 volts—however, read the manufacturers guidelines to be sure.

- Are you able to increase the difficulty of your workout as you increase your level of fitness? Check the range of stepping difficulty available on manual mode as well as the range of programs available on the machine.

- Be certain the machine is placed on a level floor.

Operation

- Is the control panel accessible and easy to read?

- Does the control panel have the capacity for manual use separate from software used for automated programming?

- Can you customize programs for yourself?

Other Considerations

- Do you have appropriate floor support for the weight of the machine? Are there rollers that allow you to move the stepper with reasonable ease?

- Does the ceiling height allow all users to use the machine safely?

- Determine your space considerations. Will you need to store the stepper periodically?

—by Hank Williford, Ed.D., FACSM,
and Michele Olson, Ph.D., FACSM

An Elliptical Trainer

Selecting A Home Elliptical Trainer

Elliptical trainers have become one of the most popular machines for cardiovascular exercise. These trainers engage the legs in a movement pattern that combines the motion of stair stepping with cross-country skiing, providing a low-impact workout. Some elliptical devices also include poles that can be maneuvered with the arms while the legs are in motion, similar to cross-country machines. This option increases the amount of muscle mass used to perform the exercise.

Following are guidelines that should be considered when purchasing an elliptical trainer. These recommendations will help you select a trainer that suits your specific needs. Before making any purchases, always be sure to try out the machine so that you can familiarize yourself with its options.

Safety

Make sure the equipment is properly fitted to your size and movement range. If the machine is motorized, there should be a safety turn-off control. When in use, the machine should be very sturdy and should neither move nor have the tendency to tip over. The side rails should also be sturdy and provide for adequate balance. Check the area around the machine for adequate headroom and space for leg and arm motion.

Maintenance And Durability

- Is the machine manufacturer reputable and reliable?
- Does the trainer come with a warranty?
- What does the warranty cover and how long is the warranty period?
- Is the machine durable, easily assembled, and easily maintained?
- Elliptical machines tend to be rather large—is the space in which it is to be used large enough?
- If it is to be stored between use, is there adequate space for storage?
- Are local technicians available for service?

Power, Performance, And Operation

- Is the trainer motorized or non-motorized?
- Does your home have the proper power supply? (Motorized machines may require 120 to 220 volts)
- Does the trainer require calibration?
- How often does the trainer have to be serviced?

- Is the noise level acceptable?

- Is the trainer sturdy and stable?

- Is there a control panel/read-out? Is it easy to read? Is it accurate?

- Does the control panel offer the information that is important for your needs (time, distance, resistance level, calories expended, etc.)?

- Is the instruction manual easy to read and follow?

Other Considerations

Make certain the pedals will comfortably accommodate the size of your feet. Pedals with a textured "non-slip" surface and high-curved ridges will also prevent your feet from sliding around or even off the pedal when exercising.

The stride length permitted by the trainer is also an important factor. Avoid purchasing a trainer if the stride length is too limited for your leg movement range. Some machines allow you to adjust the stride length.

Overall fit is very important. A good fit should allow you to move comfortably and smoothly, with a good upright posture and without the chance of your knees bumping into the console. The fixed hand-support rails should also allow you to maintain a comfortable upright posture versus a tendency to lean too far forward (which can be stressful to the back).

If the machine provides upper body handles or poles, make sure that the handles are sturdy, easy to reach, and that the handgrips are comfortable. Avoid trainers with upper body poles that infringe on your range of motion or cause contact with your knees.

Familiarize yourself with the options that increase the intensity of the workout. Some machines have elevating ramps under each pedal. Others increase the intensity through faster movement or by changing the resistance of the pedals with a tension control.

Using An Elliptical Trainer

Follow the manual regarding directions for proper set-up and use of the machine. Make certain the trainer operates properly and be sure that adequate space is available and that the power supply is nearby. Adjust the machine to suit your size and range of movement. Get comfortable with any programming features such as exercise time, distance goal, resistance level, speed level and caloric expenditure.

When exercising, maintain the correct posture by keeping your shoulder back, head up, chin straight, abdominals tight, and arms relaxed. Do not lean forward or grab and grip the balance bars tightly. The participant's weight should be supported by the lower body.

Important Points To Remember:

- **Before you start exercising on the elliptical trainer:** Make sure that you are familiar with the controls that increase speed and/or resistance. Make sure that the emergency shut-off switch or button works.

- **Maintain a good posture:** Shoulders should be back, head up and slightly forward, chin up and abdominals tight. Look forward, not down at your feet. Do not grip the handrails too tightly. Make sure that your weight is evenly distributed and that your lower body supports the majority of your weight.

- **Stride:** Relax and maintain a good stride going through your normal range of motion.

- **Make it a habit:** An elliptical trainer is only as good for your health as the frequency with which you use it. Set a specific time of day, set a specific number of minutes, and make it routine. Start out slowly, and make sure that you have checked with your doctor before beginning any exercise program.

—by Hank Williford, Ed.D., FACSM
and Michelle Olson, Ph.D., FACSM

Selecting And Effectively Using Rubber Band Resistance Exercise

About Rubber Band Resistance Exercise

Originally used to train older adults in nursing homes, flexible bands now provide exercise options for beginning to advanced exercisers and athletes.

The more you know about flexible bands, rubberized resistance cords, and the machines that use them, the better you can choose the method that's right for you. It's all about finding the resistance that matches the exercise you need.

Elastic bands offer no resistance at first, then more and more resistance as they are stretched to their limit. The resistance changes again as the bands return to resting position. This pattern—changing from extension to return—is known as hysteresis.

Rubber bands, by their nature, offer very little resistance when first stretched (for example, over the first 10–30 degrees of their range of motion.) It is important to feel resistance early in the stretch—more easily accomplished with single rubber bands than with some resistance machines.

Strength Curves

Every exercise can be illustrated by a curve showing the force used over a range of motion. The three primary strength curves are:

- **Ascending:** Force increases over the range of motion.
- **Bell:** Force is greatest in the middle of the range of motion.
- **Descending:** Force decreases over the range of motion.

Variations among exercises and individuals can affect the shape of these curves as well as the timing and degree of force used in each exercise. Exercise loading should match the strength curve to ensure that appropriate force is applied to the muscle.

Take, for example, arm curl exercises using elastic bands. Too much resistance would prevent smooth motion through the entire range. Resistance that is below the starting strength of the arm curl movement allows normal repetition of the movement.

It is important to be able to choose resistance to suit the exercise. For example, chest presses need more resistance than arm curls.

Figure 12.3 shows the resistance of an elastic band (dotted line) compared with the strength curves of two different users. Greater strength gives User 1 force greater than the band's resistance, while User 2 has insufficient force throughout the entire range of motion. Neither user is well matched with this particular band.

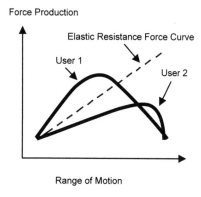

*Figure 12.3. Resistance Of An Elastic Band
Compared With Strength Curves*

Choosing Resistance Bands

When choosing from among the wide variety of rubberized resistance equipment available, ask:

- What exercises will I perform with the resistance bands? This tells you what range of resistance you'll need to adequately develop the muscle.

- What are the bands made of? Natural rubber latex, with its superior strength and elasticity, makes the best bands. Synthetic rubber is reinforced with additives that can cause the band to become harder and less elastic.

- How are the bands constructed? Understanding how bands are made can help you determine quality of construction and how they can be used in a variety of exercises. While any rubberized band provides resistance, heavier use requires a more durable product.

Some Features Of Bands Include

- **Bonded ends:** A quarter-inch strip of rubber is bonded at the ends to make a continuous band. This joint is a weak spot that can break during exercise.

- **Extruded rubber:** Strands of rubber are wound together like spaghetti, making it very strong. The bonded ends, though, are a weak spot.

- **Over-layered:** A strip of rubber is overlapped and bonded into a continuous band. The center of the overlapped section is very strong, but both ends are weak.

- **Layered on mandrills:** Bands are built in layers, forming a continuous band. The first and last layers should finish on different planes, at least three inches apart. This forms a one-piece band with no weak spots.

Exercises

Rubber band exercises can be used for a variety of drills, such as:

- Running and agility side-to-side drills;

- Power exercises such as squat jumps and conventional resistance exercises;

- Traditional exercise such as chest press, arm curl, and squats;

- As always, safety is the primary consideration. Consider band strength.

Safety Questions

Before using a resistance band or rubber band machine, ask a number of questions, especially when there are multiple users. Rubber bands should be checked at rest and then when stretched to their usable length. Examine them carefully, asking:

- Is the resistance smooth and flexible in use?

- Are there signs of wear from repetitive use, including cracks, or worn endings?

- Are there signs of weather exposure—such as sun, water, or cold— making the rubber cracked or pale?

—by William Kraemer, Ph.D., FACSM

Bosu Basics

"Bosu Basics" by Mark Eshpeter, originally published in IMPACT *Magazine, Calgary, Alberta, July/August 2005. Reprinted with permission by* IMPACT Magazine *and Mark Eshpeter.*

BOSU is an acronym for "Both Sides Up" referring to the fact that this piece of equipment can be used either on the flat "platform" side or the rounded "ball" portion. The unstable training platforms of the BOSU ensure that the user performs exercises over a constantly shifting center of balance, which makes the BOSU an ideal tool for training kinesthetic sense, balance, and proprioception.

The inherent instability of the BOSU makes it difficult for the body to "learn" movements through repetition, so the user is forced to recruit the stabilizing musculature of the trunk to maintain balance and rhythm through the entire range of motion. Straightforward exercises like push-ups and lunges take on a whole new level of difficulty when you perform them on the BOSU.

Although the BOSU is a very accessible and challenging piece of training equipment, many people do not know how to use one or incorporate it into their workouts. The exercises here are designed to highlight the versatility of the BOSU with an emphasis on big body movements. With a little imagination and some dumbbells, the BOSU can provide an excellent full body workout.

The BOSU ball is one of the most versatile and innovative yet underused training tools out there. Here are four ways you can incorporate the BOSU into your exercise regime.

✎ What's It Mean?

<u>Kinesthetic Sense:</u> The awareness of movement or activity in muscles or joints.

<u>Proprioception:</u> A sense or perception, usually at a subconscious level, of the movements and position of the body and especially its limbs, independent of vision.

Source: *Stedman's Medical Dictionary, 27th Edition*, copyright © 2000 Lippincott Williams & Wilkins. All rights reserved.

Kick-Out Push-Ups

Grasp each side of the BOSU and assume a planked position, making sure to keep your arms locked and your body straight. Take a knee and bring it to your chest, kick your leg straight back, and perform a deep push-up. Keep your leg from touching the ground throughout the entire motion. To add difficulty, try alternately lowering one side of the BOSU to the ground between each repetition. Perform two sets of 10 repetitions per leg.

Primary muscle groups used: Triceps, pectorals, abdominals, back extensors, obliques, glutes, and quadriceps.

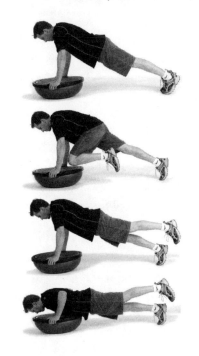

Figure 12.4. Kick-Out Push-Ups

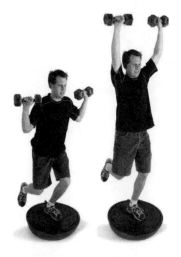

Figure 12.5. One-Legged Shoulder Presses

One-Legged Shoulder Presses

Balance on one leg in the center of the BOSU ball while holding medium weight dumbbells in both hands. Hold the dumbbells at shoulder height and perform a quarter-squat on your single leg. As you come up from the squat position press the dumbbells above your head. Lower the dumbbells back to shoulder height as you perform your next quarter-squat. To add variety, try using only a single dumbbell in the opposite arm and perform single-arm presses. Perform two sets of 10 repetitions per leg.

Primary muscle groups used: Deltoids, triceps, glutes, quadriceps, back extensors, and calves.

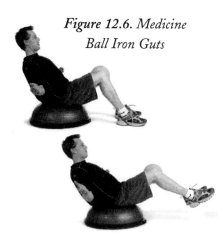

Figure 12.6. Medicine Ball Iron Guts

Medicine Ball Iron Guts

Sit just slightly forward of the very top of the BOSU ball and place a light medicine ball or yoga blocks between your knees. Lean back so that your torso makes roughly a 45-degree angle with the ground. Lift your legs off the ground and straighten them as far as you can. Try to maintain balance in this position for 10 to 30 seconds. To increase the difficulty, try holding a medicine ball at arm's length and rotating from side to side. Perform 10 repetitions holding between 10 and 30 seconds.

Primary muscle groups used: Abdominals, hip flexors, back extensors, quadriceps (*vastus medialis*), and obliques (advanced).

Lunge Curls

Place your leading foot on the center of the BOSU with the dome side up while holding medium-weight dumbbells. Move the rear leg backwards until you are in a lunge position. Keep your back straight and lower yourself while holding the weights at your sides. As you come up from the lunge, perform a biceps curl with the dumbbells. Try using the flat platform of the BOSU to make this exercise more difficult. Perform two sets of 10 to 15 repetitions per leg.

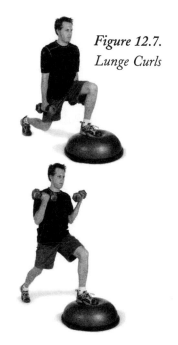

Figure 12.7. Lunge Curls

Primary muscle groups used: Biceps, back extensors, glutes, hip flexors, hamstrings, quadriceps, and calves.

—by Mark Eshpeter; photography by Senkowski Photo

Strengthen Your Abdominals With Stability Balls

Source: "Strengthen Your Abdominals with Stability Balls," is reprinted with permission from the American Council on Exercise (www.acefitness.org), © 2001. All rights reserved.

One of today's most versatile pieces of exercise equipment looks more like an overgrown beach ball than a useful fitness tool.

The stability ball—an extra-large, inflatable orb designed to improve balance while targeting specific muscle groups—has grown in popularity since it's mainstream introduction in the late 1980s and early 1990s.

The stability ball can be adapted for many uses, including developing core strength, improving posture, and facilitating stretching, among others. Its application is particularly widespread in the physical therapy industry, where it was first put to use nearly 30 years ago.

Thanks to fitness professionals' interest in the stability ball and its numerous benefits, there have been several exercise programs developed over the past few years for just about every need, desire, and body part.

The Stability Ball And Your Core

So much of the exercise we do, such as running and cycling, focuses on the lower body. Not much attention is paid to the trunk, or core, of the body. It is the muscles of the core—the abdomen, chest, and back—that stabilize the rest of the body.

Think of your core as a strong column that links the upper and lower body together. Having a solid core creates a foundation for all activities and is especially important when you add a heavy load, such as weights to your workout.

It is important when you are strengthening the core that you create balance between the muscles of the abdominal and the back. Many people will naturally have an imbalance between the strength of their abdominal muscles and the lower back muscles. Exercising with stability balls helps to develop and strengthen those muscles.

Infomercials and magazine advertisements seem to be targeting the individual who wants to strengthen their abdominal muscles. Although end results such as "toning" and "shrinking" aren't totally accurate, a handful of the techniques the equipment supports are valid.

However, you don't need an ab rocker or a special track with handles to concentrate on this area. The stability ball is well equipped to help you concentrate on your capricious core.

Here are three exercises that can be performed with a standard stability ball and target all three sections of the abdominal muscles:

- **Supine trunk curl:** Start with the top of the ball beneath the center of the back. Press the lower back into the ball and tighten the abdominals as you curl the rib cage toward the pelvis. Slowly return to the starting position.

- **Supine oblique curl:** Start with the top of the ball beneath the center of the back, then stagger feet and rotate hips to one side. Anchor the lower hip to the ball and move the rib cage at a diagonal direction toward the legs (for example, right elbow to left inner thigh). Make sure your neck and pelvis are stable.

- **Forward transverse roll:** Kneel on the floor and place your forearms on the ball, making sure your hips and arms form a 90-degree angle. From this starting position, roll the ball forward as you extend your arms and legs simultaneously. Contract your abdominals to help support your lower back, which should not be strained. Roll as far forward as possible without compressing the spine, drooping shoulders, or rounding the torso. Return to starting position.

The Benefits Of Balls

Besides providing balance training, stability balls work the trunk in almost every exercise that is performed. By concentrating on the abdominal section, your posture will improve and you will find that you are generally more balanced and aware of your body movements. Your core will be more prepared to support the rest of your body in whatever activity you choose to do.

How To Choose A Ball

It is important to buy the right size ball and maintain the proper air pressure. The firmer the ball, the more difficult the exercise will be. The softer the ball, the less difficult the exercise will be.

If you are just beginning, overweight, an older adult, or you are generally deconditioned, you may want to consider using a larger, softer ball. When sitting on the ball, your knees and hips should align at a 90-degree angle.

Following are general guidelines for buying the right size stability ball:

- Under 4'6" (137 cm): 30 cm ball (12 inches)
- 4'6"–5'0" (137-152 cm): 45 cm ball (18 inches)
- 5'1"–5'7" (155-170 cm): 55 cm ball (22 inches)
- 5'8"–6'2"(173-188 cm): 65 cm ball (26 inches)
- Over 6'2" (188 cm): 75 cm ball (30 inches)

Chapter 13

Choosing Shoes And Apparel

Selecting Athletic Shoes

Proper-fitting sports shoes can enhance performance and prevent injuries. Follow these specially designed fitting facts when purchasing a new pair of athletic shoes.

- Try on athletic shoes after a workout or run and at the end of the day. Your feet will be at their largest.

- Wear the same type of sock that you will wear for that sport.

- When the shoe is on your foot, you should be able to freely wiggle all of your toes.

- The shoes should be comfortable as soon as you try them on. There is no break-in period.

- Walk or run a few steps in your shoes. They should be comfortable.

- Always relace the shoes you are trying on. You should begin at the farthest eyelets and apply even pressure as you a crisscross lacing pattern to the top of the shoe.

About This Chapter: This chapter includes information from "Lacing Techniques For Proper Shoe Fit," © 2008 American Orthopaedic Foot and Ankle Society (www.aofas.org). Reprinted with permission; and "Selecting Athletic Shoes," © 2001 American Orthopaedic Foot and Ankle Society (www.aofas.org). Reprinted with permission.

- There should be a firm grip of the shoe to your heel. Your heel should not slip as you walk or run.

- If you participate in a sport three or more times a week, you need a sports specific shoe.

It can be hard to choose from the many different types of athletic shoes available. There are differences in design and variations in material and weight. These differences have been developed to protect the areas of the feet that encounter the most stress in a particular athletic activity.

Athletic shoes are grouped into seven categories:

- **Running, training, and walking:** Includes shoes for hiking, jogging, and exercise walking. Look for a good walking shoe to have a comfortable soft upper, good shock absorption, smooth tread, and a rocker sole design that encourages the natural roll of the foot during the walking motion. The features of a good jogging shoe include cushioning, flexibility, control, and stability in the heel counter area, lightness, and good traction.

- **Court sports:** Includes shoes for tennis, basketball, and volleyball. Most court sports require the body to move forward, backward, and side-to-side. As a result, most athletic shoes used for court sports are subjected to heavy abuse. The key to finding a good court shoe is its sole. Ask a coach or shoes salesman to help you select the best type of sole for the sport you plan on participating in.

- **Field sports:** Includes shoes for soccer, football, and baseball. These shoes are cleated, studded, or spiked. The spike and stud formations vary from sport to sport, but generally are replaceable or detachable cleats, spikes, or studs affixed into nylon soles.

- **Winter sports:** Includes footwear for figure skating, ice hockey, alpine skiing, and cross-country skiing. The key to a good winter sports shoe is its ability to provide ample ankle support.

- **Track and field sport shoes:** Because of the specific needs of individual runners, athletic shoe companies produce many models for various foot types, gait patterns, and training styles. It is always best to ask your coach about the type of shoe that should be selected for the event you are participating in.

- **Specialty sports:** Includes shoes for golf, aerobic dancing, and bicycling.

- **Outdoor sports:** Includes shoes used for recreational activities such as hunting, fishing, and boating.

Lacing Techniques For Proper Shoe Fit

Certain lacing techniques for shoes can prevent injuries, alleviate pain, and relieve foot problems. The American Orthopaedic Foot and Ankle Society urges individuals to follow these general lacing tips. Individuals with specific foot problems should follow these lacing techniques to get a good fit with their shoe:

- Loosen the laces as you slip into the shoes. This prevents unnecessary stress on the eyelets (small holes for the lace) and the backs of the shoes.

- Always begin lacing shoes at the eyelets closest to your toes, and pull the laces of one set of eyelets at a time to tighten. This provides for a comfortable shoe fit.

- When buying shoes, remember that shoes with a larger number of eyelets will make it easier to adjust laces for a custom fit.

- The conventional method of lacing, crisscross to the top of the shoe, works best for the majority of people.

Narrow Feet

Use the eyelets farthest from the tongue of the shoes. It will bring up the side of the shoe.

Wide Feet

Use the eyelets closest to the tongue of the shoe. This technique gives the foot more space.

Heel Problems

Use every eyelet, making sure that the area closest to the heel is tied tightly while less tension is used near the toes. When you have reached the next to last eyelet on each side, thread the lace through the top eyelet, making a small loop. Then, thread the opposite lace through each loop before tying it.

Narrow Heel And Wide Forefoot

Use two laces. Thread through the top half of the eyelets and the other lace through the bottom half of the eyelets. The lace closest to the heel (top eyelets) should be tied more tightly than the other lace closest to the toes (bottom eyelets).

♣ It's A Fact!!
Clothing

Comfort and safety are the key words for workout clothing.

- For outdoor, nighttime exercise, a reflective vest and light-colored clothing must be worn.

- Bikers, inline skaters, and equestrians should always wear safety devices such as helmets, wrist guards, and knee and elbow pads.

- Goggles are mandatory for indoor racquet sports.

- For vigorous athletic activities, such as football, ankle braces may be more effective than tape in preventing ankle injuries.

Source: Excerpted from "Exercise In-Depth Report," © 2008 A.D.A.M., Inc. Reprinted with permission.

Part Three

Activities To Try

Chapter 14

Aerobic Step Bench Training

Step-Bench Training For Fitness And Fun

Within the last few years, step-bench training's popularity has climbed rapidly. An estimated 10 million people have tried step training.

Could 10 million steppers be wrong? On the contrary—vigorous stepping provides the cardiovascular benefits of running but stresses the joints little more than walking. Performed to invigorating music with creative choreography, this low-impact workout is also lots of fun.

The First Step To Stepping

Before beginning a step-training class, be sure your step—the platform—is secure and at the proper height for your fitness level. If you are new to step training, or just beginning a fitness program, start with a platform height of four to six inches. (Regardless of fitness level, the platform height should not require bending your knees more than 90 degrees.)

Keep the area around your platform dry and remove objects that could interfere with your workout.

About This Chapter: This includes information from "Step-Bench Training For Fitness And Fun," reprinted with permission from the American Council on Exercise (www.acefitness.org), © 2001. All rights reserved.

✔ Quick Tip

Stepping Out

- If you initially find step training difficult to follow, focus on learning the foot patterns and omit arm movements. You can add arm movements later.

- Remember that raising your arms above shoulder level makes your heart work harder and can leave you breathless. So, if you have a hard time keeping up, lower your arms and catch your breath.

- To avoid injuries caused by too much stepping, alternate step-training classes with a variety of aerobic workouts like bicycling, walking, or other recreational activities.

- Step-training workouts may seem difficult at first, but beware—they're habit-forming! Just remember to maintain proper body alignment and stepping technique to keep you stepping injury-free for years to come.

Align Your Body

Proper body alignment during step training helps prevent injuries. While stepping:

- Relax your neck and keep it straight;
- Always keep your knees soft, don't lock the knee joints;
- Maintain good posture with shoulders back, chest lifted and pelvis tucked under;
- Lean from the ankles, not the waist, as you step onto the platform—do not bend from the hips;
- Don't arch your back.

Proper Stepping Techniques

Correct stepping technique also prevents injuries and improves your workout:

1. Always place your entire foot on the platform. No part of the foot should hang over the edge.

2. Step close to the platform, allowing the heels to contact the floor. Note: Only the ball of the foot, not the heel, should touch the floor during lunges or other rapidly repeated movements ("repeaters").

3. Step quietly. Pounding can unduly stress the ankles and knees.

4. Keep an eye on the platform at all times.

5. Don't use hand weights. They greatly increase the risk of injury and provide no benefit.

Chapter 15

Spinning And Bicycling

Spin It: What You Need To Know About Group Indoor Cycling

Some call it torturous, others exhilarating. But there's no denying the popularity of group indoor cycling. What sets these classes apart from the usual boredom of stationary cycling is the visual imagery provided by instructors. Participants are led on a "virtual" outdoor road race complete with hills, valleys, straight-aways, and finish lines. But before you reserve your spot (many classes are so popular that reservations are a must) and start composing your victory speech, there are few questions to ask yourself, as well as a few precautions to take, to make your first ride a smooth and enjoyable one.

What Kind Of Shape Am I In?

This question is crucial. Despite its heavy promotion as a workout for even the most uncoordinated, indoor cycling is by no means for everyone. The intensity levels of many classes are far beyond what most novices or part-time exercisers can achieve and maintain, particularly for 40 minutes or more.

About This Chapter: This chapter begins with information from "Spin It: What You Need To Know About Group Indoor Cycling," reprinted with permission from the American Council on Exercise (www.acefitness.org), © 2004. All rights reserved. Information under the heading "Bicycling" is from "Bicycling Activity Card," U.S. Department of Health and Human Services, Centers for Disease Control and Prevention (CDC), 2001.

It's easy to get caught up in an instructor's chant of "Faster revolutions per minute (RPMs)!" and "Don't sit down!" even if your body is telling you otherwise. And because not all fitness facilities are able to offer classes tailored for beginning exercisers, it's important that participants either be in very good cardiovascular condition or have the ability to monitor and adhere to their body's cries for moderation.

Get In Cycling Shape

Just because you may not be ready for a cycling class now doesn't mean you can't be in the very near future. Consider doing some cycling-specific training before you take your first indoor cycling class. Spend some time on a stationary bike, but make it interesting by creating your own virtual experience by "traveling" some of your favorite road trips in your mind as you listen to music. You can increase your endurance by interspersing periods of higher-intensity cycling (faster speed, greater tension) with more leisurely pedaling. In just a few short weeks you'll be ready to sign up for your first indoor cycling class.

Indoor Cycling Essentials

The following helpful tips can make your first cycling experience a positive one:

- **Don't make the dreaded mistake of showing up in running shorts or heavy sweats—there's no better way to make your ride unbearable.** Opt instead for bike shorts, preferably padded ones like most outdoor cyclists wear. While this won't eliminate the possibility of chaffing and discomfort altogether, it helps a lot.

- **Your second most important item: a full water bottle.** Get ready to consume plenty of fluids before, during, and immediately following your workout.

- **Adjust the seat to the appropriate height.** If the seat is too low, you won't be able to get enough leg extension on the downstroke and your legs will tire out faster. If it's too high, you'll be straining to reach and might injure yourself. Here's a good rule to follow: Your upstroke knee should never exceed hip level, while your downstroke knee should be about 85 percent straight. And don't grip the handlebars too tightly, as this will increase the tension in your neck and shoulders.

- **Ask your instructor about his or her training.** In addition to cycling knowledge, they should have experience teaching group exercise and have earned a primary certification from an organization such as the American Council on Exercise (ACE). Look for an instructor who encourages perceived exertion measures and/or heart-rate monitoring and is willing to get off their own bike to coach beginners.

- **Above all, concentrate on exercising at your own pace.** Don't be intimidated by the high speeds and furious intensity of your cycling mates. Listen to your body and adjust the tension and speed accordingly, and don't be afraid to slow down or take a break when necessary.

♣ **It's A Fact!!**
What A Workout!

An ACE-sponsored study revealed that exercisers in a typical group indoor cycling class reported an exertion level in the high teens (using Borg's Rating of Perceived Exertion, a scale from 6 to 20) throughout most of the class. In addition, heart-rate measurements indicated that participants were exercising close to their maximum heart rate, which validated their perceptions that they were working hard. Clearly, group indoor cycling classes provide a challenging, high-intensity workout.

Source: Reprinted with permission from the American Council on Exercise (www.acefitness.org), © 2004. All rights reserved.

Bicycling

Gear Up

To begin bicycling, you'll need two pieces of equipment:

- **A bike:** Think of the type of riding you want to do before you buy one. Mountain bikes are strong and stable and built for gravel roads and tricky trails. Racing bikes are built to go super fast on pavement, and sport bikes, a combination of both, are good for many different purposes.

- **A helmet:** Your helmet should sit right above your eyebrows and be tightly buckled so it doesn't slip while you are riding.

Play It Safe

- **Use your head and wear a helmet.** You should always wear a helmet when you ride—plus, it's the law in many states. It's also important that your helmet is approved by one of the groups who test helmets to see which ones are the best—the Consumer Product Safety Commission (CPSC) or Snell B-95 standards are best for bicycling helmets. Try not to ride at night or in bad weather, and wear brightly colored, or reflective clothes whenever you ride so you can be seen. You can even put reflectors or funky reflective stickers on your bike. Also, watch out for loose pant legs and shoelaces that could get caught in your bike chain.

> **♣ It's A Fact!!**
>
> The faster you are going, the longer it will take you to completely stop your bike once you hit the brakes. Science says that if you are going 20 MPH and you hit the brakes, it will take 15 feet to stop if you are on dry pavement, and 23½ feet if you are on wet pavement, so make sure you brake early.
>
> Source: Department of Health and Human Services, Centers for Disease Control and Prevention (CDC), 2001.

- **Be street smart.** Ride on the right side of the road, moving with traffic, and obey all traffic signs and signals. Discuss the best riding routes with your parents—they'll help you determine safe places to ride near your home.

- **When you reach an intersection, be sure to stop and look left, right, and then left again to check for cars—then go.** Use hand signals to show when you're going to turn, and be sure to keep an eye out for rough pavement ahead so you can avoid it. And although you may think you can't go out without your favorite tunes, never wear head-phones when you're on your bike.

How To Play

Bicycling can be a great competitive sport, as well as a fun activity to do with your friends. And there are plenty of different types of bicycling depending on your personality. If you love to go fast-n-furious, bicycle racing is probably more your speed. If you like to hit the rocky road, mountain biking sounds more like your taste. And if you just like to pedal for pleasure, any kind of bicycling will do. Try riding to school or to a friend's house.

Body Parts Worked

- Upper and lower legs
- Heart and lungs

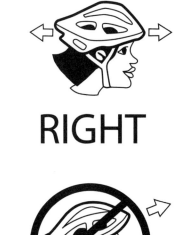

RIGHT

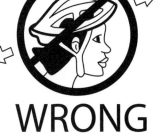

WRONG

Figure 15.1. The right way and the wrong way to wear a bicycle helmet (Source: CDC).

Chapter 16

Golf

Gearing Up For Golf

Golf is rapidly becoming the sport of choice for many Americans.

While some view the sport as slow-paced, golf actually requires a great deal of strength and stamina, not to mention skill. While you may not have to be in the best cardiovascular shape to play golf, your muscles, particularly those of the legs and upper torso, must be both strong and flexible to keep your handicap below an embarrassing level.

The Key Components

To be successful in golf there are three components of fitness that you should focus on: strength/power, flexibility, and cardiovascular endurance. These are also the three most important components of any well-rounded fitness program.

Strength And Power

Developing muscular strength and power is essential for generating club head speed, a determining factor in how far you can hit the ball. The box lists

About This Chapter: This chapter contains information from "Gearing Up For Golf," reprinted with permission from the American Council on Exercise (www.acefitness.org) © 2001. All rights reserved.

specific exercises that will help you generate more power in your upper body as well as stabilizing strength in your lower body.

One or more sets of eight to 12 repetitions of each exercise should be performed three days per week.

A recent study found this regimen to be extremely effective. As similar studies have shown, strength training brings about significant improvements in lean body weight, reduced body fat, increased leg strength and joint flexibility, and a reduction in systolic blood pressure.

But more important, at least to the golfers in this study, was the significant improvement in club head speed. The 17 exercisers increased the speed of their swing by an average of five mph. The control group experienced no such improvements.

Flexibility

Flexibility is another important key to developing a full, fluid golf swing. Simply swinging the club is not enough, but you can increase the range of motion in your shoulders, trunk, low back, and hamstrings with just a few minutes of daily stretching.

But don't save your stretching until five minutes before you tee off. Flexibility exercises must be done every day. And always warm up your muscles before you stretch them to increase your range of motion and prevent injury.

Cardiovascular Conditioning

Finally, cardiovascular conditioning is essential to help you keep your energy up during a long round of golf. That conditioning can help you deal with the stress of making a crucial putt or of getting out of a sand trap.

Try to fit in at least 20 minutes of walking, cycling, or whatever aerobic activity you prefer, three times per week.

Improving your golf game requires a bit more than simply playing a lot of golf, but it doesn't mean you have to spend hours in the gym. Try the exercises outlined in the box and you'll not only come closer to par, but you'll also reap numerous health benefits, such as increased lean body weight, reduced body fat, lower blood pressure, and increased strength and flexibility.

While it may be difficult to motivate some people to stretch or begin strength training, telling them they might lower their handicap may be just the ticket to get them to head to the gym. Or work out at home. Whichever is most convenient.

The point is to do it, regardless of whether it's for health or for a better golf score.

✔ Quick Tip
Exercises To Improve Your Golf Swing

Golfers should perform one set of eight to 12 repetitions of each of the following exercises, three days per week.

- Abdominal curl
- Biceps curl
- Chest cross
- Chest press
- Lateral raise
- Leg curl
- Leg extension

- Leg press
- Low back extension
- Neck extension
- Neck flexion
- Front lat pull
- Triceps extension
- Weight-assisted chin-up

Chapter 17

Gymnastics And Cheerleading

Gymnastics

Gear Up

Unlike some other sports, gymnastics doesn't require a lot of equipment, but there are certain things you'll need for specific events and some standard gear that all gymnasts should have.

Female gymnasts usually wear leotards (one or two piece outfits that fit snugly to the body). Boys can wear running shorts or sweatpants with fitted tops or with your shirt tucked in. Just make sure you don't wear clothing that is too loose—it could get caught on the equipment when you are performing your tricks and cause you serious problems. For those of you with long locks, you'll need to pull it back with a hair band or in a braid—this will prevent it from getting in your face during your routine, which could cause you to lose concentration and sight.

Gymnasts also wear hand guards and use chalk to prevent their hands from slipping when working on the floor mats, rings, or bars. The hand guards help prevent blisters and make it easier to swing around on the bars.

About This Chapter: This chapter includes information from "Gymnastics Activity Card," and "Cheerleading Activity Card," United States Department of Health and Human Services, Centers for Disease Control and Prevention (CDC), reviewed 2002 and 2001 respectively.

Play It Safe

The most important gymnastics rule to remember is to know what you're doing. Never attempt a trick you are not familiar with. Make sure you always have a trained spotter (someone who stands near you in case you need help while doing your tricks) just in case you lose your balance on the beam or attempt a wobbly handstand.

Before you attempt any trick or stunt, always make sure the equipment is sturdy and has been set up properly (always ask a coach or another grown-up for help). Floors should be padded with mats that are secured under every piece of equipment. Also, make sure there is enough distance between each

> ### ♣ It's A Fact!!
>
> - The first large-scale gymnastics competition was during the 1896 Olympics in Athens, Greece.
>
> - At the 1976 Olympics, Nadia Comaneci made history by becoming the first gymnast to ever score a perfect 10. At those games she received seven perfect 10s, three gold medals, one silver, and one bronze.
>
> - A standard balance beam is only four inches wide (that's about the width of a loaf of bread) and almost four feet off of the ground.

piece of equipment before you start swinging. Collisions can cause you, or others around you, to get hurt if you don't watch out. Use your head. Pay attention and be serious about your practice—horseplay and goofing around can get you into trouble. Always know what your teammates are doing and where they are.

And last but not least, never eat or chew gum while doing gymnastics—the moment you become unaware of what is in your mouth, it can easily become lodged in your throat and you could choke.

How To Play

Gymnastics is known as the sport of all sports. It's a great way to improve strength, flexibility, balance, and coordination for other types of physical activities, and it's a great way to meet new people and have fun.

It doesn't matter if you're a guy or a girl—gymnastics has a few different categories to choose from so you can find your favorite. Artistic gymnasts use lots of skills to perform on many different kinds of apparatuses (pieces of equipment). Boys participate in six events (floor, vault, parallel bars, high bar, still rings, and pommel horse) and girls in four (floor, vault, uneven parallel bars, and balance beam). Gymnasts who participate in rhythmic gymnastics jump, tumble, flip, and dance to music while using rope, hoops, bars, or ribbons as part of their routines. In gymnastics, there's something for everyone.

But, before you get started, you need to know (and master) the basics.

Hit The Mat

The handstand is one of the basic skills of gymnastics. If you're a beginner, it's a good idea to practice your handstands against a wall until you get your balance and build up your strength and confidence. And remember it is always good to have a spotter—just in case you need some help along the way.

Follow these tips to a perfect handstand:

- Face the wall.

- Get in a squatted position so that your knees are bent and your body is close to the ground.

- Put your hands on the floor with the tips of your fingers facing the wall (your hands should not be any wider than shoulder width apart).

- Bend your head down to the floor, keeping it between your arms.

- Kick your legs up putting all your weight on your hands, keeping your upper body straight and tight.

- Once your feet hit the wall, straighten out your legs.

Now that you've mastered the handstand, want to try something trickier?

Practice these steps to conquer the cartwheel:

- Stand in a ready position, your "favorite" leg in front, knees bent slightly. To find out your favorite leg, stand up and take one step. The leg you step forward with first is usually your favorite.

- Raise both of your arms.

- Reach forward with your right arm, putting your right hand on the floor/ground.

- Shift your weight to your right arm and kick your left leg up (If you're a lefty, reverse these directions).Your left hand should follow very quickly—as it touches the ground, shift your weight to your left arm. Your right leg should be off of the ground.

- Bring your left leg down, right hand up, right leg down, left hand up.

Parts Of The Body Worked

- Upper and lower legs
- Hips and butt
- Abs
- Shoulders and neck

Cheerleading

Gear Up

You'll need a good comfortable pair of sneakers that provide a lot of support and cushion for your feet. Also, many cheerleaders use spirit-raising tools such as pom-poms and megaphones.

Play It Safe

Today's cheerleading is super fun, but it's risky too—especially if you perform stunts. On this team sport, each squad member's position is key to completing the stunts safely and dazzling the crowd.

Make sure you're well conditioned for all those kicks, jumps, and splits—warm up before each practice and game and do lots of stretching. Focus on stretching your legs and back. If you do stunts and build pyramids, make sure you stretch your arms and shoulders too.

Practice safe stunts. If your squad does lifts, tosses, or builds pyramids, make sure you follow the stunt safety rules.

How To Play

When you hear the word "cheerleading," what do you think of? How about a fast-paced competitive sport for both guys and girls that involves a high level of endurance, strength, and precision? For many cheerleaders, that is exactly what cheering is. Cheerleading is coming into its own as a competitive sport. Cheer squads compete up to the national level, developing cheer and dance routines that include complex pyramids, lifts, and tosses.

If you're just starting out, here are some basic cheerleading motions:

Arm Motions

- **Goal Post:** Arms should be above your head, straight up in the air, and touching the side of your head. Your fists should be closed with your thumbs facing each other.

- **High V:** From the goal post position, move your arms out slightly wider to form a high V. Fists should be closed and thumbs facing away from your body. Your arms should be slightly in front of you so that you can see your fists out of the corner of your eyes.

- **Low V:** For this motion, the opposite of a high V, move your arms down into a v-like position by your sides. Keep your fists closed with your thumbs facing away from your body.

- **Basic T:** Your arms should be straight out on each side, in line with your shoulders. Keep your fists closed with your thumbs facing down, and your arms straight and level. Your body should look like a T.

Jump Tips

There are four main parts to a jump:

- **The Prep:** Begin with your feet together with your weight on your toes. Move your arms to a high V position and keep your shoulders back.

- **The Whip:** Next, lift your body up through your shoulders, quickly swinging your arms forward in a circle. Bend at the knees, keeping on the balls of your feet, building up to the lift.

♣ It's A Fact!!

About 98% of all female college cheerleaders are former gymnasts.

Madonna, Halle Berry, Kim Basinger, Cameron Diaz, and Kirsten Dunst were all cheerleaders.

Male celebrities who were cheerleaders include Samuel L. Jackson, Steve Martin, Aaron Spelling, and even President George W. Bush.

- **The Lift:** When your arms complete their circle to the high V position, jump off the ground, pushing through your toes. Once you are in the air, pull your legs up toward your arms. Keep your toes pointed, your arms stiff, and your head up.

- **The Landing:** Bring your legs together quickly so that your feet are together when they hit the ground. Bend your knees slightly to absorb the weight and take the pressure of your legs.

Parts Of The Body Worked

- Upper and lower legs

- Upper body

- Arms

- Knees and ankles

- Hips and butt

- Lower back

- Heart and lungs

✔ **Quick Tip**
Stunt Safety

- Always practice stunts on mats or pads.

- Never attempt a stunt unless a coach is there.

- Always use spotters for each and every stunt.

- If you are new to stunting, start with easier stunts and gradually move up to harder ones.

- Remember that if someone in the stunt yells "Down," the stunt should come down immediately.

Chapter 18

Kickboxing And Martial Arts

Kick Your Way To Fitness

Are you bored with your current fitness routine? It may be time to kick your way to one of the hottest workouts around. Kickboxing, also referred to as boxing aerobics and cardio kickboxing, is a hybrid of boxing, martial arts, and aerobics that offers an intense cross-training and total-body workout. It blends a mixture of high-power exercise routines that strengthen the body and mind, decrease stress, and hone reflexes while increasing endurance and cardiovascular power. While kickboxing's roots are in full-contact fighting, it has found a safe and very effective niche in the fitness community.

Many people are drawn to kickboxing because it increases self-esteem while burning an average of 500 to 800 calories an hour, as opposed to the 300 to 400 calories typically burned by the average hour-long step aerobics class. But before you kick down the door to the next class, take time to consider some of the basics of this sweat-intensive workout.

About This Chapter: This chapter begins with information from "Kick Your Way to Fitness," reprinted with permission from the American Council on Exercise (www.acefitness.org), © 2001. All rights reserved. Information under the heading "Martial Arts" is from "Martial Arts Activity Card," Department of Health and Human Services, Centers for Disease Control and Prevention (CDC), 2003.

What Is Your Current Fitness Level?

Keep in mind that many clubs may not offer classes that are based on progression. Even if your current routine features a hearty combination of cross-training workouts, you may want to take it easy at first, then build as your body adapts. For this reason, an hour-long session may not be the wisest choice for someone who isn't used to this level of concentrated activity.

Familiarize Yourself With The Basics

Remember, adequate warm-up and close attention to proper technique are paramount. Classes should begin with basic stretches and a light cardiovascular warm-up such as pushups and jumping jacks. A typical aerobic kickboxing routine involves a series of repetitive punches alternating with hand strikes, kicks, and then a combination of all three. The repetitions help participants focus on proper technique while engaging several muscles groups and getting a fierce cardiovascular workout. After the main section of the routine, stretches and floor exercises are commonly performed as a cooldown. Don't forget to wear loose clothing that allows freedom of movement during your kickboxing workout and drink plenty of water.

✔ Quick Tip
Basic Moves And Equipment

It may seem awkward at first, but the basic moves in a kickboxing class can be mastered with time, patience, and practice. A prepared class will have mirrors, a punching or "heavy" bag, and hit pads for participants to use. Here are two basic lower-body kickboxing moves that work the hamstrings, gluteals, and quadriceps:

- **The roundhouse kick:** Starting from a basic stance (side of body facing bag, knees slightly bent, shoulder-length apart), lift your right knee and point it just to the right of your target. Pivot on your left foot as you extend your right leg. Kick the target with the top of your foot.

- **The side kick:** From the basic stance, pull your right knee up toward your left shoulder. Pivot on your left foot as you snap your right leg into your target. Strike with either the outside edge of your foot or your heel.

Source: American Council on Exercise (www.acefitness.org), © 2001. All rights reserved.

Beginner Beware

When attending your first class, try to avoid these common mistakes:

- Wearing weights or holding dumbbells when throwing punches, which puts your joints in danger of injury

- Locking your joints when throwing kicks or punches

- Over-extending kicks (beginners should avoid high kicks until they get used to the routine and become more flexible)

- Giving in to group peer pressure and exercising beyond fatigue

And of course, you should ask your instructor about their training. Cardio kickboxing is a combination of martial arts and aerobics, and employs different techniques from a "pure" martial arts class. Many teachers may have boxing or martial arts training, but may not have the appropriate class experience or be properly certified by an organization such as the American Council on Exercise (ACE). Finally, once you understand the basics of this stress-relieving, total-body workout, you can kick your way to a new level of fitness.

Martial Arts

Gear Up

Most martial arts students wear white pants, a white jacket, and a cloth belt. For some martial arts, the belt color shows the student's skill level and personal development—from white (beginner) to black (expert).

For sparring (practice fighting), go for full gear, including a mouthpiece and padding on your head, hands, feet, and shins.

Play It Safe

Look for an instructor who's into respect and discipline, but still has plenty of patience. The class area should have lots of space and a smooth, flat floor with padding. The fewer students the better—more attention for you.

Wear all the right gear. Warm up and stretch so you're loose and ready to go. You need good instruction before launching into any moves. And when you do learn the moves, remember your limits. For example, white belt students shouldn't spar (practice fight).

How To Play

Martial arts—a special type of defense skills—started in the Orient (East Asia). Today, they're taught all over the world for self-defense and avoiding conflict, too. Body and mind control, discipline, and confidence are key. There are a lot of martial arts styles, but since certain types rough up the joints (like knees) more than others, these are some of the best for kids your age:

- Judo comes from Japan and means "gentle way." It's like Jujitsu, one of the oldest martial arts, but not as hard core. Judo has lots of wrestling moves. It also teaches participants how to make good decisions and to be mentally strong. Judokas (judo players) focus on competition.

- Karate comes from Japan, and means "empty hand." It's Japan's most popular martial art. Feet, legs, elbows, head, and fists get used for kicking, punching, defensive blocks, and more. Karate stresses defense and uses weapons.

- Tae Kwon Do comes from Korea and means "the way of the foot and fist." It's famous for high kicks. Tae Kwon Do became Korea's national sport in 1955 and is now the world's most popular martial art.

- Other martial arts include Aikido, Hwarang Do, Kung Fu, Jujitsu, Kendo, Ninjutsu, Northern and Southern Shaolin Boxing, Tai Chi, and T'an Su Do.

Interested? The first thing you need to do is to decide on the style you want to study. Do you want to enter tournaments, or simply know how to defend yourself? After that, just get into a good class.

Body Parts Worked

- Upper and lower legs
- Knees and ankles
- Abs
- Hips and butt
- Arms

Chapter 19

Pilates And Yoga

Pilates

Pilates (pronounced: puh-lah-teez) improves your mental and physical well being, increases flexibility, and strengthens muscles. Pilates uses controlled movements in the form of mat exercises or equipment to tone and strengthen the body. For decades, it's been the exercise of choice for dancers and gymnasts (and now Hollywood actors), but it was originally used to rehabilitate bedridden or immobile patients during World War I.

What Is Pilates?

Pilates is a body conditioning routine that seeks to build flexibility, strength, endurance, and coordination without adding muscle bulk. In addition, Pilates increases circulation and helps to sculpt the body and strengthen the body's "core" or "powerhouse" (torso). People who do Pilates regularly feel they have better posture, are less prone to injury, and experience better overall health.

About This Chapter: This chapter includes information from "Pilates," April 2007, reprinted with permission from www.kidshealth.org. Copyright © 2006 The Nemours Foundation. This information was provided by KidsHealth, one of the largest resources online for medically reviewed health information written for parents, kids, and teens. For more articles like this one, visit www.KidsHealth.org, or www.TeensHealth.org. Additional information from the Centers for Disease Control and Prevention (CDC) is cited separately within the chapter.

Joseph H. Pilates, the founder of the Pilates exercise method, was born in Germany. As a child he was frail, living with asthma in addition to other childhood conditions. To build his body and grow stronger, he took up several different sports, eventually becoming an accomplished athlete. As a nurse in Great Britain during World War I, he designed exercise methods and equipment for immobilized patients and soldiers. In addition to his equipment, Pilates developed a series of mat exercises that focus on the torso. He based these on various exercise methods from around the world, among them the mind-body formats of yoga and Chinese martial arts.

Joseph Pilates believed that our physical and mental health are intertwined. He designed his exercise program around principles that support this philosophy, including concentration, precision, control, breathing, and flowing movements.

There are two ways to exercise in Pilates. Today, most people focus on the mat exercises, which require only a floor mat and training. These exercises are designed so that your body uses its own weight as resistance. The other method of Pilates uses a variety of machines to tone and strengthen the body, again using the principle of resistance.

Getting Started

The great thing about Pilates is that just about everyone—from couch potatoes to fitness buffs—can do it. Because Pilates has gained lots of attention recently, there are lots of classes available. You'll probably find that many fitness centers and YMCAs offer Pilates classes, mostly in mat work. Some Pilates instructors also offer private classes that can be purchased class by class or in blocks of classes; these may combine mat work with machine work. If your health club makes Pilates machines available to members, make sure there's a qualified Pilates instructor on duty to teach and supervise you during the exercises.

The fact that Pilates is hot and classes are springing up everywhere does have a downside, though: inadequate instruction. As with any form of exercise, it is possible to injure yourself if you have a health condition or don't know exactly how to do the moves. Some gyms send their personal trainers to weekend-long courses and then claim they're qualified to teach Pilates (they're not!), and this can lead to injury. So look for an instructor who is certified by a group that has a rigorous training program. These instructors have completed several hundred hours of training just in Pilates and know the different ways to modify the exercises so new students don't get hurt.

The Pilates mat program follows a set sequence, with exercises following on from one another in a natural progression, just as Joseph Pilates designed them. Beginners start with basic exercises and build up to include additional exercises and more advanced positioning.

Keep these tips in mind so that you can get the most out of your Pilates workout.

- **Stay focused.** Pilates is designed to combine your breathing rhythm with your body movements. Qualified instructors teach ways to keep your breathing working in conjunction with the exercises. You will also be taught to concentrate on your muscles and what you are doing. The goal of Pilates is to unite your mind and body, which relieves stress and anxiety.

- **Be comfortable.** Wear comfortable clothes (as you would for yoga— shorts or tights and a T-shirt or tank top are good choices), and keep in mind that Pilates is usually done without shoes. If you start feeling uncomfortable, strained, or experience pain, you should stop.

- **Let it flow.** When you perform your exercises, avoid quick, jerky move- ments. Every movement should be slow, but still strong and flexible. Joseph Pilates worked with dancers and designed his movements to flow like a dance.

- **Don't leave out the heart.** The nice thing about Pilates is you don't have to break a sweat if you don't want to—but you can also work the exercises quickly (bearing in mind fluidity, of course) to get your heart rate going. Or, because Pilates is primarily about strength and flexibil- ity, pair your Pilates workout with a form of aerobic exercise like swim- ming or brisk walking.

Most fans of Pilates say they stick with the program because it's diverse and interesting. Joseph Pilates designed his program for variety—people do fewer repetitions of a number of exercises rather than lots of repetitions of only a few. He also intended his exercises to be something people could do on their own once they've had proper instruction, cutting down the need to remain dependent on a trainer.

Yoga

From "Yoga Activity Card," Department of Health and Human Services, Centers for Disease Control and Prevention (CDC), 2003.

Gear Up

Before you begin to relax your mind and body, make sure you suit up properly by wearing comfortable clothing that won't get in the way of your stretching. T-shirts, shorts, sweats, and tank tops are all great to wear for yoga because their fabric is movable and breaths easily. Jeans are definitely out.

Bare feet are ideal when you practice yoga, both for the traction they give you for standing poses, as well as the workout your feet will get.

One of the most important things you will need is a yoga or exercise mat to use during seated or floor postures. Don't worry if you don't have a special mat, use a firm pillow or folded up blanket—they work just as well.

✔ Quick Tip
The Hundred For Beginners

- Lie down on your back, knees bent toward your chest.

- Breathe in deeply; as you breath out, concentrate on feeling your chest and stomach sink toward the floor.

- Move your arms to the sides, palms toward the floor. Lift your head from the shoulders (not the neck) until the tips of your shoulder blades are pressing into your mat and you are looking at your belly button. Straighten your legs upward.

- Elongate your arms, as if reaching for the far side of the room, and pump your straightened arms up and down to the count of five, inhaling for five and exhaling for five. The goal is a hundred strokes, but start with fewer. Keep your belly flat and your back flat on the floor.

- Relax your head and pull your knees back to your chest.

Source: Reprinted with permission from "Pilates," www.kidshealth.org. Copyright © 2006 The Nemours Foundation, April 2007.

Play It Safe

It's important to make sure your muscles are warmed up before you begin your yoga routine. Never force your body into a posture or try to go beyond your limits—you could strain your muscles. Using the correct form is also key to getting the most out of your yoga experience, so get into a class that's right for you (whether you're a beginner or an expert). And, don't be afraid to ask your teacher for help. Learning the correct way to do each pose is important for overall mind and body development.

Feeling stiff or sore? If you are, you've overdone it. If you're just getting into yoga, it's important to start off slowly. Since yoga is not a competitive sport, your progress may be slow, but with time your body will become more flexible and you'll be able to achieve more difficult poses.

Interested in giving yoga a try, but not sure where to find classes in your area? It's important to find a class that you feel comfortable in, and has an experienced teacher. Try asking friends and family members if they know of a good place, or check out your local YMCA, county recreation centers, and fitness clubs—they sometimes have classes for all ages and skill levels. Also, don't forget about your local library—there you can find more information on yoga itself, as well as magazines or books that may have a listing of classes in your area.

How To Play

No matter what other activities you participate in, yoga can strengthen your abilities by increasing flexibility, staying power (endurance), and your ability to focus. Because yoga is a full body workout, it can help to check any imbalance in your muscles. In addition, yoga strengthens, tones, and stretches your muscles, helping to increase your flexibility.

Most yoga practices focus on physical postures called "asanas," breathing exercises called "pranayama," and meditation to bring your body and mind together through slow, careful movements. But, there's more to it than that! Yoga leads to improved physical fitness, increased ability to concentrate, and decreased stress. Yoga is an activity that helps both your body and mind work a little better.

When To Practice

Yoga can fit easily into your schedule—taking 5–10 minutes each day to practice can make a difference (just make sure to wait at least two to three hours after you've eaten.). Yoga is a perfect way to chill out and take some time just for yourself! So, set aside a special time each day and relax, release, and rejuvenate.

Where To Practice

Find a quiet spot where you won't be distracted. Look for a level area that is large enough for you to stretch upwards as well as to the sides for standing and floor positions or stretches.

How To Practice

Always warm up. Plan a well-rounded workout that includes lots of different positions from all of the major muscle groups (arms, legs, abs, back, chest). Most importantly, remember to breathe. It's a good idea to start with several arm stretches over your head and deep breaths. Inhale when you try upward and expanded movements, and exhale during downward or forward bending motions.

Concentrate on each position—move slowly making controlled movements until you feel your muscles tensing and resisting (you should feel your muscles stretching, not straining). Each pose in yoga is an experiment, so go slowly and listen to your body. Know when you are pushing yourself too hard or need to challenge yourself a little more.

Last but not least, remember to take 5–10 minutes to relax your body at the end of your workout. This will help to prevent sore muscles and is a way to unwind your body.

Parts Of The Body Worked

- Heart and lungs
- Upper and lower legs
- Hips and butt
- Lower back

Chapter 20

Play Ball: Baseball, Softball, Football, Basketball, And Soccer

Baseball

Gear Up

All ball players will need a ball, a bat, and a glove. All baseballs are pretty much the same, but bats can be either wooden or aluminum. These days, only the pros use wooden bats full time. Aluminum bats are lighter and easier to handle and don't break as often. There are a couple of different types of gloves, depending on your field position.

All batters should wear a helmet while at the plate and on base to protect the head. For better base running, try wearing baseball cleats instead of sneakers.

Catchers have a special set of protective gear that includes a helmet, a mask, shin guards, and a chest protector. All of these pieces are very important to protect you if you play behind the plate.

About This Chapter: This chapter includes information from "Baseball Activity Card," 2001, "Softball Activity Card," 2002, "Football Activity Card," 2001, "Basketball Activity Card," 2001, "Soccer Activity Card," 2001, and U.S. Department of Health and Human Services, Centers for Disease Control and Prevention (CDC).

Play It Safe

Wear your protective gear during all practices and games, especially if you're a catcher—those fast balls can pack a punch. Don't forget to warm up and stretch before each practice or game.

In the infield? Stay behind the base on any throw. You'll avoid hurting yourself—and the base runner.

In the outfield? Avoid bloopers with your teammates by calling every fly ball loudly, even if you think nobody else is close by.

In the batters' box, wear a batting helmet and use a batting glove to protect your knuckles from those inside pitches. If you think a pitch is going to hit you, turn away from the ball and take it in the back.

> **♣ It's A Fact!!**
> There are exactly 108 stitches on a baseball.
>
> In 1974, girls started playing on Little League teams.
>
> A major league pitcher can throw a baseball up to 95 miles an hour—which takes less than ½ second for the ball to cross the plate.

Throwing those fastballs can really take a toll, so if you're a pitcher, make sure to get plenty of rest between games, and don't pitch more than 4–10 innings per week.

How To Play

Baseball is known as America's favorite pastime. This sport uses many different skills from pitching, catching, and batting (which require lots of hand-eye coordination) to base running which means going from a standing start to a full sprint. To get started, you just need a bat and a ball.

How To Hit The Ball

- First, get hold of that bat by stacking your hands on the handle (right hand on top if you're a righty, left hand on top if you're a lefty), making sure the curve of the bat is in the middle of your fingers and that your knuckles are in a straight line.

- Balance on the balls of your feet, with your weight on your back foot, and bend your knees slightly. Your hands should be shoulder height, elbows in, and keep your head in line with your torso, turned toward your front shoulder. As the pitcher throws, step toward the pitch, and swivel toward the ball with your hips, keeping your arms steady as you move toward the ball.

- Keep your eye on the ball, and complete your swing by pivoting forward and shifting your weight to your front foot, following through with the bat after you hit the ball.

How To Throw The Ball

Did you know that throwing the ball accurately requires a little footwork?

- First, step toward the target with the glove side foot, making sure the toe of your shoe is pointing directly to where you want the ball to go.

- Aim the leading shoulder at the target.

- Aim the bill of your hat (the "duckbill") at the target and throw.

How To Catch The Ball

- Keep your eye on the pitch and stay low with your feet apart and knees bent so you can move quickly in any direction.

- Have your glove ready at or below knee level, pocket side out.

- When scooping up a ground ball, bend down and use both hands to scoop it to the middle of your body so you have it securely.

Parts Of The Body Worked

- Upper and lower legs
- Arms
- Back
- Shoulders and neck
- Wrist and forearm

Softball

Gear Up

You'll need a glove that fits your hand and skill level and is geared to the position you play. There's a lot of truth to the old saying, "Fits like a glove"—if your glove is too big, or small, you may have problems catching and fielding the ball. For beginners, gloves that are about 9½ to 11 inches long are a good start.

You can't play without a bat and ball. Try aluminum or other non-wooden bats—they are lighter and easier to handle. As for the ball, you can find softballs at most stores that sell sports equipment.

Also, for organized team play, you'll need a pair of shoes with rubber cleats—they dig into the ground and can give you more traction while running the bases or fielding a ball. If you're playing a pick-up game with your friends, a pair of sneakers will do. If you're a catcher, you'll need special protective gear like a helmet with a facemask, shin guards, and a chest protector.

And remember, always wear a helmet to protect your head while at the plate, or on base.

Play It Safe

Before you hit the field, warm up. Get all of your muscles ready to play by stretching before every game.

Whether you're in the field or up to bat, don't forget to wear your safety gear in games and in practices. A helmet is important when batting, waiting to bat, or running the bases. If you're a catcher, make sure you wear your protective gear during all practices and games, and wear it properly—have your coach or a parent check it out for you. Don't wear jewelry like rings, watches, or necklaces—they could cut you (or someone else) or get caught when you're running the bases.

Did you know that an umpire could call you out for throwing your bat? Well, they can. And, it's not just the out you have to worry about—it's your teammates' safety. Always drop your bat next to your side in the batters box before you head for first base.

Be a team player—always know where your teammates are before throwing the ball or swinging your bat. Make sure they are ready and have their glove up as a target before you throw the ball to them. Call loudly for every fly ball or pop up in the field, even if you don't think any of your teammates are close by.

How To Play

Softball is a game of speed, skill, and smarts. Whether you're looking to play in your backyard or at the state championships, softball is a great team sport that everyone can play.

Many of the skills in softball are similar to those in baseball, but there are some unique differences that make softball a game of its own.

Did you know that a softball isn't really soft at all and that it's almost two times bigger than a baseball? Because a softball is kind of big, it doesn't go as far when you hit it. But, keep your eye on the ball—a softball can sometimes cross the plate at a very fast speed. Even with their underhanded pitching

♣ It's A Fact!!

- Softball, including slow pitch and fast pitch, is the number one participation team sport in the United States with more than 40 million players.

- In its early stages, softball had lots of funny names such as kitten ball, mush ball, and big ball.

- The U.S. won the gold medal in softball's first Olympic appearance in the 1996 Atlanta Games.

style (unlike baseball's overhand style), softball pitchers can put a lot of heat on the ball. Most beginners play in slow pitch leagues where the "hitting game" is having a sharp eye and timing your swing . Keep your eyes peeled for pitches that are shoulder high and that drop right over the plate—they are perfect for driving into the field.

If you're interested in playing at a more competitive level, fast-pitch softball is what you'll see—you can steal bases and bunt, and you only need nine players to get a game going. If you're playing a pickup game with your friends, you'll probably play slow pitch softball. You only need ten players to field a team, but invite as many people as you want—it's more fun that way.

Parts Of The Body Worked

- Shoulders and neck
- Arms
- Back
- Upper and lower legs
- Wrist and forearm

Football

Gear Up

Obviously, you need a football to play, and you should choose the size based on your age. Always wear a helmet with a facemask and jaw pads and a mouthpiece to protect against those hard hits. Because football is a contact sport, there are many different pieces of gear you should wear to protect different areas of your body. For upper body protection, you should wear a neck roll to prevent whiplash, shoulder pads, rib pads, arm pads, and elbow pads. For leg protection, you should wear hip pads, tailbone pads, thigh pads, and knee pads. Most leagues require all this, but it's a good idea to protect yourself even in backyard games.

Play It Safe

Be sure to stretch and warm up before every practice and game and always wear your protective gear. To avoid getting hurt, learn from your coaches how to block and tackle correctly. Don't tackle with the top of your head or helmet—not only is it illegal, but it can cause injury to both players. If you play in an organized league, there are lots of rules—and they are there for a reason—to keep you safe. If you break these rules, you risk not only getting hurt, or hurting someone else, but your team will be penalized. If you're playing in the backyard with your friends, stay safe by sticking to touch or flag football and only play with kids who are around your age and size.

How To Play

There are lots of skills needed to play football—from throwing and catching the ball to blocking and tackling the other players. There's even a national Punt, Pass, and Kick contest devoted just to the main skills you need. League teams are a great way to learn all the rules and strategies of football.

Pop Warner is the most popular youth football league, but there are many others nationwide. Want the basics?

Throwing The Ball

- Grip the ball by placing each of your fingers between each lace of the ball.

- Bring your throwing arm back with your elbow bent.

- Extend your free arm (the one without the ball) in front of you and point to your target.

- Snap your throwing arm forward, releasing the ball, and follow through with your shoulders and hips.

- When you are finished, your throwing arm should be pointing toward your target with your palm facing the ground.

Catching The Ball

- Hold your arms out with your elbows slightly bent in front of your chest.

- Bring your hands together, touching the thumbs and index fingers to make a triangle with your fingers.

- Catch the nose of the ball in the triangle, and use your chest to help trap the ball.

- Bring your arms in around the ball and hold it tight against you.

Punting The Ball

- Place your feet shoulder-width apart with your kicking foot slightly in front.

- Slightly bend your knees and bend your body forward a little.

- Hold the ball out in front of you with the laces facing upward.

- Take two steps forward, beginning with your kicking foot and drop the ball toward your kicking foot.

- Kick the ball hard with the top of your foot and follow through with your leg as high as you can.

Parts Of The Body Worked

- Upper and lower legs

- Chest and back

- Arms

- Heart and lungs

♣ **It's A Fact!!**

The numbers worn on football players' uniforms represent the positions they play. For example, wide receivers and tight ends have numbers between 80–89.

A football field is 120 yards long (including the two end zones), and 53 1/3 yards wide.

Basketball

Gear Up

You'll need a basketball. Basketballs come in different sizes depending on your age and whether you're a girl or boy. There are also different basketballs for inside and outside use. If you're buying a new basketball, make sure you ask the salesperson for help to figure out what size and type ball you need.

You'll need a hoop. Basketball hoops are available in most gyms and in many parks. You can even buy a hoop and attach it to the side of your house or garage, if you have one. To create your own regulation court at your house, make sure you set your foul line 15 feet from the backboard.

Play It Safe

Basketball can really make you work, so make sure you stretch and warm up before playing. Because of all of the quick moves and jumping, it can put a lot of wear and tear on your ankles, so protect them by wearing the right pair of shoes—medium or high tops do the best job of supporting your ankles. Protect those knees by learning how to cut, stop, and land a jump safely.

Be careful not to misuse basketball equipment. It's great if you've got the skills to put up a mean slam-dunk, but hanging on the rim is dangerous and could cause you to get hurt. Also, make sure the court and sidelines are clear of any obstacles such as other basketballs or water bottles. If you're playing outside, make sure the baskets and sidelines are not too close to walls, fences, or bleachers and there are no holes on your court.

If you're a serious player, you may want to invest in a mouth guard to keep your teeth safe from flying elbows, knee and elbow pads so you don't get scraped up (especially if you're playing on an outdoor court), and sports glasses to protect your eyes.

How To Play

Basketball is fun to play in pick-up games in the yard with your pals, or you can join an organized league. Different positions rely on different skills— point guards should focus on their dribbling and passing, while centers and forwards should be powerful rebounders and shooters. Outside guards need to be quick and strong to make those three-point shots. Want some basics?

How To Dribble

- Bounce the ball on the floor with your strongest arm.

- When the ball bounces back, use your fingertips to stop the upward motion and push it back to the floor, keeping it about waist high when it bounces.

- Once you've mastered dribbling in place with one hand, switch to the other and begin to move around as you dribble.

- Practice dribbling by moving the ball in a figure eight between your legs to build your skills.

How To Pass The Ball

- Face the person you're passing to, with your head up and knees slightly bent.

- Spread your fingers wide and hold the ball at chest level, elbows out.

- Extend your arms, take a step toward the person you're passing to, and snap your wrists forward and up as you release the ball.

How To Shoot A Lay-Up

- Start about 10 feet in front of and to the right of the basket.

- Dribble toward the basket, timing it so that your last step is with your left foot.

- Holding the ball with both hands (left in front, right in back), jump off your left foot, let go with your left hand, and extend your right arm fully to release the ball at the top of your jump.

- Keep your eyes on where you want the ball to go. This really helps land the shot.

How To Cut, Stop, And Land A Jump

- Ease up on your cuts or pivots by making them less sharp to avoid rotating your knees.

- When stopping, rather than coming to a sudden stop or bringing your weight down on one foot with a single step, use the "stutter step" to slow yourself down by taking two extra steps.

> ## ♣ It's A Fact!!
>
> Former pro, Wilt Chamberlain, once scored 100 points in a single NBA game.
>
> Michael Jordan was cut from the varsity basketball team when he was in the 10th grade—and went on to be the NBA's Most Valuable Player for five seasons.

- When landing your jumps, do it softly by bending your knees over your feet (which should be pointed straight ahead) when you hit the ground.

- Instead of landing flat-footed, land on either the balls or toes of your feet and rock back toward your heels.

Parts Of The Body Worked

- Heart and lungs
- Upper and lower legs

Soccer

Gear Up

You'll need a soccer ball. Soccer balls come in different sizes depending on how old you are. Kids 8–12 should use a size four ball, and kids 13 and over should use a size five ball. Synthetic leather balls are best for beginners because they don't absorb water and get heavy.

If you play in a league, a goal will usually be provided for you, and you can buy a smaller goal if you want to play in your backyard—just make sure it is anchored to the ground. Don't have a goal? It's not a problem. Just set up any two objects (cones or water bottles are good) to shoot between.

Two pieces of equipment you need to wear at all times when playing soccer are shin guards and cleats. Shin guards are designed to protect your legs from the ball and from being kicked by other players. They are required in most leagues. The right cleats to wear for soccer are ones that are plastic or rubber. They'll help you with your quick starts, stops, and turns.

Play It Safe

Be sure to wear shin guards and appropriate soccer cleats during games as well as practices. Warming up, especially your leg muscles, is very important. To avoid headaches and dizziness, use your head and learn the proper technique for heading a ball in a game. Many leagues have strict rules about wearing jewelry, watches, and barrettes during games. Since any of these items can cause you to get hurt if you're hit with a ball, it's a good idea to not wear them when you play. Also, to protect your mouth from collisions (especially if you have braces), wear a mouthguard.

How To Play

In addition to a good strong kick, you'll want to master basic skills like passing (moving the ball to a teammate with a controlled kick), dribbling (tapping the ball with your feet to move it down the field), trapping (stopping the ball with your feet, legs, or chest), and heading (using your head to stop or pass the ball).

Here are some great passing and trapping tips.

Passing

- Pick your target out before you start the pass.

- Keep your head down to make sure you kick the ball correctly.

- Plant your non-kicking foot next to the ball and kick the ball right in the center using the inside of your foot and follow through with your leg.

Chest Trap

- As the ball comes toward you, get in front of it and let it hit your chest.

- Bring your shoulders around and slightly inward, creating a cavity for ball.

- Make sure you keep your arms down so the ball doesn't accidentally hit your hands and cause a foul.

- When the ball hits your chest, arch your back, so your chest pops the ball upward and then lands at your feet.

Parts Of The Body Worked

- Upper and lower legs
- Heart and lungs
- Knees and ankles
- Arms

♣ It's A Fact!!

- Nikolai Kutsenko of the Ukraine juggled a soccer ball for 24½ hours nonstop with his feet, legs, and head—the ball never touched the ground.

- Soccer players can run as many as six or seven miles during the course of a game.

Chapter 21

Skating And Skateboarding

Figure Skating

Gear Up

Figure skates are very thick and heavy and have a toe pick attached for tricks. Figure skates are made up of two parts, the boot and the blade. If you are just starting out, you can buy skates with both a boot and a blade, but more advanced skaters can buy each separately. The boot should be snug in the heel and supportive of the ankle. The blade is attached to the boot with screws, and is wider than the blade on an ice hockey skate, so that the edge grips the ice. You should not use figure skates to play ice hockey, because the blades extend past the boot and can cause other players to get injured.

If you are a beginning skater, along with your skates, you may want to wear a helmet to protect your head against any falls.

Be sure to wear layers so that you can put on or take off clothes depending on whether you are cold or warm. It's important to be able to move, so sweatpants or warm-up pants are perfect. You should only wear one pair of lightweight socks inside your skates, though, and remember to wear mittens and a hat to keep warm.

About This Chapter: This chapter includes information from "Figure Skating Activity Card," "Inline Skating Activity Card," and "Skateboarding Activity Card," U.S. Department of Health and Human Services, Centers for Disease Control and Prevention (CDC), 2001.

Play It Safe

Be a courteous skater—always be aware of other skaters and follow the traffic flow of the rink. Be careful not to get too close to other skaters with your exposed blades. And keep your skate laces tied tightly so that you don't trip yourself or anyone else up.

If you feel yourself beginning to fall, bring your hands, arms, and head into your body to absorb the shock of hitting the ice. And make sure you hop up quickly so that you are not in the way of other skaters.

Skating can be hard work, and puts a lot of stress on your leg and back muscles, so be sure to warm up before you skate and stretch those muscles well.

How To Play

Did you ever watch the figure skaters in the Olympics wondering how the heck they did all those jumps and spins? Well, according to the experts, the key to becoming a successful skater is one simple thing—balance. Good posture is an important part of balance, because it helps even out your weight over the skates. This keeps you from falling and helps you glide smoothly and work up some speed. Keep your head and chin up and imagine that they are connected with an imaginary line that runs down the center of your chest and connects with the toes of both of your feet.

It's also important to know how to stop. The basic stop is called a snow-plow. Keeping both knees bent, shift your weight to one foot then turn the other foot inward at an angle. Gradually shift your weight to the angled foot, which will slow you down and eventually bring you to a stop. A hockey stop is a more advanced move. To do it, quickly turn your feet sideways until they are perpendicular to the direction you were moving, putting more weight on your back foot.

Parts Of The Body Worked

- Heart and lungs
- Upper body
- Upper and lower legs
- Knees and ankles

Inline Skating

Gear Up

There are several different types of inline skates, depending on the type of skating you do. Recreational skates have a plastic boot and four wheels. These skates are best for beginners. Hockey skates have laces and are made of leather with small wheels for quick movement. Racing skates have five wheels and, usually, no brake. Freestyle skates have three wheels and a pick stop for tricks. Fitness skates have larger wheels and are used for cross-training. Aggressive skates, the kind worn by X Games competitors, are made of thick plastic with small wheels for quick movement and grind plates to protect the skate when doing tricks. No matter what kind of skates you wear, always wear a helmet, as well as wrist guards, elbow pads, and kneepads.

Play It Safe

Avoid getting hurt by making sure your helmet and pads are on correctly. Your helmet should be tightly buckled, with the front coming down to right over your eyebrow, and your pads should be on tight, so they don't slip while you are skating. It's also important that your helmet is approved by one of the groups who test helmets to see which ones are the best: the Consumer Product Safety Commission (CPSC), or Snell B-95 standards are best for inline skating helmets. Make sure you are always in control of your speed, turns, and stops; and be careful of cracks in the pavement where you are skating—they can be dangerous if your wheels get caught in them. It's best to go skating out of the way of traffic and other people (skating rinks are great places to skate).

How To Play

If you're just beginning inline skating, here are some tips to get you rolling.

- Practice balancing on your skates by walking in them on a flat, grassy area. As you move to the pavement, balance yourself without trying to move. Gradually begin to skate by moving forward, but not too fast. Keep your knees bent and flexible when you skate—it will keep you more stable. And if you fall—fall forward. Then you will fall on your kneepads—they're there to protect you.

- It's also a good idea to take lessons from a certified instructor. You can find one through the International Inline Skating Association. As you get more skilled on your skates, there are several types of competitive inline skating activities like speed skating and aggressive skating, which includes events like those at the X Games. There are also sports leagues just for those who play on wheels, such as roller hockey, roller soccer, and roller basketball.

> ## ♣ It's A Fact!!
>
> Inline skates were invented by a Minnesota hockey player so that he could skate during the off-season.
>
> California has the most inline skaters—3.6 million residents of the Golden State regularly go inline skating.
>
> Many professional skiers use inline skating to train during the off-season, because some of the skills of each activity are the same.

Parts Of The Body Worked

- Heart and lungs
- Upper and lower legs
- Hips and butt
- Lower back

Skateboarding

Gear Up

Skateboards can be bought pre-assembled, or you can buy all of the pieces and put it together yourself. Pre-assembled boards are best for beginners until you decide if skateboarding is really for you. If you are putting your own board together, you'll need a deck (the board itself), grip tape for the top of the deck so your feet don't slip, two trucks (the metal parts that are the axles of the wheels), four wheels, and two bearings per wheel (these keep the wheels spinning on the truck's axle). Before each time you ride, make sure your trucks are tightened and your wheels are spinning properly. Don't forget to wear a helmet, knee and elbow pads, and wrist guards. It's important that your helmet is approved by one of the groups who test helmets to see which ones are the best: the Snell B-95 standard is best for skateboarding helmets. Non-slippery shoes are a good idea too, so you can have better control of your board.

Play It Safe

Before you ride, make sure you give your board a safety check to make sure everything is put together right. Always wear all of your protective gear including a helmet, knee and elbow pads, and wrist guards. If you do tricks with your board, you may also want to wear gloves to protect your hands from the pavement. If you're just starting out, skate on a smooth, flat surface so you can practice keeping control of your board. And no matter how experienced you are, never hold on to the back of a moving vehicle. It's best to skate out of the way of traffic and other people (skate parks are great places to skate). But if you are skating in streets near your house, be aware of cars and people around you, and stay out of their way. Also, once the sun sets, it's a good idea to put up your board for the night, since skating in the dark can be dangerous.

How To Play

If you're just starting out, follow these steps to develop your skateboarding skills.

> **✔ Quick Tip**
>
> Skate on one foot. Practice balancing on one foot at a time while you're skating. See how long you can glide on each foot. This is a great way to work on your balance.
>
> Skate with friends. Go inline skating at the local park or skating rink, or join a skate club in your town.
>
> Combine activities. Tired of just skating around in circles? Grab some friends for a game of inline hockey, inline basketball, or even inline soccer.

- Put one foot on the board, toward the front, with the other on the ground.

- Push off the ground with your foot and put it on the rear of the board while you glide.

- Push again when you slow down.

- If you start going too fast, step off the board with your back foot.

- To turn, shift your weight to your back foot so that the front truck lifts off the ground and then move your body in the direction you want to go—the board will go with you.

If you want to find half pipes, vert ramps, and skate courses near you to practice your moves, look for a nearby skate park, designed to give skate-boarders a great ride.

There are several different styles of skateboarding:

- Street skating is skateboarding on streets, curbs, benches, and hand-rails—anything in-volving common street objects. Street skating is best left to the pros though because it is very dangerous.

♣ **It's A Fact!!**

- If you ride with your right foot for-ward, you have what's called a goofy stance. If you ride with your left foot forward, you have a regular stance.

- Professional skateboarder Tony Hawk is in the *Guinness Book of World Records* for being the only skateboarder to successfully do a "900." That's 2½ rotations in the air from a ramp.

- The first X Games competition was held in June 1995 in Rhode Island.

- Downhill skating is racing down big hills, usually on a longer skateboard called a longboard.

- Freestyle skating is more artistic, involving a series of tricks and stunts.

- Vert skating is skateboarding on mini-ramps and half pipes, which are U-shaped ramps.

Parts Of The Body Worked

- Upper and lower legs
- Knees and ankles

Chapter 22

Snow Sports: Skiing And Snowboarding

Snow Skiing

Gear Up

Are your skis the right size? If the tip of your upright ski reaches your face between your nose and chin, they are. If you're a beginner, shorter skis will be easier to control. The bindings (the part that holds your boot to the ski) are the most important parts of the ski. To make sure they don't break, get them tested regularly by a pro.

Make sure your boots fit and are comfortable. In general, ski boots are a half size smaller than your normal shoe size.

Be a trendsetter by picking up the helmet habit. Choose an American Society for Testing Materials (ASTM) approved model that fits right, is ventilated, and doesn't affect your hearing or field of vision.

Ski poles are used to give you balance and help you get up if you fall or need to side-step up a hill.

About This Chapter: This chapter includes information from "Snow Skiing Activity Card," U.S. Department of Health and Human Services, Centers for Disease Control and Prevention (CDC), 2002; and "Skiing" and "Snowboarding," President's Council on Physical Fitness and Sports, 2004.

Goggles are important to protect your eyes from flying dirt or snow, as well as stopping the sun's glare while whooshing down the slopes. Some goggles come with fun tinted lenses. If you don't have goggles, you can use sunglasses instead.

If you are renting equipment, the staff at the ski shop can help you find all the right stuff.

♣ It's A Fact!!

Competitive freestyle skiers can jump as high as a three or four-story building when performing tricks in the air.

Before it was a sport, skiing was used as a form of transportation in the mountains of Europe.

Source: CDC, 2002.

To stay warm on the slopes wear:

- Long underwear to keep you warm and absorb sweat;
- Insulated tops and pants such as sweaters and leggings—though this layer should be warm but not baggy;
- Ski pants and a jacket to protect you from snow and wetness; and
- A hat because 60 percent of heat loss is through the head.

Play It Safe

If you can, sign up for lessons from a ski school. Even if you've taken lessons before, your instructor can teach you all the right moves—for beginners as well as for more advanced students.

The key to skiing is to control your equipment and your speed. If you feel yourself start to lose control, fall onto your backside or your side and don't attempt to get up until you stop sliding.

The easiest way to get hurt while skiing is to try a run or a move that is too hard. Always ski on trails that match your skill level, and never attempt a jumping move or other trick unless taught by an instructor.

Did you know that it is just as important to drink water when you are active in the cold as in the heat? Higher altitudes and colder air can cause your body to lose water. If you experience dizziness or have dry mouth, headache, or muscle cramps take a water break. A good rule would be to drink water or sports drinks before, during, and after your ski runs.

Always check the snow conditions of the slope before you go up. You'll need to ski differently in icy conditions than you would if you were on wet snow or in deep powder.

Altitude can zap your energy, so don't push it. Ski the easier runs later in the day when you are tired. Most importantly—know when to quit.

While on the slopes, set a meeting time and place to check in with your parents or friends. Always ski with a buddy and wear plenty of sunblock because the sun's rays are strong on the mountain due to high altitude and reflection off the snow.

Tips To Get You Started

- To get on a lift, put both your poles in your inside hand. Turn to the outside and watch for the next chair. As it gets to you grab the outside pole and sit normally on the chair. Keep your skis apart, with the tips up, as you're lifted off the ground.

- To get off the lift, grab a pole in each hand, but don't put on your wrist straps. Point the pole tips toward the outside of the chair and hold them up so they don't catch on the snow. Hold the bar on the outside of the chair for balance, relax your legs, and ease yourself forward pushing off once your skis touch the snow. Don't stand up until the chair has passed over the top of the mound. When you stand up, move away from the chairlift, before you prepare to ski, so that others can get off behind you.

- To get up after a fall, make sure your skis are below you on the hill. Grab the top of both poles in one hand, grab the bottom of both poles with the other, and plant your poles in the snow just above your hip. Push up with both arms to shift yourself forward and over your skis. Make sure your weight is forward and over your skis before you stand up.

Parts Of The Body Worked

- Heart and lungs
- Upper body
- Upper and lower legs
- Knees and ankles
- Hips and butt

✔ **Quick Tip**

- Always stay in control and be able to stop or avoid other people or objects.

- People ahead of you have the right-of-way. It is your responsibility to avoid them.

- Do not stop where you obstruct a trail or are not visible from above.

- Whenever starting downhill or merging into a trail, look uphill and yield to others.

- Always use devices to help prevent runaway equipment.

- Observe all posted signs and warnings.

- Keep off closed trails and out of closed areas.

- Before using any lift, have the knowledge and ability to load, ride, and unload safely.

- Wear a t-shirt and sunscreen to make sure you don't get sunburned.

Source: CDC, 2002.

Cross-Country Skiing

Cross-country or Nordic is the oldest form of skiing. There is evidence that primitive skis were used in Norway over 5,000 years ago. As early as the tenth century, cross-country skiing was basic transportation. Vikings in northern Europe got around on skis when traversing relatively flat landscapes.

Cross-country competition was added to the Winter Olympics at Chamonix in 1924 and has been part of competition since that time. The events held at the first cross-country competition were the 15 and the 50 km. A women's cross-country event, the 10 km, was added to the program in 1952.

In competitions today, cross-country skiing is divided into two techniques—classical (diagonal stride) and freestyle—with separate events for men and women.

Classical

In the classical technique, movement is smooth and efficient—using alternate movements of the arms and legs as in walking—but with a more elongated stride. The equipment is lightweight with skinny skis and boots that look much like running shoes. In competitions, the skis remain parallel on flat ground. When going up hills, the skis are pointed outward in the shape of a "V." The bottoms of the skis are waxed for better traction.

Freestyle

In freestyle competitions, the skier can choose any style. The most common technique is skating. It is faster, more dynamic, and more physically demanding than the classical technique. Skating also requires more strength. The skis for skating are shorter and the poles longer than those used in classical competitions. Skating requires a compact surface in order to glide.

Olympic Cross-Country Competitions

During the Olympics, skiers race for a specific distance, attempting to cover that distance in the shortest possible time. Each race is measured in kilometers (about two-thirds of a mile).

In some of the longer races, skiers start at intervals (i.e., every 30 seconds), although some races call for a mass start. During the race, coaches stand along the course timing their racers and yelling out their place and time.

In relay races (four skiers with the first two using classical technique), the first group of skiers begin racing at the same time. In some of the events, skiers use a pursuit start where skiers leave the starting line one at a time. The starting order is determined by the order of finish in the previous day's race. The winner of the first race starts first, and the other racers can begin "chasing" the leader—after waiting for the same amount of time they trailed the leader at the end of the first race. The first skier across the finish line is the winner.

Wearing The Right Clothing

Wearing the right clothing is extremely important when participating in cold weather sports. Dress in layers by wearing warm, waterproof, or water-resistant clothing. Clothing for cross-country skiing should protect

✎ What's It Mean?
Cross-Country Skiing Glossary

<u>Classical Technique:</u> The traditional ski racing technique. Athletes use a diagonal stride in which both skis stay parallel to each other and do not deviate from prepared parallel tracks. The power of the stride propels the skier.

<u>Freestyle Technique:</u> The skating—or freestyle—technique, which was developed in the 1970s, closely resembles the motions of ice skating. Athletes do not keep their skis within narrow tracks but instead push off with both legs to surge forward and propel their bodies. It usually is faster than classical technique.

<u>Glide Wax:</u> Wax used to decrease the friction between the skis and the snow. It is applied to the entire ski in freestyle races, but only to the front and rear tips of the skis in classical races.

<u>Grip Wax Or Kick Wax:</u> Increases the friction between the skis and snow to improve traction. It is applied to the middle part of the skis for classical races.

<u>Harries:</u> A ski preparation technique in classical skiing used when kick wax is not appropriate for the conditions. Technicians use a wire brush to roughen the base of the skis.

<u>Mass start:</u> All competitors start together and the first skier to pass the finish line is declared the winner.

<u>Pursuit Start:</u> A starting system based on the result of the first portion of the pursuit event. The winner of the first part starts first and the competitors start behind by the amount of time they finished behind the winner in the first portion.

<u>Scramble Leg:</u> The first leg of a relay race. Named this way because relay races feature mass starts with everyone bunched together.

<u>Staggered Start:</u> A start in which skiers leave at set intervals. The winner is the athlete with the best time.

<u>Vertical:</u> An uphill climb.

Source: "Skiing," President's Council on Physical Fitness and Sports, 2004.

the participant from cold, wind, and precipitation; and should also provide ventilation. To reduce wind resistance, clothing should fit snugly to the body. Pay special attention to protecting feet, hands, face, and head. Up to 40 percent of body heat can be lost when the head is exposed. Footgear should be insulated to protect against cold and dampness.

Wearing multiple layers of varying thickness allows you to regulate your body temperature. You should flexibly layer the clothing and use proper materials so you will stay warm and still not restrict your movement. Many skiers peel off layers when cross-country skiing and replace those layers when stopping for rest or rehydration.

Wear at least three layers of clothing including a water-resistant outer layer to break the wind and allow some ventilation (nylon or other water-resistant synthetic fabric), a middle layer of wool or wool-like synthetic fabric to absorb sweat and retain insulation, and an inner layer close to the skin.

It's important to keep moisture away from your skin. Avoid cotton, which clings to perspiration. Synthetic materials such as Supplex and Coolmax are ideal because they keep you warm and dry.

Equipment

- Cross-country skis suitable for the site—track, off-track, or back country—and suitable for the technique. Lightweight or skinny skis are used for classical and shorter skis for skating. Back country (or wilderness) cross-country trips require wider skis.

- Cross-country boots that allow your heels to come off the skis or sturdier boots for back country skiing.

- Poles for balance—poles for skating are longer than poles for the classical technique.

Cross-Country Skiing Basics

Cross-country skiing is often hailed as the number one aerobic activity because the sport involves all the upper and lower body muscles in vigorous activity. The driving action of the legs strengthens those muscles while the motion of using ski poles to pull you forward uses your upper body. The gliding motion of cross-country skiing makes it a low injury, low-impact sport and easy on the joints. The sport combines family fun with fitness.

Visiting a cross-country ski resort or center is a good way to get started in this enjoyable winter sport. These facilities usually provide machine-set tracks (a consistent surface that literally guides your skis forward), which eliminates most of the balance problems plaguing beginners.

Once you can shuffle your feet while standing on the skis, you are nearly ready to begin your cross-country adventure. It's a good idea to start by taking lessons from a professional instructor. You can learn cross-country skiing in less than an hour.

The classic technique is like running up a hill and the skating technique is similar to ice skating. With both techniques, you grab the snow with your ski poles (alternating your arms in a pumping motion), kick the ski ahead of you, and then you glide. The classic technique is most easily learned in tracks, but the movement for this technique—the diagonal stride—is used by off-track skiers as well.

When skating or skate skiing, the action is to alternate your legs (pushing sideways against the snow), then gliding. Both classical and skating styles can be used on uphills, flats, and gentle downhills. Ascents can be made using the "herringbone" or the "sidestep." Backcountry cross-country skiing is more rugged and rustic than track and off-track and requires wider skis and sturdier boots.

Snowshoeing

Millions of Americans are hooked on snowshoeing, which is similar to cross-country skiing except you walk or run on snowshoes instead of gliding on cross-country skis. If you can walk, you can snowshoe. The lightweight, aluminum frames of snowshoes make it possible for you to walk and run on the snow, allowing you to enjoy hiking and hunting in a winter environment. Wide snowshoes are worn for walking and narrow ones are worn for running.

Where To Cross-Country Ski And Snowshoe

Cross-country skiing and snowshoe opportunities are as varied as the landscapes where snow falls—farmland, meadows, city parks, gentle country slopes and hills, even golf courses (if permitted). Opportunities to enjoy these activities are available at resorts, parks, and ski areas.

In the United States, ski areas and ski resorts are plentiful in the north-eastern, mid-atlantic, and western states. Canada and Europe also have many ski resorts. Some states have parks and recreation areas where cross-country skiing and snowshoeing are available. You can call your travel agent or search the internet (under "cross-country skiing") for packages and special travel fares. There is an abundance of cross-country skiing information on the web.

You'll want to check snow conditions at your chosen location. Many resorts keep their tracks and cross-country ski areas in good shape with snow machines.

Parts Of The Body Worked

- Legs
- Arms
- Abs
- Chest
- Back

☞ **Remember!!**

If you plan to go into the backwoods or wilderness to cross-country ski or snowshoe, remember to observe these safety precautions:

- Become familiar with orienteering—the use of a compass and map to find out where you are and to get where you want to go;

- Carry a day pack including a complete change of clothing and enough food and water to sustain you in an emergency;

- Be aware of avalanche dangers in your area; and

- Always take at least one buddy—never go into the backwoods alone.

Source: "Skiing," President's Council on Physical Fitness and Sports, 2004.

Common Injuries

- Sprains

- Hamstring and quadriceps strains

- Cramps

- Lower back pain (from hunching forward improperly)

- Frostbite

- Hypothermia

- Altitude sickness

Activities To Help Get/Stay In Shape

Off-Season

- Walking with poles

- Hiking (especially on hilly trails)

- Running

- Swimming

- Circuit/weight training

In Season

- Warm up

- Endurance exercises with weight training on off days

- Cool down

Snowboarding

Snowboarding is an American original. As one story goes, Sherman Poppen invented the snowboard for his daughter in 1965 when he braced a pair of skis together and tied a rope to the front to help steer. The "snurfer," as it was called when it debuted a year later, is said by some to be the world's first production snowboard. Others credit snowboarding's origins to creative efforts by surfers and skateboarders to adapt their activities, techniques, and equipment to winter recreation over the last few decades. No matter how snowboarding got started, there's no doubt that it's a native-born American sport—one that has taken the world by storm.

Olympic Snowboarding Competitions

Snowboarding competition began in the 1980s. The United States held its first national championships in 1982 and hosted the first World Championships in 1983. In 1987, a four-stop World Cup tour was established with two stops in the United States and two in Europe. In 1994, snowboarding became an officially sanctioned discipline and eligible for the Olympics.

Snowboarding made its Olympic debut in 1998 at Nagano where its two events—the giant slalom and the halfpipe—were introduced to the world.

Halfpipe: The halfpipe competition takes place in a half-cylinder-shaped course dug deep into the hill. The pipe is generally three to four meters deep and 110 meters long with an 85-degree pitch and high vertical walls on each side. Using speed gained on the slope, snowboarders come up over the rim of the pipe and perform acrobatic aerial tricks. The object of the halfpipe is to perform difficult tricks with perfect form.

The halfpipe is judged on rotations, amplitude, and overall impression. All athletes compete in the first run. The top six men and the top six women from the first run advance directly to the finals. The athletes who did not qualify in the first run do a second qualifying run. The top six men and top six women from this run advance to the finals.

Parallel Giant Slalom: An exciting version of alpine snowboarding, the parallel giant slalom, features head-to-head match ups on the mountain. After the qualification round, a 16-person tournament is established and competitors battle it out on two side-by-side courses until there is a winner. The parallel giant slalom is a series of one-on-one battles.

There are two parts of each competition—the qualifying run and the head-to-head portion. The first portion of the competition is a qualifying run. Every competitor takes one run down the course. The men race one side of the parallel course and the women race the other. The athletes are ranked in order of their times. The top 16 athletes from the qualifying round advance to the head-to-head portion of the competition.

Following the qualifying runs, the course is reset. For the head-to-head part, the athletes are seeded based on the qualifying times.

Wearing The Right Clothing

Wearing the right clothing is extremely important when participating in cold weather sports. Dress in layers—wearing warm, waterproof, or water resistant clothing. Clothing for snowboarding should protect the participant from cold, wind, and precipitation and should also provide ventilation. To reduce wind resistance, the clothing should fit snugly to the body. Pay special attention to protecting feet, hands, face, and head. Up to 40 percent of body heat can be lost when the head is exposed. Footgear should be insulated to protect against cold and dampness.

Wearing multiple layers of varying thickness allows you to regulate your body temperature. You should flexibly layer the clothing and use proper materials so you will stay warm and still not restrict your movement. Many snowboarders peel off layers while snowboarding and then replace those layers when stopping for rest and rehydration.

Wear at least three layers of clothing including a water-resistant outer layer to break the wind and allow some ventilation (nylon or other water-resistant synthetic fabric), a middle layer of wool or wool-like synthetic fabric to absorb sweat and retain insulation; and an inner layer close to the skin.

It's important to keep moisture away from your skin, so avoid cotton. It clings to perspiration. Synthetic materials such as Supplex and Coolmax are ideal because they keep you warm and dry.

Equipment

- **Helmet:** A hard plastic helmet is essential to prevent head injuries. Helmets manufactured for ski sports are required for snowboarding competition.

- **Board:** For the halfpipe, a wide flexible board should be used. For the parallel giant slalom, a stiff, narrower board should be used to allow for turns and high speed.

- **Boots:** For the halfpipe, most participants use soft boots with foot and ankle support and lace-up inner boots. For the parallel giant slalom, you'll need alpine boots with a hard plastic exterior for extensive foot and ankle support, similar to alpine ski boots.

Snowboarding Basics

When you're ready to head for the snow, the best way to get started is to sign up for snowboarding lessons at a ski resort. Classes exist for all ages and styles, from the free rider, who just wants to whoosh down the hill, to the freestyle artist, who wants to perform the dangerous jumps to thrill the audience below. Keep your expectations realistic the first day or two. Pace yourself and commit to keep trying to learn snowboarding for at least three days. By then you'll start to gain confidence and feel more control. Once you are comfortable with momentum and controlling speed, it becomes easier to balance.

Before going out on the snow, you might consider "dry land training"— practicing with the snowboard on a carpet indoors to help you become oriented and introduce you to the proper primary body alignment. The goal is an efficient foundation or stance. You should be balanced and relaxed, maintaining an athletic stance over the edge you are riding on—the heel edge (back) or the toe edge (front). You should, also, minimize tension or twisting up at the waist and your upper body should align with the angle of your feet.

Remember that you're not skiing, so you'll need to keep the upper body in somewhat of an alignment with the lower body. Your shoulders should be parallel with the board to assure that you are weighting and balancing on both feet evenly (50-50) and staying on the "sweet spot" (center) of the board.

When you are ready to take your first run down the hill, you will have to decide how you want to stand on the board. Most people stand or "board" with their left foot forward much like sliding into home plate. Others prefer to lead with their right foot. Your choice may depend on whether you are left or right-handed. Some boarders can do it either way. You'll quickly discover which side is more comfortable for you.

Next, strap your front leading foot onto the board. Your toes will inch over the edge of the board a bit with your heel against the toes of the other foot. As you balance precariously for a second or two, strap your other foot in, and start slowly down the mountainside (or bunny hill). Make sure you're facing forward with your hands in front; keeping your weight low and your knees bent. Try to maintain an even keel without catching the front or back end of your board in the snow.

✎ What's It Mean?

180 Air: An aerial maneuver in which the snowboard rotates 180 degrees— a half of a spin.

360 Air: An aerial maneuver in which the snowboard rotates 360 degrees— one full spin.

Air To Fakie: Any trick in the halfpipe in which a rider approaches the wall riding forward, no rotation is made, and the rider lands riding backwards.

Backside: The side of the snowboard on which the athlete's heels rest or the side of the snowboard to which the athlete's back faces.

Corkscrew: Sideways rotation.

Detune: To slightly dull the edges of the snowboard.

Duckfoot: A snowboard stance in which the toes point outward.

Fakie: Riding backwards.

Freeriding: Snowboarding for fun, not in a competition.

Freestyle Snowboarding: The type of snowboarding that includes tricks. Halfpipe is a type of freestyle snowboarding.

Goofy-Footed: Riding a snowboard with the right foot forward.

Invert: A trick in which the head is beneath the level of the board and the snowboarder balances on one or two hands.

Regular-Footed: Riding on a snowboard with the left foot forward.

Revert: To switch from riding fakie (backwards) to forward, or from forward to fakie.

Rolling Down The Windows: A phrase used to describe when someone is caught off-balance and they rotate their arms wildly in the air to try to recover.

Soft Boots: Boots designed for use in freestyle and freeride snowboarding. They are made soft and pliable to allow a large range of motion.

Switchstance: Performing a trick while riding backwards when the maneuver is performed exactly like it would be if you were riding forward.

Traverse: To ride perpendicular to the fall line or to ride across the halfpipe.

Source: "Snowboarding," President's Council on Physical Fitness and Sports, 2004.

Turning And Stopping

- Turns: Turns are made by leaning forward or backward and from side to side, using the toe edge (front) and the heel edge (back) of the board for steering and speed control. Similar to inline skating, the back of your board will slow you down if you press it into the snow. Many new riders find it disconcerting to travel facing the trees or the side of the slope while going down the mountain, but after a few gentle turns and twists you'll be thrilled as you gingerly pick up speed and enjoy the powder under your feet.

- Stopping: Stopping a snowboard is much like coming to a stop on ice skates—bring both feet perpendicular to the slope, then scrape to a stop. Be prepared to fall down more than a few times while learning this skill. Just as in ice skating, you have to learn how to balance your weight to scrape the snow/ice just enough to stop but not so much that you upset your position and fall.

These maneuvers will take time and practice to learn, but they are necessary skills to acquire and are fun once you master them. Finally, unbuckle your back foot from the board and push off with your foot, sliding easily to the lift for your next ride up to the top to continue snowboarding.

Where To Go Snowboarding

Snowboarding is usually done on the snowy slopes and hills of ski resorts. Opportunities to enjoy snowboarding are available at many winter resorts and ski areas.

In the United States, winter resorts are plentiful in the northeastern, mid-atlantic, and western states. Canada and Europe also have many resorts featuring winter sports. Some states have snowboarding available at park and recreation areas. You can call your travel agent or search the internet (search under "snowboarding") for packages and special travel fares. There is an abundance of information on the internet.

Of course you'll want to check snow conditions at your chosen location. Some resorts keep their slopes snow-covered with snow machines.

In addition to the cost of staying at a resort, the main expense for snowboarding is buying or renting equipment and clothing (board, helmet, boots, clothing) and purchase of lift tickets.

Parts Of The Body Worked

- Legs
- Trunk

Common Injuries

- Broken bones and other injuries from falls and collisions
- Sprains
- Hamstring and quadriceps strains
- Cramps
- Frostbite
- Hypothermia
- Altitude sickness

Activities To Help Get/Stay In Shape

Off-Season

- Walking
- Hiking
- Running
- Swimming
- Circuit/weight training

In Season

- Warm up
- Endurance exercises with strength training on off days
- Cool down

Chapter 23

Strength Training

Strength training is a vital part of a balanced exercise routine that includes aerobic activity and flexibility exercises.

Regular aerobic exercise, such as running or using a stationary bike, makes your muscles use oxygen more efficiently and strengthens your heart and lungs. When you strength train with weights, you're using your muscles to work against the extra pounds (this concept is called resistance). This strengthens and increases the amount of muscle mass in your body by making your muscles work harder than they're used to.

Most people who work out with weights typically use two different kinds: free weights (including barbells, dumbbells, and hand weights) and weight machines. Free weights usually work a group of muscles at the same time; weight machines typically are designed to help you isolate and work on a specific muscle.

For instance, you can do a squat using free weights by placing a barbell across the back of your shoulders and squatting down like a baseball catcher. (Keep your feet flat on the ground and your chest up.) This type of exercise works and tones multiple muscles, including the quadriceps (the front of the thigh), the hamstring (the back of the thigh), and even your butt. When you do a leg extension on a muscle isolation machine, you sit in a chair with your knee bent at 90 degrees and slowly straighten your leg against the padded bar. This particular exercise isolates and works the quadriceps muscle.

Most gyms or weight rooms set up their machines in a circuit, or group, of exercises that you perform to strengthen different groups of muscles.

People can also use resistance bands and even their own body weight (as in pushups) for strength training.

Many people tend to lump all types of weightlifting together, but there's a big difference between strength training, powerlifting, and competitive bodybuilding.

Strength training uses resistance methods like free weights, weight machines, resistance bands, or a person's own weight to build muscles and strength. Olympic lifting, or powerlifting, which people often think of when they think of weightlifting, concentrates on how much weight a person can lift at one time. Competitive bodybuilding involves evaluating muscle definition and symmetry, as well as size.

Powerlifting, competitive weightlifting, and bodybuilding are not recommended for people in their early teens who are still maturing. That's because these types of activity can cause serious injuries to growing bones, muscles, and joints.

Getting Started

If you've started puberty, your body will have begun making the hormones necessary to help build muscle in response to weight training. If you haven't started puberty, though, you'll still be able to get stronger—you just won't see your muscles getting bigger.

Before you start strength training, you should be checked out by your doctor to make sure it's safe for you to lift weights.

Any time you start a new sport or activity, start out slowly so that your body gets used to the increase in activity. Even if you think you're not exerting yourself

> ### ♣ It's A Fact!!
> ### Benefits Of Strength Training
>
> - Increases endurance and strength for sports and fitness activities
> - Improves focus and concentration, which may result in better grades
> - Reduces body fat and increases muscle mass
> - Helps burn more calories—even when not exercising
> - May reduce the risk of short-term injuries by protecting tendons, bones, and joints
> - Helps prevent long-term medical problems such as high cholesterol or osteoporosis (weakening of the bones) when you get older

very much, if you've never pumped iron before, your muscles may be sore when you wake up the next day. And, because of something called delayed onset muscle soreness, the pain may be at its worst two or three days after you first exercise.

Before you begin any type of strength training routine, get some guidance and expert advice. Your coach or trainer can give you advice on how many times a week you should lift and what kinds of warm-up and cool-down activities you should do before and after lifting to avoid soreness or injury. Many trainers who work at schools, gyms, and in weight rooms are knowledgeable about strength training, but it's best to get advice from someone who is a certified fitness expert and experienced working with teens.

When lifting weights—either free weights or on a machine—make sure that there's always someone nearby to supervise, or spot, you. This person, called a spotter, encourages you and also can act as your coach, telling you if you're not doing a particular exercise correctly. Having a spotter nearby is particularly important when using free weights. Even someone in great shape sometimes just can't make that last rep. It's no big deal if you're doing bicep curls; all you'll have to do is drop the weight onto the floor. But if you're in the middle of a bench press—a chest exercise where you're lying on a bench and pushing a loaded barbell away from your chest—it's easy to become trapped under a heavy weight. A spotter can keep you from dropping the barbell onto your chest.

Many schools offer weight or circuit training as units in their gym classes. Check to see if you can sign up. Don't be afraid to ask for pointers and tips about how much weight to start with, how to develop a routine, and nutrition advice.

What Are Some Dangers Of Strength Training?

You may love the challenge of lifting, especially if you and your friends do it together. You'll definitely see results over a few months in your ability to progressively lift more weight. But there are a few things to look out for.

Because your bones, joints, and tendons are still growing and developing, it's easy to overdo it and strain or even permanently damage them. When you're in the middle of a strength-training session and something doesn't feel right to you, you feel pain, or if you hear or feel a "pop" when you're in the middle of a workout, stop what you're doing and have a doctor check it out before you resume training. It's possible you may need to modify your training or even stop lifting weights for a while to allow the injury to heal.

Another danger surrounding strength training is the use of anabolic steroids or other performance-enhancing drugs and preparations that supposedly help muscles develop. Steroid use is widespread in many sports—including swimming, track and field, and baseball. But because many of their long-term effects on the body are still unknown (and because they are linked to health problems like cancer, heart disease, and sterility), resist the urge to try them. The benefit is definitely not worth the risk.

What Is A Healthy Routine?

If you take a few minutes to watch the guys and girls pump iron at your school, you'll see there are lots of different ways to train with weights. Try a few good basic routines that you can modify as you start to train harder later on.

If you're just starting out in the weight room, most fitness experts recommend you begin by training three sessions a week, ranging from 20 minutes to one hour (including warm-up and cool-down periods), allowing at least a day off between sessions. It's best to work only two or three muscle groups during each session. For example, you can work your leg muscles one day, your chest, shoulders, and triceps at the next session, and your back and biceps on the last.

Before you head for the weight bench, warm up your muscles by spending 5–10 minutes pedaling on a stationary bicycle or by taking a brisk walk around the gym. After finishing your workout, cool down by stretching all the major muscle groups to avoid injuries and keep your muscles flexible.

You can use many different exercises for each body part, but the basics— like bench presses, lat pull-downs, and squats—are great to start with. Learn proper technique first, without any added weight. Perform three sets of 8–10 repetitions (or reps) of each exercise, starting out with a light weight to warm up and increasing the weight slightly with the second and third sets. (Add more weight only after you can successfully perform 8–15 repetitions in good form.) Perform two to three different exercises for each body part to make sure you work each muscle in the group effectively.

Here are eight basic rules to follow in strength training:

1. Start with body weight exercises for a few weeks (such as sit-ups, pushups, and pull-ups) before using weights.

> ☞ **Remember!!**
> After finishing your workout, cool down by stretching all of the major muscle groups to avoid injuries and to enhance and maintain flexibility.

2. Work out with weights about three times a week. Avoid weight training on back-to-back days.

3. Warm up for 5–10 minutes before each session.

4. Stretch the muscles you plan to strengthen before each weight training session.

5. Spend no more than 40 minutes in the weight room to avoid fatigue or boredom.

6. Work more reps; avoid maximum lifts. (A coach or teacher can give you specifics based upon your needs.)

7. Ensure you're using proper technique through supervision. Improper technique may result in injuries, particularly in the shoulder and back.

8. Cool down for 5–10 minutes after each session, stretching the muscles you worked out.

Don't rely on strength training as your only form of exercise. You still need to get your heart and lungs working harder by doing some kind of additional aerobic exercise for a minimum of 20–30 minutes per session. Doctors recommend an hour a day of moderate to vigorous activity—so on days when you're not lifting weights, you may want to get more aerobic activity.

Strength training is a great way to improve strength, endurance, and muscle tone. But remember to start slowly, use proper form, avoid heavy weights, and increase workouts gradually to prevent injury. Just a few short sessions a week will really pay off—besides better muscle tone and definition, you may find that you have more energy and focus in both sports and school.

Chapter 24

Racquetball, Tennis, And Volleyball

Play Racquetball: How To Play The Game

The Game

Racquetball is a fun, fast paced action sport that can be played either on an indoor or outdoor court with anywhere from two to four players at a time. Indoor racquetball is played on a 20' x 20' x 40' court that has four walls, a ceiling, and a floor, all of which are used during play. Racquetball is also fun to practice by oneself, on a court. Outdoor racquetball is played using the same floor dimensions as an indoor court. However, there is typically no ceiling or backwall and the court may or may not include sidewalls. The sidewalls can also vary in length. Most outdoor play is referred to as "one wall" or "three wall" racquetball. The outdoor game is popular in warmer weather climates and in cities where parks and school playgrounds are present.

The sport became popular during the late 1970s and early 1980s because it was fun, easy to learn how to play, and it is one of the best workouts you

About This Chapter: This chapter begins with "Play Racquetball: How To Play The Game," by Dave George, Racquetball Manufacturers Council, © 2003. Reprinted with permission. Information under the heading "Tennis" is from "Tennis Activity Card," 2001, and information under the heading "Volleyball" is from "Volleyball Activity Card," 2002, both produced by the Department of Health and Human Services, Centers for Disease Control and Prevention (CDC).

can get in a short period of time. Today racquetball remains very strong as a sport played by over five million people each year.

The Basic Rules Of The Game: Racquetball can be played three ways. Versions include "singles play" between two players, "doubles play" between two teams of two players each, and "cut throat" which involves three players. Tournament and league play usually involves singles and/or doubles play.

The Serve: Play begins with the server standing in the "service zone" and serving to his/her opponent(s). To serve, the server must first bounce the ball and then strike it with the racquet. The ball is put into play after making contact with the front wall first and then passing into the rear half of the court before touching the floor. After the served ball hits off the front wall, it may strike one of the side walls—but it must bounce behind the short line (the line forming the back of the service box, located 20 feet from the front wall) before hitting a third wall on the fly.

The Return Of Serve: To return serve, stand in the middle of the court (equal distance between each side wall), approximately one arm and racquet's length away from the back wall. Return serve by striking the ball before the second bounce. The ball must travel to the front wall for it to be a good return. The ball may hit any surface except the floor on the return as long as it hits the front wall before the floor.

The Rally: Once the ball is in play, each player (or in doubles, each team) alternates hitting the ball. During the rally, the walls and ceiling call be used for many shot variations. The rally ends when either a ball bounces twice on the floor before being returned or on a "skip ball" when the ball makes contact with the floor before reaching the front wall after a shot. Points are scored when, after serving the ball, the server wins the rally. If the player returning serve wins the rally, the result is a "sideout" and no points are scored for either player and the player who won the rally gets to serve. Whoever wins the rally serves next. Matches are typically two games to 15 points and a tiebreaker to 11 points, if needed.

Hinders: Hinders are stoppages of play and results in the replay of the point. If there is ever a question of someone being too close or in the way, hold up from swinging and play a hinder. It is your responsibility to give your opponent enough room to hit their shot. Technically, you must give them a straight shot to the front wall as well as the angle, which would result in a crosscourt shot to the opposite back corner.

Getting Started

Safety: Racquetball is both a recreational and competitive game. It is always important to be safe. Here are some things to remember to do before and during play:

> 👉 **Remember!!**
> **Basics To Remember**
>
> Only the server scores points.
>
> The ball can only bounce once.
>
> The ball must return to the front wall after being hit.
>
> Hold up for safety reasons.
>
> Source: Racquetball Manufacturers Council, © 2003.

- Warm up before you play.

- Wear safety glasses when on the court.

- Always knock before entering a court. Players could still be playing.

- Always play using the wrist strap attached to the butt end of the racquet handle, looped around your wrist as a safety precaution.

- Watch where the ball is during play to avoid being in the way.

- Know the rules and be aware of hinders. Always stop and do not swing if a player is too close or in your way.

- Drink plenty of water to avoid dehydration.

- Wear proper athletic shoes that are appropriate for lateral movements on the court.

Equipment: The ball used to play the game is air filled, about three inches in diameter, and bounces in a lively fashion. The racquet used is a fixed frame with strings and has a grip at the end for players to hold securely during play, including a wrist tether (strap). Safety glasses are worn to help prevent eye injury. Athletic shoes, socks, and typically shorts and shirts are generally worn during play. Racquetball gloves, wristbands, and headbands are optional.

Tennis

Gear Up

What's all the racket about racquets? Well, you can't play tennis without one. If you're buying a junior racquet, choose the longest one that you can comfortably use. If you weigh more than 85 pounds you should look for an adult racquet.

When you have a racquet, you'll need to find a court. Look around at school or at parks in your neighborhood. Then, put on socks (if they're not cotton, they'll help you avoid blisters) and sneakers with good ankle support. And last, don't forget the tennis balls.

Play It Safe

Tennis is an activity that forces you to turn your body quickly in many different directions, so make sure you warm up and stretch before playing. Wear tennis shoes with good support to protect your ankles and thick (not cotton) socks that fit well to prevent blisters on your feet. To prevent hand blisters, keep your racquet handle dry by using sawdust or hand chalk. Always

♣ It's A Fact!!

Advanced players can serve a ball at more than 100 miles per hour, making it travel 80 feet across the court in less than one second.

The world's first tennis tournament took place in Wimbledon, England in 1877.

You might have heard tennis players saying the word "love" a lot around the courts. Unless it's Valentine's Day, they're probably talking about the score. In tennis, "love" means that your opponent has not scored any points yet and has a score of zero.

In tennis, one point equals 15; two points equals 30; three points equals 40; and usually, four points equals a win.

Source: CDC, 2001.

bend your arm when you swing or else it might start to hurt causing a problem known as "tennis elbow." Clip your toenails and make sure there is extra room in your shoes because "tennis toe" can be nasty too.

To protect other players, never throw your racquet or tennis balls. Try to keep loose balls off the courts too. Be courteous and keep yourself and others safe by staying off courts where other people are playing.

When you're outside waiting to play, sit in the shade and drink lots of water so you'll stay cool and won't get sunburned. While you are playing, take a break between games or sets to cool off. And you may want to keep a wet towel around your neck while you wait. Also, you can look and feel cool by wearing a cold, wet bandana on your head while you play. And always wear sunscreen.

How To Play

Tennis is a fun activity that two people (a "singles" match) or four people on two separate teams ("doubles") can play. You can play with friends at your local tennis courts or join an organized team. When you start playing tennis, some of the key strokes you should learn are: serve, forehand, backhand, two-handed backhand, volley, and smash. But first, check out these basic skills to get you started.

- **Holding The Racquet:** The racquet handle has eight side—four are flat and four are angled. Take the racquet handle between your thumb and index finger of your dominant hand (the one you write with) as if you were shaking hands. The knuckle on your index finger should be on the top right angle. Then, grip and make sure it feels comfortable. Separate your third and fourth fingers slightly.

- **Serving:** Hold the ball with the thumb, index finger, and middle finger of your free hand (hand not holding the racquet). Extend the arm with the ball just in front of you and then raise it above your head. Toss the ball gently, so it goes a few inches higher than the full height of the racquet extended above your head. Keep your eye on the ball. Bring the racquet around above your shoulder and hit the ball while it's in the air. Try to use the same toss every time.

- **Receiving And Returning The Ball:** Stand in the middle of the court and hold the racquet gently with both hands so you can run in either direction when the ball comes over the net. When the ball is hit to your forehand side (for example, right if you're right-handed), step toward the ball with your opposite leg and swing. If the ball comes to your backhand side (left if you're right-handed), go for the ball with your dominant arm in front of your chest and your other hand holding the racquet as well. Swing without moving your wrists.

Parts Of The Body Worked

- Heart and lungs
- Upper and lower legs
- Arms
- Abs

Volleyball

Gear Up

- **A Ball:** Volleyballs are about 26 inches around and weigh a bit more than half a pound.

- **A Net:** The net is stretched across the middle of the court and adjusts to different heights—7½ feet for girls and 8 feet for guys.

- **Elbow And Knee Pads:** When you're playing volleyball, you're probably going to hit the ground a few times. Protect yourself with pads.

- **Volleyball Shoes:** The bottoms of volleyball shoes are made of special rubber to keep you from slipping as you move around the court. Your shoes should also give you good ankle support and have lots of cushioning to protect your feet while you're jumping.

Play It Safe

Be sure to wear knee and elbow pads when you're playing on a hard court to protect you when you dive for the ball. When you go up for the ball, try landing on the balls of your feet with your knees bent and your hips lowered a little. Also, warm up and stretch before you play, and take off any jewelry.

Games   ✔ Quick Tip

- **Fish in the Pond:** Try tossing the ball onto your racquet or into a hula-hoop on the ground to practice aiming your toss.

- **Overhead Ball Catch:** Toss the ball up like you are about to serve and catch it just above your head.

- **Two-Handed Alligator Catch:** Stretch out your arms straight in front of you like they are the top and bottom of an alligator's mouth. Have a friend throw the ball toward you and slap your hands together to catch it. After each catch, make the alligator's mouth a little bigger.

Source: CDC, 2001.

Communicate with your teammates while you're playing to keep from running into each other. Make sure everyone on the team knows to "call" the ball by saying, "got it" or "mine" if they plan to go for it.

If you're playing outside, find a soft court made of sand or grass and clean up any sharp objects that you see. Be sure that there aren't any trees or basketball hoops in your way. Wear sunscreen and always drink plenty of water. If you're playing inside, the court should be made of wood.

If your volleyball net is held up by wires, make sure they are covered with soft materials. That way you won't get hurt if you accidentally jump or run into the net.

How To Play

Volleyball is fun to play because everybody gets involved. The game is unique because the same player isn't allowed to hit the ball twice in a row, so everyone takes turns serving, passing, and setting the ball. A team can hit the ball up to three times before they get it over then net. Before you play, check out these moves.

- **Serving The Ball:** Stand at the back of the court and face the net. Hold the ball in the palm of your non-dominant hand (for example, left if you're right-handed) and stretch out your arm at waist level.

Lean forward and swing your dominant hand (the one you write with) up toward the bottom of the ball. Now, drop the ball and hit it with your fist or the bottom of your hitting hand. Follow through, pointing your hitting arm toward your target. Finally, get ready to score. Only the team that's serving can score points. After you have practiced this underhand for a while, you can try a powerful overhead serve.

- **Passing The Ball:** Move to the place where you think the ball will land and stand with your feet shoulder-width apart. Bend your knees and put your arms straight out in front of you. Lock your hands together with your thumbs pointed forward. Watch the ball make contact with your arms and then push it forward with your forearms. Aim with your shoulders and straighten your legs, using the force from your legs to move the ball where you want it to go.

- **Setting The Ball:** Stand with your feet shoulder-width apart, facing your target. Bend your knees and raise your hands above your head with your elbows bent. Put your hands together about six inches above and in front of your forehead, and make a diamond shape with your thumbs and pointer fingers. When the ball comes to you, use only your thumbs and the tops of your fingers to push the ball up in the direction you want it to go. Your palms should not touch the ball.

Parts Of The Body Worked

- Arms
- Upper and lower legs
- Shoulders and neck
- Knees and ankles
- Hips and butt
- Back

Chapter 25

Running, Walking, Jumping, Hiking, And Climbing

Ready To Run

You see them pounding the pavement at lunch or after work, sweating away the cares of the world. They make it look so easy, as if nothing could be more natural than running for miles or minutes on end.

But the last time you tried it, all you received were blisters and shin splints for your troubles.

Sound familiar? Running (or jogging, which some see as simply a slower form of running) is one of the most effective, time-efficient workouts around, but if you, well, get off on the wrong foot, it's hard to stay motivated and easy to get discouraged.

But starting—and sticking with—a running program doesn't have to be difficult. It's simply a matter of doing the right things at the right time.

About This Chapter: This chapter begins with information from "Ready To Run?" © 2001, and "Can You Offer Some Basic Guidelines For Avoiding Overuse Injuries Associated With Running?" by Dr. Cedric X. Bryant, © 2007, both reprinted with permission from the American Council on Exercise (www.acefitness.org). All rights reserved. Information from the following documents produced by the Centers for Disease Control and Prevention (CDC) is also included: "Walking Activity Card," 2003; "Hiking Activity Card," 2002; "Jump Rope Activity Card," 2002. Additional information from Sunset Publishing Company is cited separately within the chapter.

Step By Step

First things first: check with your doctor to be sure that running is the right activity for you. Individuals who should probably bypass running in favor of walking include those with orthopedic or heart problems or those who are more than 20 percent overweight.

Nothing can derail a running program faster than sore feet. Though they often carry a hefty price tag, good-fitting running shoes can help prevent shin splints, blisters, and sore muscles. Aside from comfortable clothing, little else is required.

Once you're suited up, simply head out your front door or take a drive to a nearby park. Asphalt or dirt surfaces are preferable to concrete; be sure that where you run is safe and well lit.

✔ Quick Tip

Jog Your Memory

As a child, you probably didn't think about how you ran. You just did it. Your muscles took over while your brain concentrated on more important things, like hopscotch or baseball cards.

But as you've grown older, your muscles may have forgotten how to run effortlessly. To help jog both your and your muscles' memories, here are a few tips:

- Keep your head level, avoid bouncing, and lean forward slightly from the ankles, not the waist.
- Keep your shoulders down and relaxed.
- Strike the ground first with your heel, then roll to the ball of the foot, pushing off from the toes.

Source: American Council on Exercise (www.acefitness.org), © 2001.

F.I.T. Tip

Frequency, Intensity, and Time (FIT) are the elements you need to put together an effective beginning running program. The accompanying table offers a program for those who are less fit, but may be adapted for those who have been exercising aerobically for some time.

The best way to halt a running program in its tracks is to do too much too soon. A minimum of 20 to 30 minutes, three days per week (with days off in between) at an intensity of 50 percent to 85 percent of maximum heart rate is the standard recommendation, but may be manipulated to suit individual speed or endurance goals.

Here are a few more things to keep in mind:

• Take time to warm up before and cool down after a run.

• Never increase mileage more than 10 percent per week.

• If anything hurts, take time off until it feels better.

• Follow a strength-training program on alternate days to help reduce upper-body fatigue.

Like any activity, running isn't for everybody. If you don't enjoy it, don't do it. But if you do, take your time, progress slowly, and allow your muscles to adapt to the rigors of running.

Can You Offer Some Basic Guidelines For Avoiding Overuse Injuries Associated With Running?

Generally speaking, the vast majority of overuse injuries associated with running can be avoided by utilizing common sense and not exposing your body to sudden, high levels of orthopedic stress. Here are some basic guidelines for sidestepping running related overuse injuries:

• **Stretch before and after exercising.** Proper stretching can mean the difference between pain and enjoyment and can provide several potential benefits including improving joint flexibility, enhancing performance, and reducing injury potential. As a general rule, always precede stretching exercises with at least five minutes of low-intensity physical activity.

• **Increase your mileage sensibly.** Avoid doing too much exercise too soon. A general guideline is to limit any increase in weekly distance to 10 percent or less of the previous week's total mileage. Contrary to what some people believe, more is not always better. Instead, limit your total weekly mileage to a reasonable level according to your fitness level, body size and training experience. Exercising too much substantially

Table 25.1. Training Basics*

Week	Time	Intensity
1	20	Walk
2	22	Walk
3	22	30–60 second jog, 5 minute walk
4	24	Same as #3
5	24	30–60 second jog, 4 minute walk
6	26	Same as #5
7	26	30–60 second jog, 3 minute walk
8	28	Same as #7
9	28	30–60 second jog, 2 minute walk
10	30	Same as #8
11	30	Jog 2 minutes, walk 1 minute
12+	30	12+ 30 Gradually progress to continuous jogging

*Individuals who are in good shape may progress at a faster rate by increasing time and intensity simultaneously, while those who are less fit may opt to progress more gradually.

increases your chances of sustaining an overuse injury. Remember: Exercise quality is usually more important than quantity.

- **Don't subject your body to consecutive days of very intense exercise.** Always follow a relatively "hard" day of exercising with an easier day. If you run considerably faster and farther than usual on a particular day, take the next day off or decrease the duration and/or intensity of your next workout.

- **Incorporate an occasional "easy" week into your exercise regimen.** Keep in mind that you don't need to increase your mileage every week to continue to benefit from your training efforts. Some level of physical and/or psychological fatigue is natural following a steady diet of hard workouts. Fatigue may increase the likelihood of injury because it can diminish the precision of motor control and inhibit voluntary muscle-stabilizing activity.

- **Don't ignore sudden pain or discomfort.** Pain is the body's way of telling you that if you persist in what you're doing, you will either injure yourself or exacerbate a relatively minor injury that has already occurred. You must learn to listen to your body and respond appropriately. The acronym "RICE" (rest, ice, compression and elevation) should serve as the basis of treatment for most minor injuries (such as pulled or strained muscles and shin splits). If your acute pain does not respond to self-treatment within a reasonable period of time, see a physician, preferably a sports medicine specialist.

- **Don't try to "run through" pain.** If you alter your normal running mechanics in an effort to accommodate pain or discomfort, you may place excessive stress on your joints, muscles, and connective tissues (ligaments and tendons). Refrain from exercising until the pain subsides and no longer interferes with your natural running pattern.

- **Periodically replace your running shoes.** Proper footwear can have a significant impact on minimizing your chances of being injured. Record your mileage daily and replace your running shoes once the cumulative total exceeds 500 miles.

- **Vary your workout options.** Give your joints and muscles an occasional break from the "same old grind." Engage in other forms of low-impact, joint-friendly exercises such as elliptical cross-training, cycling, or swimming, in addition to running. Exercise variety can be both physically and mentally refreshing.

Walking

Gear Up

Shoes are the most important part of your walking gear. Good walking shoes are generally flat, but flexible, so your foot rolls with each step. They

✔ Quick Tip
Are You Up For The 10,000 Step Challenge?

How many steps do you take every day? Fitness experts say grown-ups should take at least 10,000 steps every day—that equals about five miles of walking. It's good for kids your age to take even more than 10,000 steps every day. But can you imagine counting all of those steps? Yikes!

One easy way to measure how many steps you take is to invest in a step counter. You can probably find one that doesn't cost a lot at a local sporting goods store or a store that has a sporting goods department. The step counter doesn't have to be anything fancy—it just has to count your steps.

Step counters work when you attach them to the waistband of your clothing. They count how often your hips move up and down as you walk—and that equals the number of steps you take.

It's fun to use a step counter to see how many steps you usually take in one day. To track your progress, wear your step counter all day. Then, before you go to bed, write down the number of steps shown on your step counter. Are you close to 10,000? Are you way under or over? It's OK if you're way under 10,000 steps to start with—lots of people are. Work on taking a few more steps each day until you hit the big 10,000. Then, try for even more. Wherever you start, the goal is to challenge yourself to take even more steps.

Are you ready to take the 10,000-plus step challenge? Let's get stepping. Start by counting steps in your daily routine. How many steps is it from:

- Your bedroom to the front door;
- Your locker to your homeroom or first class of the day;
- Your front door, around your house or building, and back to the front door;
- Your locker to your best friend's locker;

should fit well, but leave enough room for your feet to spread out while walking. Wear socks that are comfortable. Try socks made of cotton or other sweat-wicking materials—they will keep your feet drier and help prevent blisters. Running shoes are okay to use for walking. Don't forget to trade in the old shoes when the treads start wearing out—which is about 500 miles.

- Your home to a friend's home;
- One class to another;
- The entrance of your school to your locker or first class?

Easy ways to sneak extra steps into your day:

- Get up and walk around during commercial breaks while you're watching TV
- Get up to change the channel instead of using the remote
- If you walk to school, take a longer route (or maybe on the way home so you're not late)
- Take the stairs more often
- Become a part-time pet walker
- If you go shopping with a parent, have them park farther away from the entrance to the store
- Walk around while you're brushing your teeth or on the phone with a friend
- If you're on the computer, set a timer to remind you to get up every 30 minutes or so and walk around

Of course, taking a long walk each day with your family or a friend is a great way to meet the 10,000-step challenge. What other ideas can you come up with to take more steps? Do you feel like you're becoming more active? Do you notice that you're taking more steps each day now that you're counting them? Good.

Now keep stepping.

Source: "Are You Up For The 10,000 Step Challenge?" reprinted with permission from www.kidnetic.com, a website of the International Food Informational Council Foundation © 2006 IFIC Foundation. All rights reserved.

Wear comfortable clothing when walking. Try to dress in layers, so you can always take off something as you warm up. Layering with a t-shirt, sweatshirt, or windproof jacket is a good idea if it's windy or chilly outside.

✔ **Quick Tip**

Besides shoes and comfortable clothing, there are two other essentials you need when walking outdoors:

Sunscreen: Protects your skin from the sun.

Hat: In the summer, a hat keeps the sun out of your face. In the winter it helps to keep you warm by trapping the heat that is lost from the top of your head. A bright colored hat will also make it easy for drivers to see and avoid you.

Source: "Walking Activity Card," United States Department of Health and Human Services, Centers for Disease Control and Prevention (CDC), 2003.

Play It Safe

Before you walk out the door, talk about the best walking routes with your parents so you know your safety zones and how to avoid traffic. And, only walk in those areas so your parents will know where you are.

It's always best to walk where you can avoid traffic—like parks or even the mall. Or try to find an area where there are sidewalks. If you have to walk on a street without sidewalks, walk close to the curb facing traffic. Remember to cross the street only at marked crosswalks or at corners, keep your ears and eyes open, and watch out for traffic in front and back of you. Wear bright-colored clothing or reflectors so drivers can see you. If you are walking alone, don't wear headphones—if they are too loud, they can keep you from hearing any oncoming traffic.

It's a good idea to drink some water before you head out to walk, while you are walking, and when you get back—even if it's cold outside or you don't feel thirsty. In the summer, late afternoons (not nights) and mornings are the best times to walk to avoid the midday heat and humidity. To find out more about staying cool, click here.

It is best to warm up your muscles before stretching them. Warm up for five minutes at an easy walking pace before stretching. Then stretch by starting at the top of your body and working your way down. Make sure to cool down and stretch after your walk too.

Remember—start out slowly and gradually increase the speed and distance you walk—don't try walking a marathon your first time out! And no matter where you are walking, be aware of what is going on around you.

How To Play

You've probably been walking for about as long as you've been talking. But walking isn't just a way to get from here to there, its also a great physical activity. Walking doesn't require a lot of equipment, you can do it anywhere, it is always available by just walking out your front door, and it's a great way to relax and refresh. It's also something you can do alone or with your friends and family.

If you thought walking was just putting one foot in front of the other, you were right, but check out these tips for how to walk and breathe correctly so your walk will be safer and easier.

- **Posture.** How you hold your body is important. Stand up straight and tall. This means putting your shoulders back and relaxing them (no slouching!), and keeping your chin up and stomach in. It's a good idea to look 20 feet ahead—about the lengths of two cars. This keeps your chin up and your eyes on your path.

- **Taking your first steps.** Start out your first step with the heel first. Then roll your foot from heel to toe and push off the toes with the next step. Bringing the opposite leg forward, repeat this again. (This may feel a little funny at first but as your muscles get stronger it gets easier.)

- **Arm motion.** Moving or swinging your arms when you're walking can give you power and it balances what your legs are doing. Bend your elbow 90 degrees (so your arm looks like the letter "L"), while keeping your hands slightly curled. When you step, one foot moves forward and the arm opposite this foot should come forward too. As your foot goes back, bring back the opposite arm with it. Keep your elbows close to the body so you don't have "chicken wings."

- **Don't forget to breathe.** Your breathing should have a rhythm. Inhale one deep breath for four steps and then hold that breath for two steps. Then exhale to the count of four steps, and hold it for two steps before beginning all over again. So the rhythm is—breathe in (step 1, 2, 3, 4), hold (step 1, 2), breathe out (step 1, 2, 3, 4), and hold (step 1, 2).

Everyone's stride is different, so if you feel that four steps are too long or too short, adjust it to what is comfortable for you.

Parts Of The Body Worked

- Upper and lower legs
- Arms
- Abs
- Knees and ankles
- Hips and butt

Jump Rope

Gear Up

You'll need a jump rope. But not all jump ropes are actually made of rope. Jump ropes come in cloth (regular rope), speed (skinny cord), beaded (plastic beads that CLACK when they hit the ground), and even electric.

Play It Safe

Avoid spills—set the right length for your rope. To find out what that is, stand on the center of the cord and pull the handles up so they fit right under your arms. When you jump over the rope, the rope should just brush the floor under your feet. If it doesn't touch the floor, it's too short. If it hits the floor in front of your feet, it's too long.

How To Play

Jump rope is just a fun game that girls play in their backyards or on the playground, right? No way! Bet you didn't know that aside from being a great aerobic workout, jumpers of all ages can compete nationally in categories such as speed, freestyle, and double dutch, which is where two ropes are turned like an egg-beater by two turners, while one or two people jump within the moving ropes.

Parts Of The Body Worked

- Upper and lower legs

- Heart and lungs

- Upper arms

Hiking

First, you'll need a good pair of shoes and thick socks designed for this type of activity. You can start with some sturdy sneakers with thick bottoms. When you begin to take on more difficult trails, try a pair of hiking boots, and make sure they fit. Also, get a backpack or fanny pack to carry all of your hiking supplies. Dress in layers and bring along a waterproof jacket with a hood in case you get caught in the rain. And don't forget a hat, sunscreen, and sunglasses because the higher you hike, the more dangerous the sun's rays become.

To keep hiking fun, you always need to be prepared to beat problems that could happen while you're out, like finding the trail if you get lost or stuck in bad weather. Make sure you bring a map of the area you'll be hiking in and a sturdy compass. You'll also need to bring plenty of water and extra food, like sports bars or trail mix, in case you have to stay out late and get hungry. The adults on your hike should bring a box of waterproof matches and an Army-style knife. A flashlight and extra batteries will help you find your way if you end up out after dark.

Finally, you'll need to bring a first aid kit, in case someone gets hurt during your hike.

Play It Safe

- **Prep:** Get in shape before you head out on your hike. Try walking around your neighborhood with your pack loaded with five pounds more gear than you'll actually carry on your hike. If that goes well, plan a short hike to test your abilities on the trail.

- **Buddies:** Take a friend and an adult along on your hike. That way you can look out for each other and you'll have people to talk to. Also, be sure to let someone who's not going know where you'll be hiking and what time you'll be back.

- **Water:** Carry lots of water even if you are only planning a short hike. For warm-weather hikes, bring six to eight quarts of water per day. In the cold weather or higher elevations, you can be safe with half that amount. Whenever you are near water, make sure you wet yourself down. Dampen a bandana and wipe your face, neck, and arms or wrap it around your head while you hike.

- **Blisters and more:** To prevent blisters, try spraying your feet with an antiperspirant before heading out. Bring extra pairs of socks that you can change into if your feet get wet or sweaty—if they aren't made of cotton, they'll keep your feet drier. Once you're on the trail, stop as soon as you feel a "hot spot" on your feet and apply special type of bandage called "moleskin" to the sore area. Also, try using a hiking stick to keep some pressure off of your legs and knees.

- **Buzz:** Don't get bugged by bugs. Protect yourself from bites and stings by using a bug repellant that includes DEET. Repellents that contain DEET are the most effective, but make sure you rub them on according to the directions. A good rule of thumb from the experts is that kids should use repellents with less than 10% DEET. Get your parents to help you put it on your face so you don't get it in your mouth or eyes. And wash your hands after you apply it. Remember that stuff that smells good to you smells good to bugs too, so don't use scented shampoos or lotions before hiking.

- **Weather watcher:** When it's hot, pick trails that are shaded and run near streams. If you need to hike uphill in the sun, first soak yourself down to stay cool. You can also try wearing a wet bandana around your head or neck. Also, try to stay out of cotton clothes. Keep yourself out of bad weather by checking forecasts before you hike and watching the skies once you're out on the trail. During lightening storms, head downhill and away from the direction of the storm, and then squat down and keep your head low.

- **Keep it yummy:** To stay healthy on your hike, you'll need to know how to keep your food and water safe.

How To Play

For your first day hike (hiking for a day or less without camping overnight), choose a safe, well-marked trail that doesn't have too many steep climbs. Otherwise, you'll get tired too early and won't make it as far as you want to go. Each time you go hiking, try going a little farther and take a slightly steeper trail.

Climbing

Cliff-Hanger: A Noodle-Armed Novice Learns To Love Rock Climbing

"Cliff-hanger: A Noodle-Armed Novice Learns To Love Rock Climbing," by Samantha Schoech, Sunset Magazine, *October 2003. © 2003 Sunset Publishing Company. Reprinted with permission.*

Getting Started

I don't look like rock-climbing material. I'm only moderately athletic, I don't love heights, and I can do exactly one push-up. But now that I've learned the basics of the sport, I know that my noodle arms are not reasons to stay away from rock faces. As Mykael Lazzeri, an instructor at Mission Cliffs climbing gym in San Francisco, says: "If you can climb a ladder, you can climb a rock."

This is good news for anyone looking for an outdoor activity that is both physically challenging and mentally engaging. Steve Gerberding, an instructor at Joshua Tree Rock Climbing School and a 26-year climbing veteran, says, "Rock climbing is puzzle solving."

Climbing As An Indoor Sport

An indoor climbing gym is the best place for a novice to start. Gyms supply gear and instruction—and they have padded floors. Despite the fact that there is almost no chance of falling all the way down (known as "decking"), that padding is reassuring the first time you Spider-Man your way up a vertical surface.

The first rule of climbing is safety. So we start by learning how to put on a harness correctly and tie the rope that will be our lifeline. Minutes into my class at Mission Cliffs, I have mastered the figure-eight follow-through knot, the cornerstone of rock climbing. The next 20 minutes are devoted to belaying, in which the climber's partner uses a belay device to control the rope's slack, ensuring that the climber doesn't get injured if she loses her grip. And soon I find myself hanging 20 feet above the floor, having just climbed a wall for the very first time.

Now that I've learned how to tie in, belay, and climb, Lazzeri sets me loose to find a buddy so we can take turns as belayer and climber.

My first partner is a young woman who has been climbing indoors for about a month. She urges me to use my leg muscles to push off the small resin holds and to trust my feet. "This takes all my strength; I am working against a standard fear of heights." When I mention it to Lazzeri, he says, "Trust your fear. It's there to help you."

My second indoor class is Joel Cortez's "Basic Technique." Cortez starts by announcing that climbing is all in the legs. He teaches us to smear (use the pressure of the ball of the foot against a flat wall to step up) and match (bring both hands or feet together on the same hold), and most importantly, to position our bodies to take advantage of momentum, balance, and weight distribution. The difference is incredible. By the end of the two-hour class, I have climbed an easy intermediate route; it wouldn't impress the guys on El Capitan in Yosemite National Park, but it pleases me quite a bit.

Scaling Rocks In Joshua Tree

After just two sessions inside, I want to get outside. That is why at 8 a.m. on a Saturday I find myself standing in a parking lot in Southern California's Joshua Tree National Park, which is famous for the quartz monzonite rock that draws climbers from all over the world. Here I meet 10 other students, as well as instructors Steve Gerberding and Don Reid from the Joshua Tree Rock Climbing School.

The class is an even mixture of men and women; everyone but me is in his or her 20s. Their youth discourages me until Gerberding tells us that one of his favorite climbing students, a man who takes private lessons, is 82.

We spend the morning bouldering (moving along a rock a few feet off the ground with no ropes or harnesses). Gerberding and Reid teach us to read the rock by looking at the slope, features (any bump, ripple, or dent), and texture. They tell us how to tie our shoes (tightly), how to place our feet (with confidence). They show us that dipping our hands into powdered chalk helps our fingers grip the rock. The best way to learn, Gerberding tells us, is just to climb until we're fatigued and bleeding. "I'm not guaranteeing that you'll leave here without a little blood on you," he says.

After lunch we head for the trills. Climbing a real rock face, I realize instantly, is very different from climbing in a gym. First, there are no padded floors. For the first time in my brief climbing career, I'm scared. Ledges and holds are harder to find on a real rock than on an artificial lace, and halfway up I start to doubt that I will make it to the top. But with Gerberding and the members of my group cheering me on, I complete the route. The view at the top—of Joshua Tree's boulders looking like giant peaches beneath a sharp blue sky—is spectacular. But even better is my own sense of accomplishment.

By day's end, every student has completed at least one route. We congratulate each other with high fives. As I leave the parking lot, I am exhausted and happy. I look down and notice my battle scar: a deep scratch on my ankle. I flaunt it like a medal.

The Gear

The variety of rock-climbing gear is staggering, but there are only a few items you need to get started. All courses and gyms will rent or lend you gear to use.

- **Helmet:** Highly recommended for all outdoor climbing. It will protect you if you fall, and also protect you in the much more likely event of falling debris. From $50.

- **Chalk bag:** Not necessary, but as Steve Gerberding says, "A chalk bag will help you look cool while you're stalling on the face." From $12.

- **Harness:** The rule here is to find one that is comfortable and fits properly. Always try a harness on before purchasing. From $22.

✔ Quick Tip
Climbing Schools

To locate climbing gyms, such as Mission Cliffs (2295 Harrison St., San Francisco; www.touchstoneclimbing.com or 415-550-0515), visit www.rockclimbing.com or check your yellow pages.

Each of the well regarded climbing schools listed below offers outdoor climbing instruction to beginners. Prices for a one-day group lesson begin at about $85. For lists of reputable schools and guides, contact the American Alpine Institute (see below) or the American Mountain Guides Association (www.amga.com or 303-271-0984).

- American Alpine Institute. Bellingham, Washington; www.mtnguide.com or 360-671-1505.

- Exum Mountain Guides. Moose, Wyoming; www.exumguides.com or 307-733-2297.

- Joshua Tree Rock Climbing School. Joshua Tree, California; www.rockclimbingschool.com, 800-890-4745, or 760-366-4745.

- Moab Desert Adventures. Moab, Utah; www.moabdesertadventures.com or 877-765-6622.

- Shasta Mountain Guides. Mt. Shasta, California; www.shastaguides.com or 530-926-3117.

- Yosemite Mountaineering School and Guide Service. Yosemite National Park, California; www.yosemitemountaineering.com or 209-372-8344.

Source: *Sunset Magazine* © 2003 Sunset Publishing Company. Reprinted with permission.

- **Locking carabiner and belay device:** These pieces of hardware are belaying essentials. From about $15 each.

- **Shoes:** Rock-climbing shoes are an absolute must and are generally worn very snug. Having your own pair ensures the best fit. From $80.

—by Samantha Schoech

Chapter 26

Water Sports: Swimming, Diving, Skiing, Surfing, Kayaking, And Canoeing

The Water Well

What Is Aquatic Fitness?

Aquatic fitness is defined as activities performed in the water that promote and enhance physical and mental fitness. Aquatic Fitness is typically performed in a vertical position in shallow and/or deep water. There are numerous applications to appeal to a wide variety of participants.

The water's unique properties allow the pool to provide an environment for people of all abilities. Buoyancy creates a reduced impact exercise alternative that is easy on the joints, while the water's resistance challenges the muscles. Water lends itself to a well-balanced workout that improves all major components of physical fitness—aerobic training, muscular strength and endurance, flexibility, and body composition.

About This Chapter: This chapter begins with information from *The Water Well*, reprinted with permission from the Aquatic Exercise Association, www.aeawave.com. © 2006 Aquatic Exercise Association. All rights reserved.. Additional text under separate headings is from the following documents produced by the Department of Health and Human Services, Centers for Disease Control and Prevention (CDC): "Swimming Activity Card," 2001; "Diving Activity Card," 2002; "Water Skiing Activity Card," 2002; "Surfing Activity Card," 2002; and "Canoeing/Kayaking Activity Card," 2002.

Shallow water programming is performed in waist to chest depth. The feet remain in contact with the pool bottom during most of the workout providing a low impact training option. Deep-water programs, on the other hand, are performed in water depths that allow the participant to remain vertical (upright) and yet not touch the bottom. Flotation equipment is utilized to maintain correct alignment and provide a truly non-impact workout.

How Is Water Exercise Different?

Buoyancy: In the water your body is buoyant and the impact to the joints during exercise is significantly less than on land. Depending upon the water depth, your body "weight" is reduced in the pool due to lessened gravitational forces.

- A body immersed to the neck bears approximately 10% of its body weight.

- A body immersed to the chest bears approximately 25–35% of its body weight.

- A body immersed to the waist bears approximately 50% of its body weight.

A properly designed program in the water provides a highly effective workout in a safe and gentle environment due to the principle of buoyancy. Shallow water programs are generally best performed in water that is about mid-chest depth for maximum comfort, control of movement and optimum toning benefits for the upper body.

Resistance: Muscles must work against resistance to become developed and toned. Water provides substantially more resistance than air, because water is more viscous than air, making each movement in the pool more challenging to the muscles. Also, muscles typically work in pairs; that is, biceps and triceps or quadriceps and hamstrings. When you move your body, or your limbs, through the water you are always encountering resistance. This helps to provide a more balanced workout as opposing muscles are involved, unlike on land where you typically need to reposition the body, or select a separate exercise, to provide adequate stimulation to both muscles of the pair.

Note: If you incorporate weighted, buoyant or rubberized equipment, these muscle actions will change and it once again becomes necessary to target both muscles of a pair with separate exercises.

Cooling Effect: Water cools more efficiently than air, so when exercising in the water the body is able to eliminate excess heat more effectively. This is not to say that you will not sweat during a workout in the pool, but water helps prevent overheating and washes away the perspiration as you exercise. Because the water cools the body quickly, it is imperative that you begin every workout with a "thermal warm up" designed to elevate the body's core temperature, warm the muscles and prepare the joints for the increased workload to come. Even at the recommended temperature of 83–86 degrees Fahrenheit (28–30 degrees Celsius), a proper warm up is necessary to prevent injury and provide comfort.

Note: Special populations and specialty training may require deviations from this recommended range.

Heart Rates: Heart rate responses differ when exercising in the water than when exercising on land. Typically, aquatic exercisers experience a reduced heart rates response (that is, lowered pulse rate), but the water should not be considered less effective. Studies have shown that oxygen consumption (the true measure of the cardiovascular benefits) is comparable to a similar program on land, although the heart rate response is lower. Several factors, some of which have been previously mentioned, influence the exercising heart rate when submerged in the water to mid-chest:

- Lessened gravity allows a more efficient return of blood to the heart from the extremities. The cooling affect of water reduces the workload on the heart. (One function of the heart is to keep the body cool during sustained exercise.)

- Hydrostatic pressure, the pressure that the water exerts on the body while submerged, assists in blood flow and improves the exchange of oxygen into the blood.

How Does Water Exercise Compare To Land Exercise In Regards To Calorie Burning?

As on land, there are several variables that affect caloric consumption during vertical water exercise. Variables include:

- Water depth in which the person is exercising;

- Speed of movement through the water;

- Amount of force applied (how "hard" you work) to movements;

- Length of the person's limbs;

- Environmental factors such as water temperature, air temperature, humidity, etc.

On land, weight bearing is a primary factor for increasing calorie consumption, but in the water it appears that using the water's resistance is more of a factor. Based upon the finding of a study that compared energy expenditure (calories burned) for upper and lower body exercises performed in the water and out of the water (Cassedy 1992), one can estimate that combining upper and lower body movements in the pool would expend somewhere between 400 and 500 calories in a one hour class. This is comparable to running or walking at 10–11 minutes per mile.

Water Exercise Is Beneficial For. . .

Osteoporosis: Osteoporosis, a degenerative disease commonly referred to as adult bone loss, is associated with 1.5 million bone fractures (generally of the hip, spine or wrist) each year. Previously it was believed that only specific land-based, weight bearing activities could counteract bone loss, however research indicates that shallow water aquatic exercise is a viable method for building and maintaining bone mass. It appears that in spite of the reduction in body mass that occurs in shallow water exercise programs, the viscosity of the water offers adequate resistance to produce positive results. So in addition to walking, stair climbing and weight training, vertical water exercise can be beneficial in maintaining both strong muscular and skeletal systems. Water exercise can also enhance balance, coordination, posture and performance skills thus reducing the risk of falls and injury. [References: *Aquatic Exercise Association Aquatic Fitness Professional Manual* and *Aquatic Exercise Association Aquatic Fitness Research Journal*, 2005, Volume 2, Number 1]

Arthritis: It is estimated that some form of arthritis affects 37 million Americans. Arthritis refers to more than 100 different diseases that affect areas in or around the joints. The disease also can affect other parts of the body. Arthritis causes pain, loss of movement and sometimes swelling. Osteoarthritis affects the

Top Ten Tips For Water Safety

✔ **Quick Tip**

- **Do learn to swim.** If you like to have a good time doing water activities, being a strong swimmer is a must.

- **Do take a friend along.** Even though you may be a good swimmer, you never know when you may need help. Having friends around is safer and just more fun.

- **Do know your limits.** Get out of the water if you are too tired, too cold, too far from safety, you've had too much sun, or too much hard activity.

- **Do swim in supervised areas only.** Follow all signs and warnings.

- **Do wear a life jacket when boating , jet skiing, water skiing, rafting, or fishing.**

- **Do stay alert to currents.** They can change quickly. If you get caught in a strong current, don't fight it. Swim parallel to the shore until you have passed through it. Near piers, jetties (lines of big rocks), small dams, and docks, the current gets unpredictable and could knock you around. If you find it hard to move around, head to shore. Learn to recognize and watch for dangerous waves and signs of rip currents—water that is a weird color, really choppy, foamy, or filled with pieces of stuff.

- **Do keep an eye on the weather.** If you spot bad weather (dark clouds, lighting), pack up and take the fun inside.

- **Don't mess around in the water.** Pushing or dunking your friends can get easily out of hand.

- **Don't dive into shallow water.** If you don't know how deep the water is, don't dive.

- **Don't float where you can't swim.** Keep checking to see if the water is too deep, or if you are too far away from the shore or the poolside.

Source: Excerpted from "H2O Smarts," Department of Health and Human Services, Centers for Disease Control and Prevention (CDC), 2002.

cartilage of the joints and is seen most often in the weight bearing joints of the body such as the spine, hip, knee and ankle. This is often referred to as the "wear and tear" arthritis, however exercise, is highly recommended to increase muscular strength and flexibility, which will ultimately lessen the load placed upon the joint. Rheumatoid arthritis is an autoimmune disease, in which the joint lining becomes inflamed, particularly affecting the smaller joints such as the hands, wrists, ankles, feet, and neck. This is one of the most serious and disabling types, affecting mostly women. Water exercise—water walking, low impact aerobics, Ai Chi, Yoga, deep-water training, etc.—is highly promoted by health professionals and medical professionals. The Arthritis Foundation encourages water exercise as one of the best activities for individuals of all ages who have arthritis symptoms. [References: *The Arthritis Foundation and Fitness Empowerment of Active Adults- FEOAA*]

Diabetes: With diabetes, the body does not produce adequate insulin. Insulin helps to regulate the amount of sugar in the blood stream. There are two types of diabetes—Type 1 or insulin-dependent and Type 2 or non-insulin dependent. Most people who develop Type 2 diabetes are over 40 years of ages and many are obese. Exercising vigorously just once a week reduces your risk of Type 2 diabetes by 23%; exercising five or more times per week reduces the risk by 42%. Diabetes, like hypertension, responds well to increased physical activity. A regular exercise program is considered to be a cornerstone to diabetic care. Before initiating a fitness program, one should consult his/her physician as modifications in medications or exercise scheduling may be in order. Shoes should always be worn in and around the pool area and the diabetic should be aware that he/she might be at a higher risk for heat related illness and should avoid exercising in excessive heat. [References: *Aquatic Exercise Association Aquatic Fitness Professional Manual* and *Fitness Empowerment of Active Adults- FEOAA*]

Menopause: Women experiencing menopause will benefit from a regular exercise program, and the water provides a comfortable and enjoyable fitness option. The Melpomene Institute reports that physical activity does seem to help even the most difficult of menopausal experiences. Physiologically, everything that gets worse with aging can improve with exercise. Three significant benefits related to menopause that a women will obtain through regular exercise are listed below. [Reference: Joyce Hannah, MA, MS, *The Arthritis Foundation and Fitness Empowerment of Active Adults Newsletter*, Vol. 5 Issue 3, Summer 1998]

- Maintain muscle mass and bone density.

- Maintain a healthy weight.

- Stimulation of HDL (good cholesterol).

Pregnancy: Besides that fact that women will feel safe with regard to falls and trauma during exercise, the warm water will offer a pleasant, safe and relaxing environment. With immersion in the water, there is a reduction of the physical weight distributed to the joints. Also during pregnancy, the water may be more suitable than land-based training for prevention of overheating during exercise. Water exercise has been shown to reduce swelling often associated with pregnancy, improves circulation, provides a balanced workout, and enhances balance, coordination and posture. A pregnant woman should consult her primary caregiver regarding her exercise limitations. [Reference: J. Douglas Gil, *AKWA* letter, Vol. 12 No. 3]

Back Problems: Eighty percent of the adult population will experience, or has already experienced, back pain at some point in their life. Back injury is a leading cause of lost productivity on the job. Prevention, rather than treatment, should be the goal, and the aquatic environment is the perfect place to develop a strong, well conditioned back. Research indicates that deep-water training may be a beneficial training option for individuals with low back pain. Deep water is a non-impact environment and significantly reduces the compressive load on the spine. Deep water is also very effective for training the core muscles, which is important for proper alignment, good posture and back health. [Reference: *Aquatic Exercise Association Aquatic Fitness Professional Manual*]

Commonly Asked Questions About Water Exercise

Is it safe to exercise alone in the pool? Aquatic Exercise Association (AEA) advises against exercising alone in the pool because of the risk of drowning should something unexpected occur. Most people find it more enjoyable to exercise with a friend, so even if you plan to workout in your home pool, invite someone to join you. It is also easier to maintain a regular exercise program since you are accountable to someone other than yourself. At the least, have someone remain on deck to provide assistance. Stay safe; never exercise alone in the water.

What is the purpose of wearing shoes while exercising in the water? Although impact is greatly reduced in the pool, you will still experience some impact stress to the weight bearing joints of the body (unless you remain in a suspended position, such as deep water exercise). Therefore AEA recommends that you wear shoes for added cushion, shock absorption and comfort during bouncing movements. Shoes also provide ankle support, which is important in programs that include twisting or turning activities. Footwear can also protect your feet from rough surfaces—whether the pool bottom, pool deck or locker rooms; this is critical for individuals with diabetes. Pregnancy women are recommended to wear shoes to provide addition support as well as to prevent slipping and possible falls. The best news—water shoes can make your workout more effective.

Do I need to bring drinking water to my aquatic fitness classes? Yes. Even though the water cools the body more effectively, you will lose fluids from perspiration during a vigorous aquatic program. To prevent overheating and related problems (muscle cramps, heat exhaustion and heat stroke) it is suggested to drink water before, during and after exercise. Keep your water bottle handy at the side of the pool and your workout can continue uninterrupted.

My aquatic classes are outdoors, how do I protect my skin? Unfortunately, most all tanning has some damaging influence on your skin. Cloudy days and water submersion are not effective for preventing sun damage; up to 80% of ultraviolet radiation penetrates cloud cover and up to 50% reaches swimmers in the water. Typical cotton t-shirts can allow 30–50% of harmful ultraviolet rays through to your skin when dry—even more when wet. Special sun protective clothing is available. Wear a waterproof sunscreen with at least a SPF of 15 and apply 30–40 minutes before exposure, consider sun protective clothing and hats, and always wear your sunglasses.

What if I cannot keep up with the rest of the class during the exercise program? First of all, this is your exercise class and you need to feel comfortable listening to your own body's needs and abilities. Pace yourself and do not be afraid to do things a little differently. Also, make sure to select a class that is appropriate for your abilities. Most facilities offer a variety of programs—from special needs to advanced fitness. Observe different classes and find the one that is right for you. Also, make sure that your instructor in properly trained and certified. The instructor should be able to assist you with making necessary modifications without feeling "singled out" from the group. And finally, as you continue to exercise you will see your energy, enthusiasm and abilities continue to advance.

I love exercising in the water, but my skin gets so dry. What can I do? The best way to prevent dry skin is to drink—yes, drink—plenty of water everyday. However, being submerged in the pool for an hour or more will tend to dry the skin. Do not put on lotions (except waterproof sunscreens) before your class; it will simply wash off, waste your money, and adversely affect the pool's water quality. Immediately after class, shower and apply a good quality moisturizing lotion to your damp skin (now is a good time to moisturize the hair too). Your swim suit will also last longer if you rinse thoroughly immediately after exercising in the pool, chlorine and other chemicals necessary to provide a safe environment will gradually deteriorate the material of your suit. Products are available to help remove the chlorine residue from your skin/hair and suit, and some companies manufacturer chlorine resistant swim wear/exercise wear.

I am young and athletic. Can water exercise really provide the workout I need? Definitely! Water fitness programming has progressed and diversified over the past several years, which is one of the reasons, we are seeing such a big "wave" of participation. Although a significant part of the workout intensity is up to the individual (that is, you can employ various training principles to alter the intensity), the type of program selected is also very important. Most facilities offer a variety of options for water exercise participants—just as they do for land-based group exercise. Check out aquatic programs featuring kick boxing, sports specific training, intervals, and circuits. Or, if you prefer the one-on-one approach, consider aquatic personal training to more specifically target your goals and needs. And don't forget specialized aquatic fitness equipment can further enhance your training results.

Water exercise provides a safe, effective, and fun option for all ages and all abilities. So jump in and begin enjoying the benefits of this exciting fitness option that is making a splash across the globe.

Swimming

Gear Up

Pick out a swimsuit that fits your style. If you plan to swim competitively, you'll need a suit that is lightweight and stretchy. It should also fit snugly so it won't slow you down when you're racing or slip off as you dive into the water.

A pair of goggles will allow you to see where you are going underwater without your eyes feeling itchy and irritated. They even make prescription goggles so you can see underwater if you wear glasses.

Finally, if you're outside, you'll want to guard against the sun. So, rub on some sunscreen.

How To Play

Swimming is more than a great way to cool off when it's hot, it's also a fun activity that helps you work out your whole body. If you don't know how to swim, or you want to brush up your skills, you'll want to take some lessons at your local pool. There, you'll master the basics to help keep your head above water.

Floating

Our bodies have a natural tendency to float—so go with it. Relax and let the water support your body. Lie back with your arms stretched out to the side. Turn your palms up and keep the backs of your hands in the water. Arch your back, stretch out your legs (some gentle kicking will help you float easier), and take short breaths to stay relaxed. Floating is a great way to rest, or rest while you call for help if you don't have enough energy to swim to shore or the side of a pool.

Treading Water

Another way to keep afloat is to tread water. Get into the water and pretend you are gently riding a bicycle, with your back straight and your arms straight out in front of you. Sweep your arms together with your palms facing down and in. Then, sweep them back out with your palms facing down and away from each other.

Now that you know how to keep your head above the water, try swimming with your head below water.

Swimming Underwater

Breathe in as much air as you can and then let it all out, take one more breath and hold it, and slide under the water. Even though it seems like taking lots of quick breaths before going underwater could help you, doing that is called "hyperventilating" and it can actually make you pass out underwater. Stretch out your body with your legs together and your arms straight out a little bit above your head. Pull your legs up then kick them apart to start gliding. Next, bring your legs together and kick in a scissor motion to move around. While you kick, put your arms out to your sides and push them back towards your legs. Glide as far as you can, and then come back up when you need a breath. Try to stay relaxed and don't push yourself too far. The more you practice, the stronger your lungs will become.

Once you've got the basics, to be a strong swimmer and enjoy lots of water activities, you'll need to learn these strokes: backstroke, breaststroke, freestyle, and butterfly—to name a few.

♣ It's A Fact!!

Elephants can swim up to 20 miles a day.
They stick their trunks above the water like snorkels.

It takes about 800,000 gallons of water to fill up an Olympic-size pool.

Source: Excerpted from "Swimming Activity Card," Department of Health and Human Services, Centers for Disease Control and Prevention (CDC), 2001.

Play It Safe

- Learn to swim and always swim with a friend. It's more fun and having a friend there if you need one is just plain smart.

- Make sure to respect rules and lifeguards. Pool rules like "no running" or beach rules like "no swimming outside the flags" are there to protect you. (And lifeguards enforce them so that you can stay safe, not to ruin your fun.) Make sure a lifeguard or an adult can see you just in case you need help.

- Don't try to keep up with stronger or more experienced swimmers, especially if they swim out further than you think you can swim back.

- Swimming is real workout. So, take breaks. If you get tired while you're in the water, float on your back for a few minutes until you get your power back.

- Make sure to keep an eye on mother nature. If you spot bad weather (dark clouds, lightening), it's time to take the fun inside.

- And when you get out of the water, tilt and shake your head to let all of the water drain out of your ears. Swimmer's ear can be a real pain.

- Diving makes a splash, but make sure you know how deep the water is before you leap.

Parts Of The Body Worked

- Upper and lower legs
- Arms
- Shoulders and neck
- Heart and lungs
- Back

Games

Wet T-Shirt Relay: All you need to play this relay game is two t-shirts, some friends, and some pool time.

- Divide into two teams.
- Half of each team should line up on opposite sides of the pool.
- When you're ready to go, the first player on each team puts on the wet t-shirt and jumps into the pool.
- The players swim across to the other side as fast as they can and tag the next person in their team's line. Then they take off the wet t-shirt

and give it to their teammate to put on. As soon as it's on, the next swimmer can jump in and go.

- The first team to have all of its swimmers finish the relay wins.

Diving

Gear Up

All you'll need is a swimsuit and a pool with a diving board. Check out your neighborhood or a community center in your area for a pool you can use.

How To Play

Diving is about precision, flexibility, and strength. Experienced divers leap 5–10 meters (about 16–33 feet) into the air from a springboard or platform, do stunts like somersaults or twists, and then plunge into the water below.

A certified diving instructor can help you master the diving board, but for now, try this beginners' dive:

- Point your arms straight over your head, with your shoulders by your ears.
- Keep your head between your arms and tuck your chin to your chest.
- Bend at the waist, but don't bend the knees.
- Keep your legs straight.
- Fall towards the water, making sure not to lift your head or shoulders.
- Follow through with your fingers into the water.

Be water wise. Check the depth before you dive.

Play It Safe

Before you dive, you'll need to follow these safety tips.

- Know how to swim well before stepping on the board.
- Always dive with someone else.
- Know the water depth before you dive, and never ever dive into shallow water. Check around for signs or ask a lifeguard. Diving areas are usually marked.

♣ **It's A Fact!!**

Platform diving became an Olympic
event in 1904. Springboard diving made it in 1908.

In January 1991, Fu Mingxia from China became the
world's youngest platform champion. She was only 12.

Divers hit the water at speeds of up to 34 miles per hour.

Source: "Diving Activity Card," Department of Health
and Human Services, Centers for Disease
Control and Prevention (CDC), 2002.

- Above-ground pools are not designed for diving. They're way too shallow. Lots of in-ground pools aren't deep enough either, so check out the water before you dive.

- When you are on the board, enter the water straight on and make sure there's nothing in your way before you leap.

- If people come into the diving area from other parts of the pool, wait until they're gone, or just ask the lifeguard to clear the area for you. If you jump when there is someone else in the diving area, or even just mess around while diving, you could land on top of someone and get hurt.

- Don't run up to a dive. Always stand at the edge of the board or pool and then dive. And dive straight ahead—not off to the side.

- Warm-up and stretch before diving, and then cool down after your plunge session.

- Only try dives that are in your comfort zone. Leave fancy or stunt leaps to experienced divers. An adult can help you decide which dives are safe to try.

Parts Of The Body Worked

- Heart and lungs
- Arms
- Abs
- Upper and lower legs

Water Skiing

Gear Up

First you'll need water skis. There are four types: combination pairs, slalom, tick, and jump skis. New skiers should start with combination pairs, since they are wider and easiest to learn on. Make sure your skis have been checked and that they fit properly. You will also need a flexible towrope that has a floating handle.

All water skiers wear life vests, also known as personal floatation devices (PFDs). You should wear a special water skiing life vest that is approved by the Coast Guard. You and your parents should check this out to get the official word on which life vest is right for you.

Finally, since you're outside, you need to guard against the sun.

How To Play

Want to walk on water? Try water skiing. Water skiers hold onto a rope and are pulled on their skis behind a boat going fast. They glide across the water with the wind in their faces. It's a great activity that you can do with your family or friends and it can be competitive. Check out these tips and you'll be skiing in no time.

Getting Started: Before you get in the water to ski, make sure you're wearing a life vest that is the right size and is on the right way. Get in the water with your skis. Wet your ski bindings before you put on your skis, and keep the bindings loose enough that the skis will come off if you fall. Bend your knees up towards your chest with your arms straight out in front of you. As the boat pulls the rope toward you, grab the rope handle with both hands and hold it between your knees. You should almost be sitting on the skis. Facing the boat, lift the tips of your skis a bit above the water, keep your skis shoulder width apart, and keep your arms straight. Nod your head to let the boat driver know you are ready to go, and begin straightening your legs as you are pulled out of the water. If you stand too soon you'll fall down, so take it slow and be patient.

Steering: To turn, just lean in the direction you want to go. Move your weight to the edge of the skis on the side you want to turn toward while you keep the skis pointed forward. If you want to turn faster, crouch down while you lean.

Play It Safe

- Water skiers need to be good swimmers and always wear a life jacket that fits properly.

- Safe water skiing requires three people: the skier, an experienced boat driver, and the spotter to look out for the skier's signals.

- Since the noise from the boat is so loud, it's important that everyone agrees on and understands the hand signals to use so you can talk without saying a word. Remember that you need to master hand signals before you begin cutting across the water on your skis.

- When you're out on the water, be sure you're in a safe area to ski. Don't ski near docks, boats, rocks, or in shallow water. The only place to start is in the water—dock or land starts should be left to the pros.

- If you start to lose your balance while skiing, just bend your knees and crouch down so you don't fall.

- If you do fall—and everyone does—remember to let go of the rope. Then, find your skis and hold one of them up to signal you're okay and to let other boaters know you're in the water.

Parts Of The Body Worked

- Arms
- Upper and lower legs
- Heart and lungs
- Knees and ankles
- Hips and butt
- Upper body

Surfing

Gear Up

All you really need is a bathing suit or a wetsuit (for cold water or if it's cold out), and of course, a surfboard. You may want to get a used or inexpensive board at first. It wouldn't be smart to mess up a cool new board making beginner's mistakes. The fins should be in good condition, and it should have a place to attach a leash (cord that hooks your ankle to the board so it doesn't get away). Long boards are easier to ride and control. Your board should be 12 to 14 inches taller than you are. Also, put two

✔ **Quick Tip**
Boating And Jet Skiing Safety

Stay alert. When you're riding, keep a lookout for other boats, jet skiers, water skiers, divers, and swimmers.

Know who has the right-of-way. Generally, drivers should keep to their right when they are passing other boats—just like you do when you are walking in the hall at school.

Always ride at a speed that will let you stay in control. This way you can stop or go another way if you need to.

Don't jump wakes or speed through choppy water. Wakes (tracks in the water left by other boats or jet skis) and choppy water can cause you to loose control.

Stay safe. Do not ride with a driver who has been drinking alcohol. Also, make sure you know and practice what to do if someone falls out of the boat.

Source: Excerpted from "H2O Smarts," Department of Health and Human Services, Centers for Disease Control and Prevention (CDC), 2002.

coats of wax on your board if the deck (top) doesn't have a pad that keeps you from slipping.

Play It Safe

- First, you have to be a strong swimmer. As a beginner, you are going to be in the water more than riding your board. Always surf with someone else.

- While you're a beginner, stick to waves no bigger than three feet. If you are a real beginner, surf only broken (white) waves. Never paddle out farther than you can swim back with your board. Most of all, if it doesn't feel right or you are too scared, just don't go.

- Always leash your board to control it. When you begin the wipeout (fall at the end of a ride), kick your board out and away from you.

- Did you know that surfers have rules for who "owns" a wave? Surfers riding waves have to get out of the way of those paddling out, and everyone has to stay clear of swimmers. A surfer who is standing and riding a wave gets to keep it—no one should "drop in" (try to catch the same wave).

- Finally, make sure to wear sunscreen and never surf in bad weather.

How To Play

What do surfing and walking a dog have in common? Well, surfboards don't bark, but they still need a "leash" to keep them from getting away. Surfing takes lots of practice, but when you're riding that wave, it's incredible. Learn these basic surfing techniques to get you started.

- **Regular Or Goofy-Footed Stance:** Put your best foot forward—find out whether you are regular or goofy-footed. Try sliding across a smooth floor with socks on. If you lead with your left foot, you're regular-footed and the left foot goes near the front of the board when you're surfing. If your right foot goes first, you're goofy-footed and the right foot goes up front.

- **Paddling:** To get around in the water, lay chest-down on your board, keeping your legs straight behind you. With each arm, make an overhand swimming stroke that starts at the front of the board and finishes under the board near your legs. (It's like swimming the crawl stroke, except you're on top of the board.) As you finish the stroke with one hand, the other hand is just starting. Try practicing in shallow water or a pool first.

- **Catching The Wave:** When you see white water (breaking waves) coming, turn around to face the shore, aim your board the direction the wave is coming, and start to paddle in. When the wave reaches you, it will push you forward. Stop paddling, grab the side of the board, push up your body, and quickly get your feet under you. Both should land at the same time, toes pointing sideways. Move your lead (regular or goofy) foot in front. Now you're surfing.

Parts Of The Body Worked

- Upper and lower legs
- Hips and butt
- Knees and ankles
- Shoulders and neck
- Lower back

Canoeing And Kayaking

Gear Up

You'll need a kayak (boat that's almost completely closed on top with space for just one person) or a canoe (open boat that can fit you and a friend or two) plus the right kind of paddle. Kayak paddles have a blade on both sides, but canoe paddles have one blade. Be sure to pick the right size paddle— the stick part of a canoe paddle should be about six to eight inches longer than the length of your arm with your fingers out. Don't forget another essential: the life vest. Water shoes or sneakers—not sandals—that grip on the bottom will help your feet stay put when you are pulling the paddle through the water. Keep a whistle attached to your life vest so you are always ready to get attention if trouble strikes.

Play It Safe

You need to be a strong swimmer because you might have to swim underwater, or in moving water. Always go paddling with another person—not just for times of trouble, but because someone should help you carry, load, and launch your boat, right?

Make sure your life jacket fits. Since paddling is an activity that you can do all through the year, leave enough room to put clothes under it when it is cold out. Be prepared to get wet. Take along extra dry clothing, just in case. Remember to keep sun proof with sunscreen.

Save paddling for good weather days. Since you don't know what mother nature will throw at you, know where your float trip will take you, spots where you can get out or camp for the night, and different ways to go in case

---

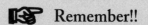 **Remember!!**

Use Sun Protection

It's key to get outside and get active—just make sure you're protected. For outdoor activity, you may need a helmet, a ball, or a club, but you always need sun protection. It's just another part of your gear. Protecting yourself against the sun is the smart choice that kids like you are making these days.

Source: Excerpted from "Sun Proof," the Department of Health and Human Services, Centers for Disease Control and Prevention (CDC), 2002.

---

unexpected trouble strikes your route. Avoid whitewater rapids, dams, and falls—only experienced whitewater paddlers should take these on.

Sure, you want all your friends and their stuff to come along, but don't put too much weight in the boat—you should have more than six inches of side between the top of the fully loaded boat and the water. Spread out the weight (including people) so the boat will stay balanced.

Take lessons to help you learn ways to get yourself back in your boat if it tips over—before you take your first trip. And then practice them. The main thing to remember is not to panic. If you can't get back in, stay with your boat and flip it back over—it'll float—and try to swim the boat to shore.

How To Play

Canoeing: Hold the paddle with your inside hand on top and your waterside hand two to three feet down. Your knuckles should be facing out. Without stretching, insert the blade of the paddle all the way in the water as far forward as you can reach. Push your top hand forward and pull your bottom hand back, turning your shoulders to move the paddle blade straight through the water to your hip. Keep the top of the paddle handle lower than your eyes and don't follow the curve of the canoe. Have a friend paddle on the other side of the canoe, or switch sides as you paddle, to keep the boat gliding along straight.

Kayaking: Kayak paddles have a blade on each side. Lift your paddle with both hands and hold it across your chest. Place your hands the same distance from each blade, just outside your shoulders. Hold the paddle out in front of you, just a few inches above the kayak. Keeping your left elbow straight, bring your right hand straight back, and letting your right elbow bend back toward your body. Your body will twist to the right a bit. Paddle. Now, use the other arm.

Canoeing And Kayaking Tips

Kayakers and canoers should follow these tips so they don't annoy other people or the environment.

- **Be polite.** Only get to the water through marked paths—not through someone else's property. Take your paddling breaks in public places too.

- **Keep lunch spots and campsites clean.** Don't leave garbage in the water or lying around. If there's nowhere to put your trash, take it with you and dump it when you get home.

- **Be considerate of people who are fishing.** Give people fishing plenty of room and try not to disturb the water too much where they are—it'll scare the fish off.

✔ **Quick Tip**

Oops! I Got Too Much Sun. What Do I Do Now?

If you've been in the sun too long, use these tips to make your skin feel better.

- Take a cool bath.
- Use unscented moisturizer (lotion, no petroleum jelly).
- Use hydrocortisone cream.
- Sit in cool water.
- Stay out of the sun. An adult may choose to give you medicine that stops pain. When your burn is severe and you have a headache and chills or a fever, too, an adult may need to take you to a doctor.

Source: Excerpted from "Sun Proof," the Department of Health and Human Services, Centers for Disease Control and Prevention (CDC), 2002.

- **Keep away from the wildlife.** Don't disturb animals and birds even if they are as cute as pets.

Parts Of The Body Worked

- Back

- Arms

- Abs

- Shoulders and neck

♣ **It's A Fact!!**

- Native Americans used animal skins and a variety of tree barks to make canoes. The very best canoe covering was made from paper birch bark because it was lightweight and very strong.

- Thirty thousand years ago, canoes helped ancient people move to new places along the Pacific Ocean: first in Asia, then along the coasts of Canada, the U.S., and South America.

Source: "Canoeing/Kayaking Activity Card," the Department of Health and Human Services, Centers for Disease Control and Prevention (CDC), 2002.

Chapter 27

Activities For Kids With Physical Challenges

Meet The Challenge: You Can Do It Too

Nearly five million U.S. kids have activity limitations. That means it's tough for them to do things that other kids take for granted like playing, going to school, and participating in physical activity. Other challenges, such as learning disabilities, may prevent people from getting involved too.

Fortunately, it's becoming much easier for people with all kinds of disabilities to take part in physical activities. Lots of groups across the U.S. help out by providing information and chances to compete.

Special equipment uses the latest materials (such as light plastics) and improved design to let people with disabilities hold their own in almost any activity. For example, today's wheelchairs for racing, tennis, and basketball are lighter and easier to control than ever. Some wheelchairs weigh only 15 pounds. That's about as much as a book bag with two or three textbooks in it.

Check out what some athletes with disabilities have done.

• Down hill skiers with one leg have been clocked at over 74 miles per hour while Olympic skiers with two legs usually go 80–85 miles per hour.

About This Chapter: This chapter contains information from "Meeting the Challenge: U Can Do It 2," the Department of Health and Human Services, Centers for Disease Control and Prevention (CDC), 2001.

- Joseph Bishop won at the Special Olympics when he tried the softball throw, long jump, and 100 meter dash.

- Rudy Garcia-Tolson uses his gear and his unbeatable attitude to get in the game. He runs, swims, bikes, and skateboards.

- Waterskier, Mark "the Animal" Turner and judo stars Lisa Newton and Lynn Manning have excelled at their sports.

What do these athletes have in common? They live as athletes first and people with disabilities second.

♣ It's A Fact!!
Check Out The Playground
In Your School And Neighborhood

Look around your school and neighborhood playgrounds to see how many barriers need to be changed to help kids with disabilities play. If you can't answer "yes" to both of the questions, kids who have difficulty moving around may not have the same opportunities to be athletes as kids without disabilities.

1. Would kids who have difficulty moving around be able to play on the playground equipment in your neighborhood? Or are there steps, rough pathways, or narrow doorways that get in their way?

2. If you were in a wheelchair, could you swing in the swings?

If you answered "no" to either one of these questions, you may want to check out these websites on accessibility guidelines.

- **Boundless Playgrounds:** A non-profit program providing technical assistance to communities to help them build accessible playgrounds. Their website can be found at www.boundlessplaygrounds.org.

- **A Guide To The ADA Accessibility Guidelines For Play Areas:** This website gives you information about how to make your playground accessible at www.access-board.gov/play/guide/intro.htm.

Source: "Kids Quest on Disabilities and Health," National Center on Birth Defects and Developmental Disabilities, Centers for Disease Control and Prevention (CDC), September 2006.

♣ It's A Fact!!
Videos About Kids With Disabilities

Ask your parents or teachers if you can get these videos about kids who have difficulty moving around to watch in the classroom or at home.

- **A Winner Never Quits (1986):** During World War II, a baseball player (Pete Gray, outfielder for St. Louis Browns) plays with only one arm lost as a child and becomes an inspiration for a young boy also with one arm. Gray went into the sport of baseball after his brother became brain damaged while boxing. Initially he got his first job in minor league with the Memphis Chicks because of his oddity value. He proves his worth and, with the drain of many major league players to the war, he earns promotion. The boy, Nelson Gary Jr., who he encourages, also became a minor league player. (TV Film/Rated G)

- **The Mighty (1998):** This is the story of a boy who has difficulty getting around. He has a taste for adventure stories and befriends his neighbor who is physically strong but mentally challenged. (Rated PG-13)

- **Simon Birch (1998):** This is a story about a young boy who is short and has difficulty getting around. Follow his story as he tries to figure out his place in the world. (Rated PG)

Source: "Kids Quest on Disabilities and Health," National Center on Birth Defects and Developmental Disabilities, Centers for Disease Control and Prevention (CDC), September 2006.

What's In It For You?

Physical activity has the same benefits for everyone, whether or not they have a disability. It builds your endurance. It keeps your body strong, including your heart, lungs, muscles, and bones. Exercise is a must for staying healthy.

Physical activity also helps increase your flexibility and coordination. It can keep your weight at a healthy level too. If your disability makes moving a challenge, these are especially great benefits. If you get upset or frustrated at times, physical activity also lets you work out your stress. You can prove to yourself that you can do whatever you set out to achieve.

The keys to being an athlete are choosing the right sport, getting the right gear, and keeping at it. In many cases, colleges have athletic programs for people with disabilities, so you may be able to continue to compete in your favorite activity through college and beyond. The activity that's best for you and the gear you may need depend on your personality and what type of disability you have.

Part Four

Maintaining Health And Fitness

Chapter 28

Take Charge Of Your Health

You may feel stressed from school, after-school activities, peer pressure, and family relationships. Your busy schedule may lead you to skip breakfast, buy lunch from vending machines, and grab whatever is in the refrigerator for dinner when you get home. Yet healthy behaviors like nutritious eating and regular physical activity may help you meet the challenges of your life. In fact, healthy eating and regular exercise can help you feel energized, learn better, and stay alert in class. These healthy habits may also lower your risk for diseases such as diabetes, asthma, heart disease, and some forms of cancer.

Dieting Is Not The Answer

The best way to lose weight is to eat healthfully and be physically active. It is a good idea to talk with your health care provider if you want to lose weight.

Many teens turn to unhealthy dieting methods to lose weight including eating very little, cutting out whole groups of foods (like grain products), skipping meals, and fasting. These methods can leave out important foods you need to grow. Other weight loss tactics such as smoking, self-induced vomiting, or using diet pills or laxatives can lead to health problems.

About This Chapter: This chapter includes information from "Take Charge Of Your Health," NIH Publication No. 06-4328, Weight-control Information Network, an information service of the National Institute of Diabetes and Digestive and Kidney Diseases (NIDDK), September 2006.

♣ It's A Fact!!
Did You Know?

From 2003 to 2004, approximately 17.4 percent of
U.S. teens between the ages of 12 and 19 were overweight.

Overweight children and teens are at high risk for developing serious
diseases. Type 2 diabetes and heart disease were considered adult
diseases, but they are now being reported in children and teens.

Source: Weight-control Information Network,
September 2006.

In fact, unhealthy dieting can actually cause you to gain more weight because it often leads to a cycle of eating very little, then overeating or binge eating. Also, unhealthy dieting can put you at greater risk for growth and emotional problems.

Take Charge

This information is designed to help you take small and simple steps to keep a healthy weight. It gives you basic facts about nutrition and physical activity, and offers practical tools that you can use in your everyday life, from reading food labels and selecting how much and what foods to eat, to replacing TV time with physical activities.

Healthy Eating

Eating healthfully means getting the right balance of nutrients your body needs to perform every day. You can find out more about your nutritional needs by checking out the 2005 Dietary Guidelines for Americans. Published by the U.S. Government, this publication explains how much of each type of food you should eat, along with great information on nutrition and physical activity. The guidelines suggest the number of calories you should eat daily based on your gender, age, and activity level.

According to the guidelines, a healthy eating plan includes a variety of foods.

- Fruits and vegetables

- Fat-free or low-fat milk and milk products

- Lean meats, poultry, fish, beans, eggs, and nuts

- Whole grains

In addition, a healthy diet is low in saturated and trans fats, cholesterol, salt, and added sugars.

When it comes to food portions, the Dietary Guidelines use the word "servings" to describe a standard amount of food. Serving sizes are measured as "ounce" or "cup" equivalents." Listed below are some tips based on the guidelines that can help you develop healthy eating habits for a lifetime.

Eat fruits and vegetables every day. When consumed as part of a well-balanced and nutritious eating plan, fruits and vegetables can help keep you healthy. You may get your servings from fresh, frozen, dried, and canned fruits and vegetables. Teenagers who are consuming 2,000 calories per day should aim for two cups of fruit and 2½ cups of vegetables every day. You may need fewer or more servings depending on your individual calorie needs, which your health care provider can help you determine.

Count your calcium. Calcium helps strengthen bones and teeth. This nutrient is very important since getting enough calcium now can reduce the risk for broken bones later in life. Yet most teens get less than the recommended 1,200 mg of calcium per day. Aim for at least three one-cup equivalents of low-fat or fat-free calcium-rich foods and beverages each day.

Power up with protein. Protein builds and repairs body tissue like muscles and organs. Eating enough protein can help you grow strong and sustain your energy levels. Teens need 5½ one-ounce equivalents of protein-rich foods each day.

Go whole grain. Grain foods help give you energy. Whole-grain foods like whole-wheat bread, brown rice, and oatmeal usually have more nutrients than refined grain products. They give you a feeling of fullness and add bulk to your diet. Try to get six one-ounce equivalents of grains every day, with at least three one-ounce equivalents coming from whole-grain sources.

Know your fats. Fat is also an important nutrient. It helps your body grow and develop, and it is a source of energy as well—it even keeps your skin and hair healthy. But be aware that some fats are better for you than others. Limit your fat intake to 25–35 percent of your total calories each day. Unsaturated fat can be part of a healthy diet—as long as you do not eat too much since it is still high in calories. Good sources include olive, canola, safflower, sunflower, corn, and soybean oils; fish like salmon, trout, tuna, and whitefish; and nuts like walnuts, almonds, peanuts, and cashews. Limit saturated fat, which can clog your arteries and raise your risk for heart disease. Saturated fat is found primarily in animal products and in a few plant oils.

- Butter
- Full-fat cheese
- Whole milk
- Fatty meats
- Coconut, palm, and palm kernel oils

Limit trans fat, which is also bad for your heart.

- Baked goods like cookies, muffins, and doughnuts
- Snack foods like crackers and chips
- Vegetable shortening
- Stick margarine
- Fried foods

Look for words like "shortening," "partially hydrogenated vegetable oil," or "hydrogenated vegetable oil" in the list of ingredients. These ingredients tell you that the food contains trans fat. Packaged food products are required to list trans fat on their Nutrition Facts.

Replenish your body with iron. Teen boys need iron to support their rapid growth—most boys double their lean body mass between the ages of 10 and 17. Teen girls also need iron to support growth and replace blood lost during menstruation. To get the iron you need, eat iron-rich foods.

- Fish and shellfish

- Lean beef

- Iron-fortified cereals

- Enriched and whole-grain breads

- Cooked dried beans and peas like black beans, kidney beans, black-eyed peas, and chickpeas (also known as garbanzo beans)

- Spinach

Control your food portions. The portion sizes that you get away from home at a restaurant, grocery store, or school event may contain more food than you need to eat in one sitting. Research shows that when people are served more food, they eat more food. Use these tips to control your food portions.

- When eating out, share your meal, order a half-portion, or order an appetizer as a main meal. Be aware that some appetizers are larger than others and can have as many calories as an entree.

- Take at least half of your meal home.

- When eating at home, take one serving out of a package (read the Nutrition Facts to find out how big a serving is) and eat it off a plate instead of eating straight out of a box or bag.

- Avoid eating in front of the TV or while you are busy with other activities. It is easy to lose track of how much you are eating if you eat while doing other things.

- Eat slowly so your brain can get the message that your stomach is full.

- Do not skip meals. Skipping meals may lead you to eat more high-calorie, high-fat foods at your next meal or snack. Eat breakfast every day.

Read food labels. When you read a food label, pay special attention to serving size, calories and nutrients, and the percentage daily value (%DV).

- **Serving size:** Check the amount of food in a serving. Do you eat more or less? The "servings per container" line tells you the number of servings in the food package.

It's Your Lunch. Get Involved.

Help out with your lunch. Work out a menu for the week so you can choose different foods that you like and are still good for you. When your parents go to the grocery store, ask them to get the stuff you need. To keep things simple, try snack-size packs or get big packages of your favorite foods, repack enough for each day in sandwich bags, and then grab them when it's time to throw lunch together. If mornings get hectic, try packing your lunch the night before. Just make sure you keep the cold stuff in the fridge until it's time to go.

Get creative. Try to jazz up your lunch by using different kinds of breads like whole-grain pita pockets, tortilla wraps, raisin bread, or English muffins. Make kabobs with cut-up fruits and vegetables and bring along yogurt or salad dressing as a dip. Toss in a salad with some chicken on top. Pack dry cereal or granola to mix into yogurt, or snack on pretzels or trail mix. Choose low-fat or non-fat foods whenever you can—like low-fat yogurt, cheese, or milk.

Use pyramid power. Here's a lunch formula for the power and energy you need to make it through the day.

- Lots of fruits and vegetables (like carrot sticks, celery, or apples)

- A container of milk or yogurt or some cheese

- Some whole-grain bread for a sandwich, cereal mix, or pasta (like spaghetti)

- Some meat (like ham or chicken), tuna fish, hard-boiled eggs, beans (like a bean burrito), or nuts/trail mix

- A little bit of dessert (like pudding or graham crackers)

It's not as tough as it sounds. A turkey and cheese wrap with lettuce and tomato, plus an apple or banana, and some milk would cover all this. Lunch doesn't have to be hard or boring. Take charge. Pack yourself stuff that makes you love lunchtime, and gives you energy to make it through school, practice, and homework—all the way until dinner.

Source: "Power Packing," Department of Health and Human Services, Centers for Disease Control and Prevention (CDC), 2002.

- **Calories and other nutrients:** Remember, the number of calories and other listed nutrients are for one serving only. Food packages often contain more than one serving.

- **Percent Daily Value:** Look at how much of the recommended daily amount of a nutrient (% DV) is in one serving of food—five-percent of the daily value or less is low and 20-percent daily value or more is high. For example, if your breakfast cereal has a 25-percent daily value for iron, it is high in iron.

Plan meals and snacks. You and your family have busy schedules, which can make eating healthfully a challenge. Planning ahead can help. Think about the meals and snacks you would like for the week—including bag lunches to take to school—and help your family make a shopping list. You may even want to go grocery shopping and cook together.

Jump-start your day with breakfast. Did you know that eating breakfast can help you do better in school? By eating breakfast you can increase your attention span and memory, have more energy, and feel less irritable and restless. A breakfast that is part of a healthy diet can also help you maintain an appropriate weight now and in the future.

Pack your lunch. Whether you eat lunch from school or pack your own, this meal should provide you with one-third of the day's nutritional needs. A lunch of chips, cookies, candy, or soda just gives you lots of calories, but not many nutrients. Instead of buying snacks from vending machines at school, bring food from home. Try packing your lunch with a lean turkey sandwich on whole-grain bread, healthy foods like fruits, vegetables, low-fat yogurt, and nuts.

Snack smart. A healthy snack can contribute to a healthy eating plan and give you the energy boost you need to get through the day. Try these snack ideas, but keep in mind that most of these foods should be eaten in small amounts.

- Fruit—any kind—fresh, canned, dried, or frozen
- Peanut butter on rice cakes or whole-wheat crackers
- Baked potato chips or tortilla chips with salsa
- Veggies with low-fat dip
- String cheese, low-fat cottage cheese, or low-fat yogurt

♣ It's A Fact!!

Power Packing

Did you know germs that grow on food can make lots more germs in a little over two hours? Without smart packing, some of your sandwiches and snacks could end up making you sick. You can make sure your lunch gives you the energy you need—not a bellyache you don't need—with these simple tips.

Super Storage

Those puffy, insulated lunch boxes or bags keep cold food cold and hot food hot, so germs can't multiply like crazy. Regular lunch boxes and paper bags are okay too, but you have to help them keep stuff the right temperature. So, if you've got one of those, follow these cool rules.

Double bag your lunch. The layers of paper and air help keep the cold in. Or, put an ice pack or frozen juice box in a plastic sandwich bag (a zip-up one so your sandwich doesn't get soggy) to make your lunch bag a mini cooler. If you go for the juice box, get the real stuff—100% juice. Don't worry, your drink will thaw by lunchtime. And depending on how cold your locker or classroom is, you might even get a slushy. If you make sandwiches the night before, keep them in the refrigerator or freezer until you pack up to go in the morning.

Make hot bites. On cold days, nothing can warm you up like hot soup, pasta, or chili. The key is to keep the hot lunch hot until it's time to eat—making it hard for germs to grow in it. Try using a thermos.

- Frozen fruit bars, fruit sorbet, or low-fat frozen yogurt
- Vanilla wafers, graham crackers, animal crackers, or fig bars
- Popcorn (air popped or low-fat microwave)

Eat dinner with your family. For many teens, dinner consists of eating on the run, snacking in front of the TV, or nonstop munching from after school to bedtime. Try to eat dinner as a family instead. Believe it or not, when you eat with your family you are more likely to get more fruits, vegetables, and other foods with the vitamins and minerals your body needs. Family meals also help you reconnect after a busy day. Talk to your family about fitting in at least a few meals together throughout the week.

Pack it light and tight. Keep your food wrapped up and make sure to wrap each part separately so that they don't leak onto each other. Use zipper plastic bags, plastic containers made for carrying food, or get one-serving packs (like yogurt, pudding, or fruit cups). You can skip wrapping up fruits like apples, oranges, and bananas—Mother Nature already did it for you! Just be sure to wash your fruits and veggies before you take a bite. If you peel them, though, wrap them up and chill them. Here are some foods that are good to go all of the time.

- Fruits
- Vegetables
- Bread
- Crackers
- Peanut butter
- Jelly

- Pickles
- Nuts
- Pretzels
- Graham crackers
- Trail mix
- Fruit cups

Wash it or toss it. Food is not the only thing that can carry germs—you can too. So, wash your hands with soap and water before you make your lunch, before you eat, and after you're finished. Also, wash fruits and vegetables under cold, running water before packing them in your lunch. Pack your lunch with only the amount of food you think you'll eat and toss out any leftovers. Make sure that you wash your containers and lunch box every day, or get yourself a new paper bag.

Source: "Power Packing," the Department of Health and Human Services, Centers for Disease Control and Prevention (CDC), 2002.

Limit fast food and choose wisely. Like many teens, you may eat at fast food restaurants often. If so, you are probably taking in a lot of extra calories from added sugar and fat. Just one value-sized fast food meal of a sandwich, fries, and sweetened soda can have more calories, fat, and added sugar than anyone should eat in an entire day. The best approach is to limit the amount of fast food you eat. If you do order fast food follow the listed suggestions.

- Skip "value-sized" or "super-sized" meals

- Choose a grilled chicken sandwich or a plain, small burger

- Use mustard instead of mayonnaise

- Limit fried foods or remove breading from fried chicken, which can cut half the fat
- Order garden or grilled chicken salads with light or reduced-calorie dressings
- Choose water, fat-free, or low-fat milk instead of sweetened soda

Rethink your drinks. Soda and other sugary drinks have replaced milk and water as the drinks of choice for teens and adults alike. Yet these drinks are actually more like desserts because they are high in added sugar and calories. In fact, soda and sugar-laden drinks may contribute to weight problems in kids and teens. Try sticking to water, low-fat milk, or fat-free milk.

Physical Activity

Like eating well, physical activity may help you feel good. Physical activity also helps your body in other ways.

- It helps you control your weight, build lean muscle, and reduce your body fat
- It strengthens your bones
- It increases flexibility and balance
- It reduces your risk for chronic diseases like type 2 diabetes, heart disease, and high blood pressure

Physical activity also has possible emotional and social benefits.

- It improves self-esteem and mood
- It decreases feelings of anxiety and depression
- It helps you do better in school
- It improves you teamwork skills through sports

Be Active Every Day

Physical activity should be part of your daily life, whether you play sports, take physical education or other exercise classes, or even get from place to place by walking or bicycling. Teens should be physically active for 60 minutes or more on most, preferably all, days of the week.

✔ Quick Tip
Turn Off The TV And Get Moving

Can too much TV contribute to weight problems?
Several research studies say yes. In fact, one study noted
that boys and girls who watched the most TV had more body
fat than those who watched TV less than two hours a day.

Try to cut back on your TV, computer, and video game time and get
moving instead. Here are some tips to help you break the TV habit.

Tape your favorite shows and watch them later. This cuts down on TV
time because you plan to watch specific shows instead of zoning out
and flipping through the channels indefinitely.

**Replace after-school TV watching and video game use
with physical activities.** Get involved with activities at
your school or in your community.

Source: Weight-control Information
Network, September 2006.

Making It Work

Look for chances to move more and eat better at home, at school, and in
the community. It is not easy to maintain a healthy weight in today's environment. Fast food restaurants on every corner, vending machines at schools,
and not enough safe places for physical activity can make it difficult to eat
healthfully and be active. Busy schedules may also keep families from fixing
and eating dinners together. Understanding your home, school, and community is an important step in changing your eating and activity habits.

Old habits are hard to break and new ones, especially those related to
eating and physical activity, can take months to develop and stick with, so
make changes slowly. Do not expect to change your eating or activity habits
overnight. Changing too much too fast can hurt your chances of success.

Chapter 29

Exercise And Weight Control

Just about everybody seems to be interested in weight control. Some of us weigh just the right amount and others need to gain a few pounds. Most of us "battle the bulge" at some time in our life. Whatever our goals, we should understand and take advantage of the important role of exercise in keeping our weight under control.

Carrying around too much body fat is a major nuisance. Yet excess body fat is common in modern-day living. Few of today's occupations require vigorous physical activity, and much of our leisure time is spent in sedentary pursuits.

Recent estimates indicate that 34 million adults are considered obese and 20 percent are above desirable weight. Also, there has been an increase in body fat levels in children and youth over the past 20 years. After infancy and early childhood, the earlier the onset of obesity, the greater the likelihood of remaining obese.

Excess body fat has been linked to such health problems as coronary heart disease, high blood pressure, osteoporosis, diabetes, arthritis, and certain forms cancer. Some evidence now exists showing that obesity has a negative effect on both health and longevity.

About This Chapter: This chapter includes information from "Exercise And Weight Control," from The President's Council on Physical Fitness and Sports, October 2004.

Exercise is associated with the loss of body fat in obese and normal weight persons. A regular program of exercise is an important component of any plan to help individuals lose, gain, or maintain their weight.

Overweight Or Overfat?

Overweight and overfat do not always mean the same thing. Some people are quite muscular and weigh more than the average for their age and height. However, their body composition, the amount of fat versus lean body mass (muscle, bone, organs, and tissue), is within a desirable range. This is true for many athletes. Others weigh an average amount yet carry around too much fat. In our society, however, overweight often implies overfat because excess weight is commonly distributed as excess fat. The addition of exercise to a weight control program helps control both body weight and body fat levels.

A certain amount of body fat is necessary for everyone. Experts say that the percentage of body fat for women should about 20 percent, 15 percent for men. Women with more than 30 percent fat and men with more than 25 fat are considered obese.

How much of your weight that is fat can be assessed by a variety of methods including underwater (hydrostatic) weighing, skinfold thickness measurements, and circumference measurements. Each requires a trained person to administer the test and perform correct calculations. From the numbers obtained, a body fat percentage is determined. Assessing body composition has an advantage over the standard height-weight because it can help distinguish between "overweight" and "overfat."

An easy self-test you can do is to pinch the thickness of the fat folds at your waist and abdomen. If you can pinch an inch or more of fat (make sure no muscle is included) chances are you have too much body fat.

People who exercise appropriately increase lean body mass while decreasing their overall fat level. Depending on the amount of fat loss, this can result in a loss of inches without a loss of weight, since muscle weighs more than fat. However, with the proper combination of diet and exercise, both body fat and overall weight can be reduced.

Energy Balance: A Weighty Concept

Losing weight, gaining weight, or maintaining your weight depends on the amount of calories you take in and use up during the day, otherwise referred to as energy balance. Learning how to balance energy intake (calories in food) with energy output (calories expended through physical activity) will help you achieve your desired weight.

Although the underlying causes and the treatments of obesity are complex, the concept of energy balance is relatively simple. If you eat more calories than your body needs to perform your day's activities, the extra calories are stored as fat. If you do not take in enough calories to meet your body's energy needs, your body will go to the stored fat to make up the difference. (Exercise helps ensure that stored fat, rather than muscle tissue, is used to meet your energy needs.) If you eat just about the same amount of calories to meet your body's energy needs, your weight will stay the same.

On the average, a person consumes between 800,000 and 900,000 calories each year. An active person needs more calories than a sedentary person does, as physically active people require energy above and beyond the day's basic needs. All too often, people who want to lose weight concentrate on counting calorie intake while neglecting calorie output. The most powerful formula is the combination of dietary modification with exercise. By increasing your daily physical activity and decreasing your caloric input you can lose excess weight in the most efficient and healthful way.

Counting Calories

Each pound of fat your body stores represents 3,500 calories of unused energy. In order to lose one pound, you would have to create a calorie deficit of 3,500 calories by either taking in 3,500 less calories over a period of time than you need or doing 3,500 calories worth of exercise. It is recommended that no more than two pounds (7,000 calories) be lost per week for lasting weight loss.

Adding 15 minutes of moderate exercise, say walking one mile, to your daily schedule will use up 100 extra calories per day. (Your body uses approximately 100 calories of energy to walk one mile, depending on your body weight.) Maintaining this schedule would result in an extra 700 calories per week used up, or a loss of about 10 pounds in one year, assuming your food intake stays the same. To look at energy balance another way, just one extra slice of bread or one extra soft drink a day—or any other food that contains approximately 100 calories—can add up to ten extra pounds in a year if the amount of physical activity you do does not increase.

If you already have a lean figure and want to keep it you should exercise regularly and eat a balanced diet that provides enough calories to make up for the energy you expend. If you wish to gain weight you should exercise regularly and increase the number of calories you consume until you reach your desired weight. Exercise will help ensure that the weight you gain will be lean muscle mass, not extra fat.

The Diet Connection

A balanced diet should be part of any weight control plan. A diet high in complex carbohydrates and moderate in protein and fat will complement an exercise program. It should include enough calories to satisfy your daily nutrient requirements and include the proper number of servings per day from the basic four food groups.

- Vegetables and fruits (4 servings)
- Breads and cereals (4 servings)
- Milk and milk products (2–4 servings, depending on age)
- Meats and fish (2 servings)

Experts recommend that your daily intake not fall below 1200 calories unless you are under a doctor's supervision. Also, weekly weight loss should not exceed two pounds.

Remarkable claims have been made for a variety of "crash" diets and diet pills. And some of these very restricted diets do result in noticeable weight loss in a short time. Much of this loss is water and such a loss is quickly regained when normal food and liquid intake is resumed. These diet plans are often expensive and may be dangerous. Moreover, they do not emphasize lifestyle that will help you maintain your desired weight. Dieting alone will result in a loss of valuable body tissue, such as muscle mass, in addition to a loss in fat.

How Many Calories

The estimates for number of calories (energy) used during a physical activity are based on experiments that measure the amount of oxygen consumed during a specific bout of exercise for a certain body weight.

The energy costs of activities that require you to move your own body weight, such as walking or jogging, are greater for heavier people since they have more weight to move. For example, a person weighing 150 pounds would use more calories jogging one mile than a person jogging alongside who weighs 115 pounds. Always check to see what body weight is referred to in caloric expenditure charts you use.

Exercise And Modern Living

One thing is certain. Most people do not get enough exercise in their ordinary routines. All of the advances of modern technology—from electric can openers to power steering—have made life easier, more comfortable, and much less physically demanding. Yet our bodies need activity, especially if they are carrying around too much fat. Satisfying this need requires a definite plan and a commitment. There are two main ways to increase the number of calories you expend.

1.   Start a regular exercise program if you do not have one already.

2.   Increase the amount of physical activity in your daily routine.

The best way to control your weight is a combination of the above. The sum total of calories used over time will help regulate your weight as well as keep you physically fit.

Active Lifestyles

Before looking at what kind of regular exercise program is best, let's look at how you can increase the amount of physical activity in your daily routine to supplement your exercise program.

• **Pursue recreational pursuits.** Gardening on weekends, bowling in a league, family outings, an evening of social dancing, and many other activities provide added exercise. They are fun and can be considered an extra bonus in your weight control campaign.

- **Add more "action" to your day.** Walk to the neighborhood grocery store instead of using the car. Park several blocks from school and walk the rest of the way. Walk up the stairs instead of using the elevator. Start with one flight of steps and gradually increase the steps over time.

- **Change your attitude toward movement.** Instead of considering an extra little walk or trip an annoyance, look upon it as an added fitness boost. Look for opportunities to use your body. Bend, stretch, reach, move, lift, and carry. Timesaving devices and gadgets eliminate drudgery and are a bonus to mankind, but when they substitute too often for physical activity they can demand a high cost in health, vigor, and fitness.

These little bits of action are cumulative in their effects. Alone, each does not burn a huge amount of calories. When added together, though, they can result in a sizable amount of energy used over the course of the day. Plus, they will help improve your muscle tone and flexibility at the same time.

What Kind Of Exercise?

Although any kind of physical movement requires energy (calories), the type of exercise that uses the most energy is aerobic exercise. The term "aerobic" is derived from the Greek word meaning "with oxygen." Jogging, brisk walking, swimming, biking, cross-country skiing, and aerobic dancing are some popular forms of aerobic exercise.

Aerobic exercises use the body's large muscle groups in continuous, rhythmic, sustained movement, and require oxygen for the production of energy. When oxygen is combined with food (which can come from stored fat) energy is produced to power the body's musculature. The longer you move aerobically, the more energy needed and the more calories used. Regular aerobic exercise will improve your cardiorespiratory endurance. It will also improve the ability of your heart, lungs, blood vessels, and associated tissues to use oxygen to produce energy needed for activity. You'll build a healthier body while getting rid of excess body fat.

In addition to the aerobic exercise, supplement your program with muscle strengthening and stretching exercises. The stronger your muscles, the longer you will be able to keep going during aerobic activity and the less chance of injury.

Tips To Get You Started

✔ Quick Tip

Hopefully, you are now convinced that in order to successfully manage your weight you must include exercise in your daily routine. Here are some tips to get you started.

- **Check with your doctor first.** Since you are carrying around some extra baggage, it is wise to get your doctor's OK before embarking on an exercise program.

- **Choose activities that you think you'll enjoy.** Most people will stick to their exercise program if they are having fun, even though they are working hard.

- **Set aside a regular exercise time.** Whether this means joining an exercise class or getting up a little earlier every day, make time for this addition to your routine and don't let anything get in your way. Planning ahead will help you get around interruptions in your workout schedule, such as bad weather and vacations.

- **Set short term goals.** Don't expect to lose 20 pounds in two weeks. It has taken awhile for you to gain the weight and it will take time to lose it. Keep a record of your progress and tell your friends and family about your achievements.

- **Vary your exercise program.** Change exercises or invite friends to join you to make your workout more enjoyable. There is no "best" exercise— just the one that works best for you. It won't be easy, especially at the start. As you begin to feel better, look better, and enjoy a new zest for life, you will be rewarded many times over for your efforts.

How Much? How Often?

Experts recommend that you do some form of aerobic exercise at least three times a week for a minimum of 20 continuous minutes. Of course, if that is too much, start with a shorter time span and gradually build up to the minimum. Gradually progress until you are able to work aerobically for 20–40 minutes. If you need to lose a large amount of weight, you may want to do your aerobic workout five times a week.

It is important to exercise at an intensity vigorous enough to cause your heart rate and breathing to increase. How hard you should exercise depends to a certain degree on your age and is determined by measuring your heart rate in beats per minute. The heart rate you should maintain is called your target heart rate and there are several ways you can arrive at this figure. The simplest is to subtract your age from 220 and then calculate 60 to 80 percent of that figure. Beginners should maintain the 60 percent level, more advanced can work up to the 80 percent level. This is just a guide, however, and people with any medical limitations should discuss this formula with their physician.

You can do different types of aerobic activities like walking one day and riding a bike the next. Make sure you choose an activity that can be done regularly and is enjoyable for you. The important thing to remember is not to skip too many days between workouts or fitness benefits will be lost. If you must lose a few days, gradually work back into your routine.

The Benefits Of Exercise In A Weight Control Program

The benefits of exercise are many, from producing physically fit bodies to providing an outlet for fun and socialization. When added to a weight control program these benefits take on increased significance.

We already have noted that proper exercise can help control weight by burning excess body fat. It also has two other body-trimming advantages.

1. Exercise builds muscle tissue and muscle uses calories up at a faster rate than body fat.

2. Exercise helps reduce inches and a firm, lean body looks slimmer even if your weight remains the same.

Remember, fat does not turn into muscle, as is often believed. Fat and muscle are two entirely different substances and one cannot become the other. However, muscle does use calories at a faster rate than fat, which directly affects your body's metabolic rate or energy requirement. Your basal metabolic rate (BMR) is the amount of energy required to sustain the body's functions at rest and it depends on your age, sex, body size, genes, and body composition. People with high levels of muscle tend to have higher BMRs and use more calories in the resting stage.

Some studies have even shown that your metabolic rate stays elevated for some time after vigorous exercise, causing you to use even more calories throughout your day. Additional benefits may be seen in how exercise affects appetite. A lean person in good shape may eat more following increased activity, but the regular exercise will burn up the extra calories consumed. On the other hand, vigorous exercise has been reported to suppress appetite, making physical activity a positive substitute for between meal snacking.

✔ **Quick Tip**

Adopt a specific plan and write it down.

Keep setting realistic goals as you go along and remind yourself of them often.

Keep a log to record your progress and make sure to keep it up-to-date.

Include weight and/or percent body fat measures in your log. Extra pounds can easily creep back.

Upgrade your fitness program as you progress.

Enlist the support and company of your family and friends.

Update others on your successes.

Avoid injuries by pacing yourself and including a warm-up and cool-down period as part of every workout.

Reward yourself periodically for a job well done.

Better Mental Health

The psychological benefits of exercise are equally important to the weight conscious person. Exercise decreases stress and relieves tensions that might otherwise lead to overeating. Exercise builds physical fitness, which in turn builds self-confidence, enhanced self-image, and a positive outlook. When you start to feel good about yourself, you are more likely to want to make other positive changes in your lifestyle that will help keep your weight under control.

In addition, exercise can be fun, provide recreation, and offer opportunities for companionship. The exhilaration and emotional release of participating in sports or other activities are a boost to mental and physical health. Pent-up anxieties and frustrations seem to disappear when you're concentrating on returning a serve, sinking a putt or going that extra mile.

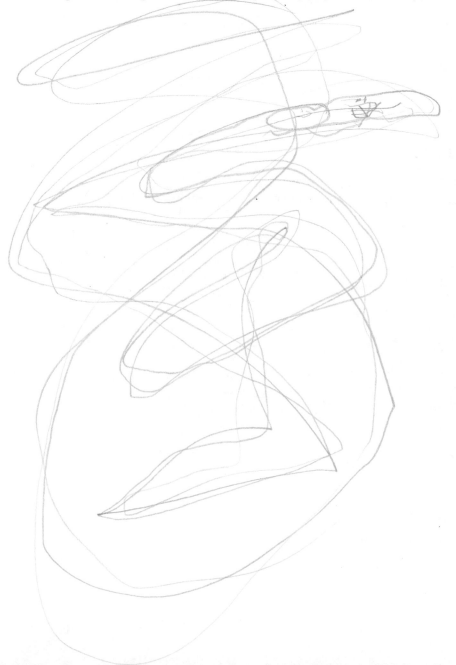

Chapter 30

Water: An Essential Nutrient

Fluids

Do you pass by water stations in road races or skip water breaks during practice because you are not thirsty? Have you ever felt fatigued, dizzy, or cramps while exercising in hot weather? If you answered yes to either of these questions, read on to learn how important fluids are for optimal health and performance. If your answers were no, read on to make sure you are following fluid recommendations that will optimize your health and performance.

Role In The Body

Water is key to life. Humans can survive more than a month without food, but only a few days without water. Water is found inside and outside cells and circulates in the blood. Our body consists of about 60–65% of water. For a 150-pound person, this represents approximately 90–98 pounds of water. Water plays many important roles in the body including:

Transportation

- Water transports glucose, oxygen, and fat to working muscles.

- Water transports waste products, such as carbon dioxide and lactic acid away from working muscles.

About This Chapter: "Fluids," © 2007 Iowa State University Extension Service. Reprinted with permission.

Body Temperature Regulation

- The body wants to keep a constant temperature of approximately 98.6° F or 37° C. If the body temperature increases to more than 106° F or 41° C, cells will die.

- Working muscles generate heat. In fact, the body can generate 20 times more heat when working, than when at rest.

- To prevent overheating, the body regulates temperature by sweating. Water absorbs heat from the working muscles and dissipates this heat to circulating blood and ultimately through the skin.

- Sweat evaporates from the skin, which cools it down. This cools down the blood and the rest of the body.

Urine

- Water transports and eliminates waste-products in the urine.

- The darker the urine indicates a greater concentration of waste-products and less water—this indicates dehydration.

- Vitamin/mineral supplementation can result in dark urine. Since supplements of individual vitamins or minerals (such as, Vitamin C, selenium, or chromium) may contain more than the body can absorb, they are excreted in the urine.

> ♣ **It's A Fact!!**
> **Steamy Situation**
> When your body temperature gets hotter than normal—98.6 degrees—your brain sends out a distress signal that causes you to sweat, which cools you down. Think of it this way—your body, like an air conditioner, has an internal thermostat that helps control its temperature. Whenever your body heats up from physical activity or the hot weather outside, your internal air conditioner turns on and you begin to sweat. And remember, now that your air conditioner is using its coolant (your sweat), it is important to refill the tank—by drinking lots of water.
>
> Source: Excerpted from "Keeping Your Cool," Department of Health and Human Services, Centers for Disease Control and Prevention, 2002.

Digestion

- Water is an important component of saliva and gastric juices, which help digest food.

Lubrication

- Water is a good lubricator of joints, organs, and tissues.

Role In The Diet

Water comes from more than just fluids. It is a major component of many foods. In fact, it is estimated that 20% of our water needs are met through food, not fluids. Foods with high water content add volume but minimal calories to the diet. Thus, these foods high in water are known to promote a feeling of fullness.

Fruits and vegetables are two food groups that have generally high water content. Even meat, bread, and dairy products contain some water.

Example of fruits and vegetables high in water include:

Dehydration

Athletes need to stay hydrated for optimal performance. Many athletes drink when they are thirsty and fail to hydrate before they become dehydrated. Thirst is a biological indicator of dehydration; however, dehydration has already occurred when an athlete becomes thirsty. Even a small drop in body fluids (one percent of body weight or 1.5 pounds in a 150-pound person) can impair performance.

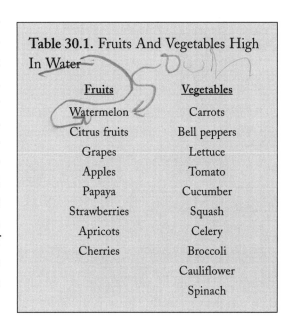

Table 30.1. Fruits And Vegetables High In Water

Fruits	Vegetables
Watermelon	Carrots
Citrus fruits	Bell peppers
Grapes	Lettuce
Apples	Tomato
Papaya	Cucumber
Strawberries	Squash
Apricots	Celery
Cherries	Broccoli
	Cauliflower
	Spinach

Causes Of Dehydration

- Inadequate fluid intake

- Profuse sweating

- Failure to replace losses after exercise

- Exercising in hot weather, regardless of fluid consumption

- Relying on thirst to hydrate

Dehydration, or excessive fluid loss, causes the blood volume to drop. This increases heart rate as it tries to compensate for the decreased blood supply to the organs. Muscle cramps, dizziness, and fatigue are caused by dehydration and can increase the risk for injury.

Dehydration can lead to heat illness, which impacts physical performance. Signs of heat illness are:

- Headache, dizziness;

- Nausea, vomiting;

- Weakness, reduced performance;

- Irritability;

- Irrational behavior;

- Inability to concentrate;

- Fatigue;

- Muscle Cramps;

- Confusion/disorientation.

♣ **It's A Fact!!**
The daily recommended fluid intake is 10–15 glasses (8-ounce glass) depending on your age and sex. Females and younger people are at the lower end of the range while males are at the upper end of the range. Foods contribute 20% of the fluids so actual fluid recommendations are 8–13 glasses (8-ounce glass) daily. Focus on fruits and vary your veggies to help with fluid intake.

Source: © 2007 Iowa State University Extension Service.

Signs of dehydration and heat illness directly related to performance include reduced muscular strength and endurance.

Even a two to four percent loss of body water (3–6 pound loss for a 150-pound person) will reduce muscular strength and endurance. Studies have shown reduced isometric and isotonic muscular contraction of 20–25% with four-percent dehydration. In addition, 24–36 hours are needed to fully recover muscular strength and endurance after dehydration. This is noteworthy because wrestlers commonly use dehydration to make weight. This practice compromises their muscular strength and endurance and there is not enough time between weigh-in and competition to adequately rehydrate.

👉 **Remember!!**

Athletes have greater fluid needs related to the role of water in physical activity. Thirst alone does not adequately supply these fluid needs, it will only supply 50% of fluid needs.

Source: © 2007 Iowa State University Extension Service.

Urine volume and color are good indicators of hydration. A light colored urine indicates adequate hydration. In addition, a larger volume of urine indicates better hydration. Since vitamin supplements can make the urine darker, volume may be the better indicator for those taking vitamin supplements.

Prevention

It is important to adequately hydrate before, during, and after exercising to prevent dehydration. Keep in mind the following factors that will influence your fluid needs:

- **Altitude:** Fluid requirements are greater at high altitudes.

- **Climate:** If the temperature is warm you will need to consume more water. Even during a cold day when you may not sweat as readily. It is very important to hydrate.

- **Sweat:** Individuals who sweat easily and in large quantities are at greater risk for dehydration. Estimate your sweat rate per hour by weighing yourself before and after.

  1. If you lose two pounds in one hour, you lose 32 ounces of fluid. This translates into a consumption of 8 ounces of water every 15 minutes.

  2. To make fluid replacement easy, measure eight ounces of water and then count how many gulps it takes to drink. Then use the number of gulps as a guideline.

- **Type and length of activity:** The intensity and length of duration of an activity will determine the need for fluids. Endurance athletes who exercise for hours will lose more water and may be more sensitive to dehydration for optimal performance than a sprinter. Swimmers may not feel the heat and the extent of sweating from exercise due to the cooling effect of the water thus are at increased risk for dehydration. Wrestlers who dehydrate themselves before weigh-ins will impair their performance and place themselves at risk for health problems related to dehydration.

Pre, During, And Post Exercise Hydration

Adequate fluid consumption before, during, and after exercise is very important for optimal athletic performance and health.

Pre-Exercise Hydration

- 17–20 fluid ounces, two to three hours before practice or competition
- 7–10 fluid ounces after the warm-up (10–15 min before practice/competition)

During Exercise

- 7–10 fluid ounces every 10–15 minutes of practice or competition
- Drink a fluid replacement drink after 15–30 minutes of practice or competition if exercise will last more than 90 minutes.
- Carbohydrate content should not exceed eight percent (about 19 grams per cup).

Post-Exercise Hydration

- Replace fluid loss.
- Weigh yourself before and after practice to estimate the water loss.
- Drink three cups of water for every one pound lost.
- Drink a carbohydrate containing sports drink within 15 minutes post exercise to begin restoring glycogen and optimize performance for the following event.

♣ It's A Fact!!

How Much Water Is Too Much?

While dehydration is a more common concern for exercisers, some experts think the public should be aware of the danger of drinking too much water, which can lead to a potentially fatal condition called hyponatremia.

Characterized by an abnormally low blood concentration of sodium, it is most often seen at extremely high-endurance events such as ultra-marathons.

Hyponatremia is more common among women than men, and was responsible for the death of a 43-year-old woman running in the Chicago Marathon last year.

Symptoms include nausea, vomiting, muscle weakness, headache and disorientation, and bloating in the face and hands.

Research suggests that drinking about two cups of fluid two hours before exercise and another six to eight ounces every 20 minutes can help optimize performance.

Some exercisers may opt to measure the amount of fluid they lose by weighing themselves before and after exercise to determine the number of pounds lost through perspiration. For every pound lost, experts recommend drinking one pint of fluid during exercise.

Sports drinks may also be a good choice because they help replace lost sodium and have been shown to enhance performance during prolonged exercise.

Source: "How Much Water Is Too Much?" © American Council on Exercise (www.acefitness.org). All rights reserved. Reprinted with permission. Accessed May 2008.

Overhydration (Hyponatremia)

Although rare, overhydration, also known as hyponatremia, can occur in athletes. Athletes with a high concentration of sodium in their sweat, who consume large/excessive quantities of water, or exercise long periods of time (4–6 hours) are at greatest risk for hyponatremia. Hyponatremia is a serious condition, which in worst cases can be fatal. Hyponatremia occurs when plasma sodium concentrations reach less than 135 mmol/L (normal levels are 138–142 mmol/L).

Hyponatremia can cause gastrointestinal problems (bloating, nausea, etc.), wheezy breathing, swollen hands and feet, unusual fatigue, and incoordination. Life-threatening problems include swelling of the brain, which can result in throbbing headache, confusion, seizures, coma, and death.

Determine if you are at risk...

- Do you have high sweat volumes and high sweat salt concentrations?

- If you sweat large amounts and notice white salt on your skin, or if your sweat stings your eyes, the sodium concentration is high.

- Do you exercise for hours?

- Do you eat a low sodium diet and consume excessive amounts of water?

Chapter 31

Sports Nutrition

What diet is best for athletes?

It's important that an athlete's diet provides the right amount of energy, the 50-plus nutrients the body needs and adequate water. No single food or supplement can do this. A variety of foods are needed every day. But, just as there is more than one way to achieve a goal, there is more than one way to follow a nutritious diet.

Do the nutritional needs of athletes differ from non-athletes?

Competitive athletes, sedentary individuals, and people who exercise for health and fitness all need the same nutrients. However, because of the intensity of their sport or training program, some athletes have higher calorie and fluid requirements. Eating a variety of foods to meet increased calorie needs helps to ensure that the athlete's diet contains appropriate amounts of carbohydrate, protein, vitamins, and minerals.

Are there certain dietary guidelines athletes should follow?

Health and nutrition professionals recommend that 55–60% of the calories in our diet come from carbohydrate, no more than 30% from fat, and the remaining 10–15% from protein. While the exact percentages may vary

About This Chapter: This chapter includes information from "Questions Most Frequently Asked About Sports Nutrition," The President's Council on Physical Fitness and Sports, U.S. Department of Health and Human Services, October 2004.

slightly for some athletes based on their sport or training program, these guidelines will promote health and serve as the basis for a diet that will maximize performance.

How many calories do I need a day?

This depends on your age, body size, sport, and training program. For example, a 250-pound weight lifter needs more calories than a 98-pound gymnast. Exercise or training may increase calorie needs by as much as 1,000 to 1,500 calories a day. The best way to determine if you're getting too few or too many calories is to monitor your weight. Keeping within your ideal competitive weight range means that you are getting the right amount of calories.

☞ **Remember!!**

Your calorie needs depend on your age, body size, sport, and training program.

The best way to make sure you are not getting too many or too few calories is to check your weight from time to time.

If you're keeping within your ideal weight range, you're probably getting the right amount of calories.

Source: "Fast Facts About Sports Nutrition," from The President's Council on Physical Fitness and Sports, U.S. Department of Health and Human Services, October 2004.

Which is better for replacing fluids—water or sports drinks?

Depending on how muscular you are, 55–70% of your body weight is water. Being "hydrated" means maintaining your body's fluid level. When you sweat, you lose water, which must be replaced if you want to perform your best. You need to drink fluids before, during, and after all workouts and events. Whether you drink water or a sports drink is a matter of choice. However, if your workout or event lasts for more than 90 minutes, you may benefit from the carbohydrates provided by sports drinks. A sports drink that contains 15–18 grams of carbohydrate in every eight ounces of fluid should be used. Drinks with a higher carbohydrate content will delay the absorption of water and may cause dehydration, cramps, nausea, or diarrhea. There are a variety of sports drinks on the market. Be sure to experiment with sports drinks during practice instead of trying them for the first time the day of an event.

What are electrolytes?

Electrolytes are nutrients that affect fluid balance in the body and are necessary for our nerves and muscles to function. Sodium and potassium are the two electrolytes most often added to sports drinks. Generally, electrolyte replacement is not needed during short bursts of exercise since sweat is approximately 99% water and less than one-percent electrolytes. Water, in combination with a well-balanced diet, will restore normal fluid and electrolyte levels in the body. However, replacing electrolytes may be beneficial during continuous activity of longer than two hours, especially in a hot environment.

What do muscles use for energy during exercise?

Most activities use a combination of fat and carbohydrate as energy sources. How hard and how long you work out, your level of fitness, and your diet will affect the type of fuel your body uses. For short-term, high-intensity activities like sprinting, athletes rely mostly on carbohydrate for energy. During low-intensity exercises like walking, the body uses more fat for energy.

What are carbohydrates?

Carbohydrates are sugars and starches found in foods like breads, cereals, fruits, vegetables, pasta, milk, honey, syrups, and table sugar. Carbohydrates are the preferred source of energy for your body. Regardless of origin, your body breaks down carbohydrates into glucose that your blood carries to cells to be used for energy. Carbohydrates provide four calories per gram, while fat provides nine calories per gram. Your body cannot differentiate between glucose that comes from starches or sugars. Glucose from either source provides energy for working muscles.

Is it true that athletes should eat a lot of carbohydrates?

When you are training or competing, your muscles need energy to perform. One source of energy for working muscles is glycogen, which is made

♣ It's A Fact!!
Fast Facts About Sports Nutrition

Water: You can survive for a month without food, but only a few days without water.

Sports Drinks: Water is a fine choice for most workouts. However, during continuous workouts of greater than 90 minutes, your body may benefit from a sports drink.

Carbohydrates: Carbohydrates are your body's main source of energy.

Protein: It is a myth that eating lots of protein and/or taking protein supplements and exercising vigorously will definitely turn you into a big, muscular person.

Vitamins and Minerals: Eating a varied diet will give you all the vitamins and minerals you need for health and peak performance.

Iron: Iron supplies working muscles with oxygen.

Calcium: Many people do not get enough of the calcium needed for strong bones and proper muscle function.

Source: "Fast Facts About Sports Nutrition," from The President's Council on Physical Fitness and Sports, U.S. Department of Health and Human Services, October 2004.

from carbohydrates and stored in your muscles. Every time you work out, you use some of your glycogen. If you don't consume enough carbohydrates, your glycogen stores become depleted, which can result in fatigue. Both sugars and starches are effective in replenishing glycogen stores.

When and what should I eat before I compete?

Performance depends largely on the foods consumed during the days and weeks leading up to an event. If you regularly eat a varied, carbohydrate-rich diet you are in good standing and probably have ample glycogen stores to fuel activity. The purpose of the pre-competition meal is to prevent hunger and to provide the water and additional energy the athlete will need during competition. Most athletes eat two to four hours before their event. However, some athletes perform their best if they eat a small amount 30 minutes before competing, while others eat nothing for six hours beforehand. For many athletes, carbohydrate-rich foods serve as the basis of the meal. However, there is no magic pre-event diet. Simply choose foods and beverages that you enjoy and that don't bother your stomach. Experiment during the weeks before an event to see which foods work best for you.

Will eating sugary foods before an event hurt my performance?

In the past, athletes were warned that eating sugary foods before exercise could hurt performance by causing a drop in blood glucose levels. Recent studies, however, have shown that consuming sugar up to 30 minutes before an event does not diminish performance. In fact, evidence suggests that a sugar-containing pre-competition beverage or snack may improve performance during endurance workouts and events.

What is carbohydrate loading?

Carbohydrate loading is a technique used to increase the amount of glycogen in muscles. For five to seven days before an event, the athlete eats 10–12 grams of carbohydrate per kilogram body weight and gradually reduces the intensity of the workouts. (To find out how much you weigh in kilograms, simply divide your weight in pounds by 2.2.) The day before the event, the athlete rests and eats the same high-carbohydrate diet. Although carbohydrate loading may be beneficial for athletes participating in endurance sports which require 90 minutes or more of non-stop effort, most athletes needn't worry about carbohydrate loading. Simply eating a diet that derives more than half of its calories from carbohydrates will do.

As an athlete, do I need to take extra vitamins and minerals?

Athletes need to eat about 1,800 calories a day to get the vitamins and minerals they need for good health and optimal performance. Since most athletes eat more than this amount, vitamin and mineral supplements are needed only in special situations. Athletes who follow vegetarian diets or who avoid an entire group of foods (for example, never drink milk) may need a supplement to make up for the vitamins and minerals not being supplied by food. A multivitamin-mineral pill that supplies 100% of the Recommended Dietary Allowance (RDA) will provide the nutrients needed. An athlete who frequently cuts back on calories, especially below the 1,800 calorie level, is not only at risk for inadequate vitamin and mineral intake, but also may not be getting enough carbohydrates. Since vitamins and minerals do not provide energy, they cannot replace the energy provided by carbohydrates.

Will extra protein help build muscle mass?

Many athletes, especially those on strength-training programs or who participate in power sports, are told that eating a ton of protein or taking protein supplements will help them gain muscle weight. However, the true secret to building muscle is training hard and consuming enough calories. While some extra protein is needed to build muscle, most American diets

---

♣ It's A Fact!!

Fuel Up For Fun

Whether you hit the court, the field, the track, the rink, or your back yard to get some physical activity, you'll need some fuel to keep you going. Here are some great snacks to munch on to keep your body moving and your stomach silent.

- Fresh veggies like carrots and celery sticks
- Snack-sized boxes of raisins
- Pretzels
- Low-fat yogurt
- Crackers—try graham crackers, animal crackers, or saltines
- Bagels
- Fig bars
- Fruit juice boxes (make sure you choose 100% pure fruit juice or, for an added boost, try orange juice with added calcium)
- Small packages of trail mix
- Fresh fruits such as bananas, oranges, grapes (try freezing your grapes for a new taste sensation), and berries

Source: "Fuel Up For Fun," the U.S. Department of Health and Human Services, Centers for Disease Control and Prevention (CDC), 2001.

provide more than enough protein. Between one and one-and-a-half grams of protein per kilogram body weight per day is sufficient if your calorie intake is adequate and you're eating a variety of foods. For a 150-pound athlete, that represents 68–102 grams of protein a day.

Why is iron so important?

Hemoglobin, which contains iron, is the part of red blood cells that carries oxygen from the lungs to all parts of the body, including muscles. Since your muscles need oxygen to produce energy, if you have low iron levels in your blood, you may tire quickly. Symptoms of iron deficiency include fatigue, irritability, dizziness, headaches, and lack of appetite. Many times, however, there are no symptoms at all. A blood test is the best way to find out if your iron level is low. It is recommended that athletes have their hemoglobin levels checked once a year. The RDA for iron is 15 milligrams a day for women and 10 milligrams a day for men. Red meat is the richest source of iron, but fish and poultry also are good sources. Fortified breakfast cereals, beans, and green leafy vegetables also contain iron. Our bodies absorb the iron found in animal products best.

Should I take an iron supplement?

Taking iron supplements will not improve performance unless an athlete is truly iron deficient. Too much iron can cause constipation, diarrhea, and nausea and may interfere with the absorption of other nutrients such as copper and zinc. Therefore, iron supplements should not be taken without proper medical supervision.

Why is calcium so important?

Calcium is needed for strong bones and proper muscle function. Dairy foods are the best source of calcium, however, studies show that many female athletes who are trying to lose weight cut back on dairy products. Female athletes who don't get enough calcium may be at risk for stress fractures and, when they're older, osteoporosis. Young women between the ages of 11 and 24 need about 1,200 milligrams of calcium a day. After age 25, the recommended intake is 800 milligrams. Low-fat dairy products are a rich source of calcium and also are low in fat and calories.

Chapter 32

Dietary Supplements: Facts Vs. Fads

You've seen the ads: "Natural herbs melt pounds away—without diet or exercise!" or "Amazing new discovery boosts athletic performance!" They usually claim that a doctor has discovered a new dietary supplement, a miracle substance that will make you thinner, stronger, smarter, or better at whatever you do. Best of all, you're told, this supplement works without any real effort. All you have to do is send in your money and swallow what they send you.

Having trouble believing these ads? You're right to be skeptical. There's little evidence that dietary supplements have the effects that they claim—and there is evidence that some supplements can cause serious damage to a user's health, especially when that user is a young person.

What are dietary supplements?

Dietary supplements are products that include vitamins, minerals, amino acids, herbs, or botanicals (plants)—or any concentration, extract, or combination of these—as part of their ingredients. You can purchase dietary supplements in pill, gel capsule, liquid, or powder forms.

How safe are they? In many cases, no one really knows. The U.S. Food and Drug Administration (FDA), which normally checks out the safety of foods and medicines before they come on the market, does not check on the safety of dietary supplements before they're sold. The FDA has to wait until it receives reports of problems caused by supplements before it can investigate and ban a dietary supplement. This is what happened with the herb ephedra (also called ma huang or herbal Fen-Phen) in 2003 when the FDA pulled the supplement from the U.S. market after it was linked to the death of a well-known baseball player.

This means that if you take an untested supplement, you are serving as the manufacturer's unpaid guinea pig and risking your own health.

Can supplements make me a better athlete?

Some athletes take dietary supplements believing that they improve performance. However, claims for these improvements are often exaggerated or not based on scientific evidence.

And some supplements may be hazardous. Anabolic steroids (manmade hormones similar to the male hormone testosterone) are unsafe and illegal. That's because the large quantities of these steroids that are found in the supplements can have devastating side effects on the body, including heart damage, kidney damage, and bone problems. Studies also show that steroids may be addictive, and that even small doses can interfere with growth.

Because sports supplements like creatine are unregulated, there is no standard dose. So users have no way of knowing what levels, if any, are safe, especially for teens who are still growing. The same goes for androstenedione, the supplement that gained attention because professional baseball player Mark McGwire used it. Research suggests that this hormone supplement may lead to health problems such as acne, gynecomastia (breast enlargement in guys), and heart problems.

Some people think that taking amino acid powders is helpful for increasing their muscle mass, but these powders don't actually have any special muscle-building effects. Amino acids are the building blocks of protein. Although it's scientifically true that they're necessary to build muscle (along with enough exercise), the human body can easily get all the amino acids it needs from the protein in food. So, if you work out properly and eat a balanced diet with enough protein, taking amino acid supplements won't actually do anything for you—except maybe empty your wallet.

Energy bars are also often used as a dietary supplement. These high-calorie, fortified treats should be used with caution, though. They may serve a purpose for athletes who burn lots of calories in high-intensity activities, like competitive cycling. But for most people they can add unwanted calories to the diet, and they're not particularly filling as a meal replacement.

Can supplements help me lose weight?

If you'd like to lose a few pounds, you might be tempted to try some of the many herbal weight-loss products available today. But none of these herbal remedies work. And some (like ephedra) can have serious side effects.

Herbs like chickweed, ginseng, kelp, and bee pollen, often included in diet aids, do nothing to promote weight loss—and some can be harmful or deadly in large doses. The only safe and effective way to take off excess pounds remains healthy eating and exercise. If you are concerned about your weight, talk to a doctor or dietitian. He or she can help you get to a healthy weight.

What about vitamin and mineral supplements?

The best way to get your daily dose of vitamins and minerals is from food. Although there's usually nothing wrong with a teen taking a basic multivitamin, if you're eating well, you probably don't need one. If you do choose to take a multivitamin, stick with a basic supplement and avoid brands that contain higher doses than 100% of the Recommended Daily Allowance (RDA) for any vitamin or mineral. Some vitamins can build up in the human system and cause problems when taken in excess amounts.

Talk to your doctor about additional vitamin and mineral supplements. If you can't eat dairy products for example, you might need a calcium supplement. Vegetarians might want to take vitamin B12 (a vitamin that is found mainly in food that comes from animals and may be missing in a vegetarian diet). People whose doctors have put them on weight-loss diets of less than

1,200 calories a day or those with food allergies should also discuss vitamin and mineral needs with their doctors.

✔ **Quick Tip**
Supplement Warning Signals

Check with your doctor before you take any dietary supplement, including vitamins and minerals. If your doctor starts you on a supplement, watch for warning signals that could indicate problems: stomach discomfort, pain, headache, rashes, or even vague symptoms like tiredness, dizziness, or lethargy.

Because it's not always clear what goes into some supplements, people with food allergies should be particularly wary. Some supplements contain ingredients from shellfish and other potential allergens, and you just don't know how you'll react to them.

When it comes to supplements, be a skeptical consumer. We'd all love to think there's a quick fix. But if it looks too easy, it probably is.

Chapter 33

Mental Wellness

Eating Disorders: Facts For Teens

What is an eating disorder?

An eating disorder is an obsession with food and weight that harms a person's well-being. Although we all worry about our weight sometimes, people with an eating disorder go to extremes to keep from gaining weight. There are two main eating disorders: anorexia nervosa and bulimia.

What causes eating disorders?

We don't know exactly. Possible causes include feeling stressed out or upset about something in your life, or feeling like you need to be "in control." Society also puts a lot of pressure on people to be thin. This pressure can contribute too.

What is anorexia?

People with anorexia are obsessed with being thin. They don't want to eat, and they are afraid of gaining weight. They may constantly worry about how many calories they take in or how much fat is in their food. They may take diet pills, laxatives, or water pills to lose weight. They may exercise too much. Anorexics usually think they're fat even though they're very thin. People with anorexia may get so thin that they look like they're sick.

What is bulimia?

Bulimia is eating a lot of food at once (called bingeing) and then throwing up or using laxatives to remove the food from the body (called purging). After a binge, some bulimics fast (don't eat) or overexercise to keep from gaining weight. People with bulimia may also use water pills, laxatives, or diet pills to "control" their weight. People with bulimia often try to hide their bingeing and purging. They may hide food for binges. Bulimics are usually close to normal weight, but their weight may go up and down.

Can eating disorders be treated?

Yes. For anorexics, the first step is getting back to a normal weight. If you're malnourished or very thin, you may be put in the hospital. Your doctor will probably want you to see a dietitian to learn how to pick healthy foods and eat at regular times. For both anorexics and bulimics, family and individual counseling (talking about your feelings about your weight and problems in your life) is helpful.

What are the warning signs?

The following are possible warning signs of anorexia and bulimia:

- Unnatural concern about body weight (even if the person is not overweight)

- Obsession with calories, fat grams, and food

- Use of any medicines to keep from gaining weight (diet pills, laxatives, and water pills)

More serious warning signs may be harder to notice because people who have an eating disorder try to keep it secret. Watch for these signs:

♣ It's A Fact!!
What's wrong with trying to be thin?

It's healthy to watch what you eat and to exercise. What isn't healthy is worrying all the time about your weight and what you eat. People with eating disorders do harmful things to their bodies because of their obsession about their weight.

If it isn't treated, anorexia can cause the following health problems:

- Stomach problems
- Heart problems
- Irregular periods or no periods
- Fine hair all over the body, including the face
- Dry, scaly skin

If it isn't treated, bulimia can cause the following health problems:

- Stomach problems
- Heart problems
- Kidney problems
- Dental problems (from throwing up stomach acid)
- Dehydration (not enough water in the body)

Source: Reprinted with permission from "Eating Disorders: Facts for Teens," November 2006, Family Doctor.org. Copyright © 2006 American Academy of Family Physicians. All Rights Reserved.

- Throwing up after meals
- Refusing to eat or lying about how much was eaten
- Fainting
- Over-exercising
- Not having periods
- Increased anxiety about weight
- Calluses or scars on the knuckle (from forced throwing up)
- Denying that there is anything wrong

Teens And Stress: Who Has Time For It?

What is stress?

Stress is what you feel when you react to pressure, either from the outside world (school, work, after-school activities, family, friends) or from inside yourself (wanting to do well in school, wanting to fit in). Stress is a normal reaction for people of all ages. It's caused by your body's instinct to protect itself from emotional or physical pressure or, in extreme situations, from danger.

Is stress always bad?

No. In fact, a little bit of stress is good. Most of us couldn't push ourselves to do well at things—sports, music, dance, work, and school—without feeling the pressure of wanting to do well. Without the stress caused by a deadline, most of us also wouldn't be able to finish projects or get to work or school on time.

If stress is so normal, why do I feel so bad?

With all the things that happen at your age, it's easy to feel overwhelmed. Things that you can't control are often the most frustrating. Maybe your parents are fighting, or your social life is a mess. You can also feel bad when you put pressure on yourself—like pressure to get good grades or to get promoted at your part-time job. A common reaction to stress is to criticize yourself. You may even get so upset that things don't seem fun anymore and life looks pretty grim. When this happens, it's easy to think there's nothing you can do to change things. But you can. See the tips.

Signs You're Stressed Out

- Feeling depressed, edgy, guilty, tired
- Having headaches, stomachaches, trouble sleeping
- Laughing or crying for no reason
- Blaming other people for bad things that happen to you
- Only seeing the down side of a situation
- Feeling like things that you used to enjoy aren't fun or are a burden
- Resenting other people or your responsibilities

Things That Help Fight Stress

- Eating well-balanced meals on a regular basis
- Drinking less caffeine
- Getting enough sleep
- Exercising on a regular basis

How can I deal with stress?

Although you can't always control the things that are stressing you out, you can control how you react to them. The way you feel about things results from the way you think about things. If you change how you think, you can change the way you feel. Try some of these tips to cope with your stress:

- **Make a list of the things that are causing your stress.** Think about your friends, family, school, and other activities. Accept that you can't control everything on your list.

- **Take control of what you can.** For example, if you're working too many hours and you don't have time to study enough, you may need to cut back your work hours.

- **Give yourself a break.** Remember that you can't make everyone in your life happy all the time. And it's okay to make mistakes now and then.

- **Don't commit yourself to things you can't do or don't want to do.** If you're already too busy, don't promise to decorate for the school dance. If you're tired and don't want to go out, tell your friends you'll go another night.

- **Find someone to talk to.** Talking to your friends or family can help because it gives you a chance to express your feelings. However, problems in your social life or family can be the hardest to talk about. If you feel like you can't talk to your family or a friend, talk to someone outside the situation. This could be your priest or minister, a school counselor or your family doctor.

I've tried dealing with my stress, but I just feel like giving up.

This is a danger sign. Stress can become too much to deal with. It can lead to such awful feelings that you may think about hurting—or even killing—yourself. When you feel like giving up, it may seem like things will never get better. Talk to someone right away. Talking about your feelings is the first step in learning to deal with them and starting to feel better.

Anxiety And Panic: Gaining Control Over How You're Feeling

What is anxiety?

Anxiety can be a normal "alarm system" alerting you to danger. Imagine coming home and finding a burglar in your living room. Your heart beats fast. Your palms get sweaty. Your mind races. In this situation, anxiety can provide an extra spark to help you get out of danger. In more normal but busy situations, anxiety can give you the energy to get things done.

> **♣ It's A Fact!!**
>
> There are safe and unsafe ways to deal with stress. It's dangerous to try to escape your problems by using drugs and alcohol. Both can be very tempting, and your friends may offer them to you. Drugs and alcohol may seem like easy answers, but they're not. Using drugs and alcohol to deal with stress just adds new problems, such as addiction, or family and health problems.
>
> Source: Reprinted with permission from "Teens and Stress: Who Has Time For It?" December 2006, Family Doctor.org. Copyright © 2006 American Academy of Family Physicians. All Rights Reserved.

But sometimes anxiety can be out of control, giving you a sense of dread and fear for no apparent reason. This kind of anxiety can disrupt your life.

Are there different types of anxiety?

Yes. Anxiety can be a general feeling of worry, a sudden attack of panicky feelings, or a fear of a certain situation or object.

What is generalized anxiety disorder?

Generalized anxiety disorder is ongoing worry or fear that isn't related to a particular event or situation, or is out of proportion to what you would expect—for instance, constantly worrying about a child who is perfectly healthy.

Symptoms of generalized anxiety disorder include muscle tension, trembling, shortness of breath, fast heartbeat, dry mouth, dizziness, nausea, irritability, loss of sleep, and not being able to concentrate.

What is panic disorder?

Panic disorder is another type of anxiety. It occurs when you have repeated periods of extreme panic called panic attacks.

Suppose one day you're getting out of your car to go to work. Suddenly, your chest feels tight. Your heart races. You begin to feel dizzy and faint. You start to choke. You feel as if the end is near. Was it all in your head? No. Most likely, you had a panic attack.

Panic attacks last about five to 30 minutes and may include any of the symptoms listed. Panic attacks can lead to phobias if they aren't treated.

Panic Attack Symptoms

- Feeling like you're going to choke

- Chest pressure or chest pain

- Pounding heart

- Racing pulse

- Dizziness or lightheadedness

- Shortness of breath or tightness in the throat

- Sweating

- Trembling or shaking

- Nausea

- Tingling or numbness in the hands or feet

- Hot flashes or chills

- Sense of unreality or dreamlike sensations

- Extreme fear of losing control, doing something embarrassing, going "crazy" or dying

What is a phobia?

A phobia is an extreme, unreasonable fear in response to something specific. There are lots of different phobias, including fear of crowds, bridges, snakes, spiders, heights, open places, or social embarrassment.

A phobia is only considered a problem when it keeps you from living a normal life. An example is being afraid to leave home because you are afraid of one of the things listed.

What causes anxiety disorders?

Suppose the fire alarm goes off in your home. You race around frantically to find the fire. Instead, you find that there is no fire—the alarm just isn't working properly.

It's the same with anxiety disorders. Your body mistakenly triggers your alarm system when there is no danger. This may be due to a chemical imbalance in your body. It may also be related to an unconscious memory, a side effect of a medicine, or to an illness.

Can anxiety disorders be treated?

Yes. Talk to your family doctor if you think you have an anxiety disorder. He or she can help you form a plan to develop skills to cope with your anxiety. Your doctor may also suggest counseling and prescribe medicine if needed. The following are some tips on coping with anxiety:

- **Control your worry.** Pick a place and time to do your worrying. Make it the same place and time every day. Spend 30 minutes thinking about your concerns and what you can do about them. Try not to dwell on what "might" happen. Focus more on what's really happening. Then let go of the worry and go on with your day.

- **Learn ways to relax.** These may include muscle relaxation, yoga, or deep breathing exercises. Muscle relaxation is simple. Start by choosing a muscle and holding it tight for a few seconds. Then relax the muscle. Do this with all of your muscles. Try starting with your feet muscles and working your way up your body.

> **✔ Quick Tip**
> **Steps To Deep Breathing**
>
> 1. Lie down on a flat surface.
>
> 2. Place one hand on your stomach, just above your navel. Place the other hand on your chest.
>
> 3. Breathe in slowly and try to make your stomach rise a little.
>
> 4. Hold your breath for a second.
>
> 5. Breathe out slowly and let your stomach go back down.
>
> Source: Reprinted with permission from "Anxiety and Panic: Gaining Control Over How You're Feeling," September 2006, Family Doctor.org. Copyright © 2006 American Academy of Family Physicians. All Rights Reserved.

- **Exercise regularly.** People who have anxiety often quit exercising. But exercise can give you a sense of well-being and help decrease feelings of anxiety.

- **Get plenty of sleep.**

- **Avoid alcohol and drug abuse.** It may seem that alcohol or drugs relax you. But in the long run they make anxiety worse and cause more problems.

- **Avoid caffeine.** Caffeine is found in coffee, tea, soft drinks, and chocolate. Caffeine may increase your sense of anxiety because it stimulates your nervous system. Also avoid over-the-counter diet pills and cough and cold medicines the contain a decongestant.

- **Confront the things that have made you anxious in the past.** Begin by just picturing yourself confronting these things. By doing this, you can get used to the idea of confronting the things that make you anxious before you actually do it. After you feel more comfortable picturing yourself confronting these things, you can begin to actually face them. If you feel yourself getting anxious, practice a relaxation technique or focus on a simple task, such as counting backward from 100 to zero. Although feelings of anxiety are scary, they won't hurt you. Label the level of your fear from zero to 10 and keep track as it goes up and down. Notice that it doesn't stay at a very high level for more than a few seconds. When the fear comes, accept it. Wait and give it time to pass without running away from it.

- **Use medicine if it helps.** Your doctor may give you medicine to help reduce your anxiety while you learn new ways to respond to the things that make you anxious. Many types of medicine are available. Your doctor will decide which medicine is right for you.

- **Talk about your anxiety with your doctor.** Your doctor can help you make a plan to cope with anxiety. Counseling can help you learn to express your needs and wants so you can feel more in control and hold in less of your anger and anxiety.

The most important thing is to take action. Any action you take will help you gain a sense of control over your anxiety.

Depression

What is depression?

When doctors talk about depression, they mean the medical illness called major depression. Someone with major depression has symptoms like those listed nearly every day, all day, for two weeks or longer.

If you're depressed, you may also have headaches, other aches and pains, digestive problems, and problems with sex. An older person with depression may feel confused or have trouble understanding simple requests.

Symptoms Of Depression

- Feeling sad, hopeless and having frequent crying spells
- Losing interest or pleasure in things you used to enjoy
- Feeling guilty, helpless, or worthless
- Thinking about death or suicide

- Sleeping too much or having problems sleeping

- Loss of appetite and unintended weight loss or gain

- Feeling very tired all the time

- Having trouble paying attention and making decisions

- Having aches and pains that don't get better with treatment

- Feeling restless, irritated, and easily annoyed

What causes depression?

Depression seems to be related to a chemical imbalance in the brain that makes it hard for the cells to communicate with one another. Depression also seems to be hereditary (to run in families).

Depression can be linked to stressful events in your life, such as the death of someone you love, a divorce, or loss of your job. Taking certain medicines, abusing drugs or alcohol or having other illnesses can also lead to depression. Depression isn't caused by personal weakness, laziness, or lack of willpower.

How is depression diagnosed?

If you're having symptoms of depression, be sure to tell your doctor so you can get help. Don't expect your doctor to be able to guess that you're depressed just by looking at you. The sooner you seek treatment, the sooner the depression will lift.

Once you tell your doctor how you're feeling, he or she may ask you some questions about your symptoms, about your health, and about your family

---

♣ It's A Fact!!
Reasons To Get
Help For Depression

- Early treatment helps keep depression from getting worse or lasting a long time.

- Thoughts of suicide are common in people with depression. The risk of suicide is higher if you don't get treatment for your depression. When depression is successfully treated, the thoughts of suicide will go away.

- Treatment can help you return to your "normal" self, enjoying life.

- Treatment can help prevent depression from coming back.

Source: Reprinted with permission from "Depression," November 2007, Family Doctor.org. Copyright © 2007 American Academy of Family Physicians. All Rights Reserved.

history of health problems. Your doctor may also give you a physical exam and do some tests.

How is depression treated?

Depression can be treated with medicines, with counseling, or with both.

What about medicines?

Many medicines can be used to treat depression. These medicines are called antidepressants. They correct the chemical imbalance in the brain that causes depression.

Antidepressants work differently for different people. They also have different side effects. So, even if one medicine bothers you or doesn't work for you, another may help. You may notice improvement as soon as one week after you start taking the medicine, but you probably won't see the full effects for about eight to 12 weeks. You may have side effects at first but they tend to decrease after a couple of weeks.

> **✔ Quick Tip**
>
> People who have depression sometimes think about suicide. This thinking is part of the depression. If you have thoughts about hurting yourself, tell your doctor, your friends, your family, or call your local suicide hot line, such as the National Suicide Prevention Lifeline at 1-800-273-8255.
>
> Get help right away. The good news is that there are people who can help you, and depression can be treated.
>
> Source: Reprinted with permission from "Depression," November 2007, Family Doctor.org. Copyright © 2007 American Academy of Family Physicians. All Rights Reserved.

How long will I need medicine?

How long you'll need to take the medicine depends on your depression. Your doctor may want you to take medicine for four to six months or longer. You need to take the medicine long enough to reduce the chance that the depression will come back. Talk with your doctor about any questions you have about your medicine.

✔ Quick Tip

Getting Through Depression

- **Pace yourself.** Don't expect to do everything you normally can. Set a realistic schedule.

- **Don't believe negative thoughts** you may have, such as blaming yourself or expecting to fail. This thinking is part of depression. These thoughts will go away as your depression lifts.

- **Get involved** in activities that make you feel good or feel like you've achieved something.

- **Avoid making big life decisions while you are depressed.** If you must make a big decision, ask someone you trust to help you.

- **Avoid drugs and alcohol.** Both make depression worse. Both can cause dangerous side effects with your antidepressants.

- **Physical activity** seems to cause a chemical reaction in the body that may improve your mood. Exercising four to six times a week for at least 30 minutes each time is a good goal. But even less activity can be helpful.

- **Try not to get discouraged.** It will take time for your depression to lift fully.

Source: Reprinted with permission from "Depression," November 2007, Family Doctor.org. Copyright © 2007 American Academy of Family Physicians. All Rights Reserved.

What is psychotherapy?

In psychotherapy, you talk with your family doctor, a psychiatrist, or a therapist about things that are going on in your life. The focus may be on your thoughts and beliefs or on your relationships. Or the focus may be on your behavior, how it's affecting you, and what you can do differently. Psychotherapy often lasts for a limited time, such as eight to 20 visits.

Will I need to go to the hospital?

Depression can usually be treated through visits to your doctor. Treatment in the hospital may be needed if you have other medical conditions that could affect your treatment or if you're at high risk of suicide.

How long will the depression last?

This depends on how soon you get help. Left untreated, depression can last for weeks, months or even years. The main risk in not getting treatment is suicide. Treatment can help depression lift in eight to 12 weeks or less.

Handling Sports Pressure And Competition

"Handling Sports Pressure And Competition," August 2007, reprinted with permission from www.kidshealth.org. Copyright © 2006 The Nemours Foundation. This information was provided by KidsHealth, one of the largest resources online for medically reviewed health information written for parents, kids, and teens. For more articles like this one, visit www.KidsHealth.org, or www.TeensHealth.org.

Most people play a sport for the thrill of having fun with others who share the same interest, right? But it's not always fun and games. Most student athletes who play competitive sports have had thoughts that go like this at one time or another: "Man, I can't believe I let the ball in the goal, and I know from the look in coach's eyes he wasn't happy."

There can be a ton of pressure in high school sports. A lot of the time it comes from the feeling that a parent or coach expects you to always win. But sometimes it comes from inside, too. Some players are just really hard on themselves. And individual situations can add to the stress: Maybe there's a recruiter from your number one college scouting you on the sidelines. Whatever the cause, the pressure to win can sometimes stress you to the point where you just don't know how to have fun anymore. Perhaps it could even be the reason why you haven't been playing as well lately.

How can stress affect sports performance?

Stress is a feeling that's created when we react to particular events. It's the body's way of rising to a challenge and preparing to meet a tough situation with focus, strength, stamina, and heightened alertness. A little stress or the right kind of positive stress can help keep you on your toes, ready to rise to a challenge.

The events that provoke stress are called stressors, and they cover a whole range of situations—everything from outright danger to stepping up to take the foul shot that could win the game. Stress can also be a response to change or anticipation of something that's about to happen—good or bad. People can feel stress over positive challenges, like making the varsity team, as well as negative ones.

Distress is a bad type of stress that arises when you must adapt to too many negative demands. Suppose you had a fight with a close friend last night, you forgot your homework this morning, and you're playing in a tennis match this afternoon. You try to get psyched for the game but can't. You've hit stress overload. Continuous struggling with too much stress can exhaust your energy and drive.

Eustress is the good type of stress that stems from the challenge of taking part in something that you enjoy but have to work hard for. Eustress pumps you up, providing a healthy spark for any task you undertake.

What can I do to ease pressure?

When the demands of competition start to get to you, try these relaxation techniques:

- **Deep breathing:** Find a quiet place to sit down. Inhale slowly through your nose, drawing air deep into your lungs. Hold your breath for about five seconds, then release it slowly. Repeat the exercise five times.

- **Muscle relaxation:** Contract (flex) a group of muscles tightly. Keep them tensed for about five seconds, then release. Repeat the exercise five times, selecting different muscle groups.

- **Visualization:** Close your eyes and picture a peaceful place or an event from your past. Recall the beautiful sights and the happy sounds. Imagine stress flowing away from your body. You can also visualize success. People who advise competitive players often recommend that they imagine themselves completing a pass, making a shot, or scoring a goal over and over. Then on game day, you can recall your stored images to help calm nerves and boost self-confidence.

- **Mindfulness:** Watch out for negative thoughts. Whether you're preparing for a competition or coping with a defeat, repeat to yourself: "I learn from my mistakes!" "I'm in control of my feelings!" "I can make this goal!"

When sports become too stressful, get away from the pressure. Go to a movie or hang out with friends. Put your mind on something completely different.

How can I keep stress in check?

If sports make you so nervous that you get headaches, become nauseated, or can't concentrate on other things, you're experiencing symptoms of unhealthy, potentially chronic (which means long-lasting and continuous) stress. Don't keep such stress bottled up inside you. Suppressing your emotions might mean bigger health troubles for you later on.

Talk about your concerns with a friend. Simply sharing your feelings can ease your anxiety. Sometimes it may help to get an adult's perspective— someone who has dealt with stress over and over like your coach or fitness instructor. Here are some other things you can do to cope with stress:

☞ Remember!!
Enjoy The Game

Winning is exhilarating, but losing and some amount of stress are part of almost any sports program— as they are in life. Sports are about enhancing self-esteem, building social skills, and developing a sense of community. And above all, sports are about having fun.

Source: Copyright © 2006 The Nemours Foundation.

- **Treat your body right.** Eat well and get a good night's sleep, especially before games where the pressure's on.

- **Learn and practice relaxation techniques,** like those described in the previous section.

- **Get some type of physical activity other than the sport you're involved in.** Take a walk, ride your bike, and get completely away from the sport that's stressing you out.

- **Don't try to be perfect.** Everyone flubs a shot or messes up from time to time (so don't expect your teammates to be perfect either). Forgive yourself, remind yourself of all your great shots, and move on.

It's possible that some anxiety stems only from uncertainty. Meet privately with your coach or instructor. Ask for clarification his or her expectations seem vague or inconsistent. Although most instructors do a good job of fostering athletes' physical and mental development, you may need to be the one who opens the lines of communication. You may also want to talk with your parents or another adult family member.

If you're feeling completely overscheduled and out of control, review your options on what you can let go. It's a last resort, but if you're no longer enjoying your sport, it may be time to find one that's less stressful. Chronic stress isn't fun—and fun is what sports are all about.

Recognizing when you need guidance to steer yourself out of a stressful situation doesn't represent weakness; it's a sign of courage and wisdom. Don't stop looking for support until you've found it.

Chapter 34

Adolescent Sleep Needs And Patterns

Introduction

Sleep is a basic drive of nature. Sufficient sleep helps us think more clearly, complete complex tasks better and more consistently, and enjoy everyday life more fully. Although many questions regarding the role of sleep remain unanswered, scientific studies have shown that sleep contributes significantly to several important cognitive, emotional, and performance-related functions.

Sleep is, in essence, food for the brain, and insufficient sleep can be harmful, even life-threatening. When hungry for sleep, the brain becomes relentless in its quest to satisfy its need and will cause feelings of "sleepiness," decreased levels of alertness or concentration, and, in many cases, unanticipated sleep. Excessive sleepiness is also associated with reduced short-term memory and learning ability, negative mood, inconsistent performance, poor productivity, and loss of some forms of behavioral control.

Researchers have identified several changes in sleep patterns, sleep/wake systems and circadian timing systems associated with puberty. These changes contribute to excessive sleepiness that has a negative impact on daytime functioning in adolescents, including increasing their risk of injury. Findings are similar in North America and in industrialized countries on other continents.

Scientists hypothesize that these sleep-related problems are due largely to conflicts between physiologically-driven sleep needs and patterns and behavioral and psychosocial factors that influence sleep habits.

Key changes in sleep patterns and needs that are associated with puberty include:

Physiological Patterns

- **Adolescents require at least as much sleep** as they did as pre-adolescents (in general, 8.5 to 9.25 hours each night).

- **Daytime sleepiness increases**—for some, to pathological levels—even when an adolescent's schedule provides for optimal amounts of sleep.

- **Adolescents' sleep patterns undergo a phase delay,** that is, a tendency toward later times, for both sleeping and waking. Studies show that the typical high school student's natural time to fall asleep is 11:00 p.m. or later.

Behavioral And Psychosocial Patterns

- **Many U.S. adolescents do not get enough sleep,** especially during the week. Survey data show that average total sleep time during the school week decreases from 7 hours and 42 minutes in 13 year olds to 7 hours and four minutes in 19 year olds. Only 15 percent of adolescents reported sleeping 8.5 or more hours on school nights, and 26 percent of students reported typically sleeping 6.5 hours or less each school night.

- **Adolescents have irregular sleep patterns;** in particular, their weekend sleep schedules are much different than their weekday schedules, to some extent as a direct consequence of weekday sleep loss. These differences include both the quantity and the timing of sleep. One study of more than 3,000 adolescents showed that the average increase of weekend over weekday sleep across ages 13–19 was one hour and 50 minutes. In 18-year-olds, the average discrepancy was more than two hours. In addition, 91 percent of the surveyed high school students reported going to sleep after 11:00 p.m. on weekends, and 40 percent went to bed after 11:00 p.m. on school nights. Irregular sleep schedules—including significant discrepancies between weekdays and weekends—can contribute to a shift in sleep phase (that is, a tendency toward morningness or eveningness), trouble falling asleep or awakening, and fragmented (poor quality) sleep.

Consequences Of Poor Sleep In Adolescents

Data on children, teens, and adults confirm that sleep loss and sleep difficulties can have serious detrimental effects. Research specifically on adolescents and young adults is relatively new and limited, but scientists believe that many effects demonstrated in studies and clinical observations of adults are similar in adolescents. Sleep researchers, therefore, believe that insufficient sleep in teens and young adults is linked to:

- **Increased risk of unintentional injuries and death.** As noted, drowsiness or fatigue has been identified as a principle cause in at least 100,000 traffic crashes each year. In addition, about one million, or one-sixth, of traffic crashes in the United States are believed to be attributable to lapses in the driver's attention. Sleep loss and fatigue significantly increase the chances of such lapses occurring. A North Carolina state study found that drivers age 25 or younger cause more than one-half (55 percent) of fall- asleep crashes. The same symptoms of sleepiness that contribute to traffic crashes can also play a role in non-traffic injuries, such as those associated with handling hazardous equipment in the workplace or in the home. Furthermore, adolescents who have not received sufficient sleep and who consume even small amounts of alcohol are at greater risk of injury than those who are not lacking sleep because sleep loss has been shown to heighten the effects of alcohol.

- **Low grades and poor school performance.** High school students who describe themselves as having academic problems and who are earning C's or below in school report getting less sleep, having later bedtimes and having more irregular sleep schedules than students reporting higher grades. (Note: A causal relationship has not yet been established.)

- **Negative moods** (for example, anger, sadness, and fear), difficulty controlling emotions and behavior problems. In one study, female high school students who went to sleep on the weekend two or more hours later than their typical weeknight bedtime reported feeling more depressed than those who did not stay up late on the weekends. Studies also suggest that sleep loss may be associated with a decreased ability to control, inhibit or change emotional responses. Some signs of sleepiness, such as inability to stay focused on a task, impulsivity, difficulty "sitting still," and problems completing tasks, resemble behaviors common also in attention deficit hyperactivity disorder (ADHD). In addition, a 1995 study of students in transition from junior high to senior high school found that conduct/aggressive behaviors were highly associated with shorter sleep times and later sleep start time.

- **Increased likelihood of stimulant use** (including caffeine and nicotine), alcohol and similar substances.

Teens who are heavily involved in school and community activities, their jobs, and other responsibilities appear to be at greater risk for the above effects of sleepiness than those who are less involved in activities and who either do not hold jobs or who work fewer hours.

What Can Be Done

The consequences of insufficient sleep among adolescents are particularly important to understand because they appear to be closely tied to key elements of human development. Achieving developmental goals during adolescence is essential for lifelong success and for what psychologists call social competency. In addition, the transition from childhood to adulthood is a critical time for "seeding" the values and habits that will shape their lives. Therefore, intervention to improve the sleep patterns of adolescents is important.

Influencing Physiological Sleep Patterns

Sleep researchers have established that basic sleep needs within individuals generally remain the same throughout their lifetime. Furthermore, insufficient sleep accumulates into a sleep debt that can ultimately be relieved only through additional sleep.

Tips For Teens   ✔ **Quick Tip**

1. **Sleep is food for the brain.** Lack of sleep can make you look tired and feel depressed, irritable, or angry. Even mild sleepiness can hurt your performance—from taking school exams to playing sports or video games. Learn how much sleep you need to function at your best—most adolescents need between 8.5 and 9.25 hours of sleep each night—and strive to get it every night. You should awaken refreshed, not tired.

2. **Keep consistency in mind.** Establish a regular bedtime and waketime schedule, and maintain this schedule during weekends and school (or work) vacations. Don't stray from your schedule frequently, and never do so for two or more consecutive nights. If you must go off schedule, avoid delaying your bedtime by more than one hour. Awaken the next day within two hours of your regular schedule, and, if you are sleepy during the day, take an early afternoon nap.

3. **Get into bright light as soon as possible in the morning, but avoid it in the evening.** The light helps to signal to the brain when it should wake up and when it should prepare to sleep.

4. **Understand your circadian rhythms.** Then you can try to maximize your schedule throughout the day according to your internal clock. For example, to compensate for your "slump (sleepy) times," participate in stimulating activities or classes that are interactive. Try to avoid lecture classes and potentially unsafe activities, including driving.

5. **After lunch (or after noon), stay away from caffeinated coffee and colas as well as nicotine, which are all stimulants.** Also avoid alcohol, which disrupts sleep.

6. **Relax before going to bed.** Avoid heavy reading, studying, and computer games within one hour of going to bed. Don't fall asleep with the television on—flickering light and stimulating content can inhibit restful sleep.

Circadian timing systems are also very resistant to change. Behavioral methods, such as controlled light exposure and chronotherapy, can sometimes help shift circadian timing to more socially appropriate sleep and wake times. Because the circadian rhythms in teenagers are typically highly sensitive to erratic schedules, to effectively adjust them requires making gradual, persistent and consistent changes. Adapting to an early school schedule following summer or other vacation periods during which very late schedules are typically kept, for example, can take several days to several weeks.

It is important to recognize that excessive sleepiness during the day and other sleep problems can be an indication of an underlying biological sleep disorder. Accurate diagnosis of disorders such as narcolepsy, sleep apnea, and periodic limb movement disorder usually requires examination by a qualified sleep specialist and an overnight stay in a sleep laboratory. In most cases, symptoms of sleep disorders can be eliminated or minimized through the use of appropriate behavior modifications, medication or other therapies.

Creating Sleep-Friendly Schools

School systems can help positively influence adolescent sleep patterns in several ways. Suggestions include:

- **Educate** teachers, school health providers, and other school personnel about adolescent sleep needs and patterns and about the signs of sleep loss and other sleep or alertness difficulties. Teachers and school staff should also be informed about accommodations that might be needed by some students with chronic sleep disorders.

🖘 Remember!!
Changing Sleep Habits

Perhaps the most significant behavioral change that adolescents can make—and that their parents can encourage them to make—is to establish and maintain a consistent sleep/wake schedule. This is a good practice for people at all ages, but may be especially important for adolescents.

Understanding and practicing other behaviors that are considered good sleep habits are also important. These include getting enough sleep, avoiding caffeine and other stimulants late in the day and alcohol at night, gaining exposure to bright light at appropriate times to reinforce the brain's circadian timing system, relaxing before going to sleep and creating an environment conducive to quality sleep.

- **Integrate** sleep-related education in curricula so that students can learn about the physiology and benefits of sleep and the consequences of sleep deprivation. Relevant academic subjects include, for example, biology, health, and psychology. In addition, driver's education courses should cover the prevalence and prevention of crashes related to drowsy driving.

- **Structure** the school schedule and related activities to accommodate adolescents' sleep needs and behaviors and circadian rhythm at this developmental stage. One approach is to start daily high school schedules when students are most likely to be alert and able to learn. Several school districts in the nation have adopted later school start times—countless more are considering doing so.

Preliminary findings and focus group studies conducted by the Center for Applied Research and Educational Improvement (CAREI) at the University of Minnesota reveal that after schools shifted from early to later start times, students from both urban and suburban high schools reported that they felt more rested and alert during the first hour of class and, in general, throughout the day.

In addition, students in the suburban Edina high school district whose schools delayed their start times reported increased hours of sleep, less erratic sleep behaviors and less depressive feelings and behaviors, better grades and little restriction in time spent in extracurricular activities. Findings in urban (Minneapolis) schools with later start times varied from the suburban schools somewhat; in particular, student mood appeared unchanged and schedule conflicts with extracurricular activities and employment were more pronounced.

Establishing Public Policies

Governmental and organizational policies significantly influence social change. In addition to federal agencies, national medical and health care specialty organizations, education and parent associations, and youth groups can play a key role in developing and implementing recommendations, policies and cooperative initiatives.

Furthermore, state, district, and local efforts may be spearheaded through voluntary, professional, and governmental organizations such as school boards and parent-teacher associations, state or district medical societies, motor vehicle administration departments, public health departments, and social service agencies.

Below are some examples of policy-related approaches that have been or could be used to better match adolescent sleep patterns and needs with cultural expectations and external demands, thereby increasing teens' overall safety and well-being.

- Legislation to encourage starting high schools no earlier than 9:00 a.m., and appropriations to help defray the school or school district's costs of changing school schedules.

- Legislation or policies to include age-appropriate sleep information in school curricula, grades K through 12.

- Initiatives to include information about the effects of drowsiness on driving ability in drivers' education courses and licensing tests.

- Graduated licensing regulations to reduce the number of adolescents driving unsupervised at night.

- Child labor laws to restrict the number of hours and the time of day that adolescents are permitted to work.

- Funding to support public education and scientific research on topics such as the interrelationships among sleep loss and injury, learning and performance, as well as epidemiological data. Relevant federal oversight of funded agencies include the National Center for Sleep Disorders Research and other agencies of the National Institutes of Health, the Food and Drug Administration, the Department of Transportation, the Department of Education, the Centers for Disease Control and Prevention, and military branches.

- Initiatives to educate key adults who have frequent and regular contact with adolescents (for example, caregivers and authoritarians) about sleep, the signs and hazards of sleepiness, and appropriate interventions for children and adolescents showing signs of sleep difficulties or disorders. Constituents include parents, teachers, school administrators, school nurses and counselors, coaches, employers, health providers (family practitioners, adolescent medicine special-ists, and those who specialize in mental health or learning disabili-ties), and voluntary group leaders of youth-oriented organizations. In addition, police and emergency care personnel should be trained to recognize problem sleepiness and distinguish its signs from those associated with drug or alcohol use.

♣ It's A Fact!!
Making New Discoveries

Sleep research has established clear relationships between sleepiness, health, safety, and productivity. However, the sleep research field in general is relatively young, and scientists still have much to learn about the role of sleep and the effects of sleep loss in hu-mans. Additional studies on the neurobiology, genetics, epidemiology, and neurobehavioral and functional consequences of sleepiness are needed. More studies specifically on the adolescent population are also needed, including interdisciplinary research to further examine sleep's role in ado-lescent development, health, and behavior.

Chapter 35

Locker Room Hygiene

Lurking In The Locker Room

Do you know where nasty things like bacteria and fungi may be hiding? Come on into the locker room to see what's lurking under foot and behind closed doors.

- **Clothing:** Loose-fitting clothes are best for physical activity. If you have acne on your arms, back, or shoulders keeping clothing loose cuts down on the amount of friction on your body. Friction can make your acne worse.

- **Sweatbands:** It's best not to wear them. Sweatbands can trap sweat in your pores and provide a perfect place for bacteria to grow and cause acne.

- **Sneakers:** Air out your sneakers between wears to prevent athlete's foot.

- **Towels:** When you're in the gym, using two towels can help to cut down on the spread of bacteria. Use one to wipe off the equipment before and after you use it and one to wipe the sweat from your skin.

- **Water Bottles:** Clean out your water bottle after each time you use it. This will prevent bacteria from growing inside.

About This Chapter: This chapter contains information from "Lurking In The Locker Room," BAM! (Body And Mind), Centers for Disease Control and Prevention (CDC), 2001.

- **Water:** Drink plenty of water before, during, and after you are physically active to stay hydrated. In addition to keeping your body working right, it can help prevent acne by flushing out your pores.

- **Flip-Flops:** Wear flip-flops to walk around the locker room. Wet floors are a popular hangout for fungi.

- **Wash Your Face:** Keeping your pores clean helps prevent acne, so wash your face right after you work out to get rid of sweat.

- **Makeup:** Girls, be sure to take off your makeup before you work out. This will keep your pores clear and help prevent acne.

- **Locker Room Benches:** When sitting in the locker room, sit on a clean towel. Damp benches harbor bacteria and fungi that can easily be spread from person to person. If you can, get dressed first before you sit down.

- **Gym Bag And Locker:** Storing damp or wet workout clothes in your locker or gym bag is an invitation for fungus to grow. Hang your clothes up to dry before cramming them into your locker, and take them home at least once a week to be washed.

♣ It's A Fact!!
Additional Information For Boys

- **Athletic Supporter:** Always wear a clean, dry athletic supporter or pair of underwear when you participate in sports or your regular activity. Otherwise, you might be at risk for a nasty case of jock itch.

- **Shower:** Take a shower immediately after your workout and dry off well. This will remove sweat and fungi from your skin and will reduce the risk of getting athlete's foot and jock itch.

- **Powder And Talc:** use an anti-fungal or talc powder on your feet and groin area after you shower to prevent athlete's foot and jock itch.

Part Five

Avoiding Fitness Busters

Chapter 36

Overcome Barriers:
Make Physical Activity Easy And Safe

Overcoming Barriers To Physical Activity

Given the health benefits of regular physical activity, we might have to ask why two out of three (60%) Americans are not active at recommended levels. Many technological advances and conveniences that have made our lives easier and active, many personal variables, including physiological, behavioral, and psychological factors, may affect our plans to become more physically active. Understanding common barriers to physical activity and creating strategies to overcome them may help you make physical activity part of your daily life.

Suggestions For Overcoming Physical Activity Barriers

Lack Of Time: Identify available time slots. Monitor your daily activities for one week. Identify at least three 30-minute time slots you could use for physical activity. Add physical activity to your daily routine. For example, walk or ride your bike to school or shopping, organize school activities around physical activity, walk the dog, exercise while you watch TV, or park farther away from your destination. Make time for physical activity.

About This Chapter: This chapter begins with excerpts from "Overcoming Barriers To Physical Activity," Department of Health and Human Services, Centers for Disease Control and Prevention (CDC), May 2007. Excerpts from "The Nolan Ryan Fitness Guide," President's Council on Physical Fitness and Sports, October 2004, are also included.

Social Influence: Explain your interest in physical activity to friends and family. Ask them to support your efforts. Invite friends and family members to exercise with you. Plan social activities involving exercise. Develop new friendships with physically active people. Join a group, such as the YMCA or a hiking club.

Lack Of Energy: Schedule physical activity for times in the day or week when you feel energetic. Convince yourself that if you give it a chance, physical activity will increase your energy level—then, try it.

Lack Of Motivation: Plan ahead. Make physical activity a regular part of your daily or weekly schedule and write it on your calendar. Invite a friend to exercise with you on a regular basis and write it on both your calendars. Join an exercise group or class.

Fear Of Injury: Learn how to warm up and cool down to prevent injury. Learn how to exercise appropriately considering your age, fitness level, skill level, and health status. Choose activities involving minimum risk.

Lack Of Skill: Select activities requiring no new skills, such as walking, climbing stairs, or jogging. Exercise with friends who are at the same skill level as you are. Find a friend who is willing to teach you some new skills. Take a class to develop new skills.

Lack Of Resources: Select activities that require minimal facilities or equipment, such as walking, jogging, jumping rope, or calisthenics. Identify inexpensive, convenient resources available in your community.

Weather Conditions: Develop a set of regular activities that are always available regardless of weather (indoor cycling, aerobic dance, indoor swimming, calisthenics, stair climbing, rope skipping, mall walking, dancing, or gymnasium games). Look on outdoor activities that depend on weather conditions (cross-country skiing, outdoor swimming, outdoor tennis, etc.) as bonus activities when weather and circumstances permit.

Travel: Put a jump rope in your suitcase and jump rope. Walk the halls and climb the stairs in hotels. Stay in places with swimming pools or exercise facilities. Join the YMCA or YWCA (ask about reciprocal membership agreement). Visit the local shopping mall and walk for half an hour or more. Bring a small tape recorder and your favorite aerobic exercise tape.

♣ It's A Fact!!
Ten Common Reasons For Not Adopting A Physically Active Lifestyle

- Do not have enough time to exercise

- Find it inconvenient to exercise

- Lack self-motivation

- Do not find exercise enjoyable

- Find exercise boring

- Lack confidence in their ability to be physically active (low self-efficacy)

- Fear being injured or have been injured recently

- Lack self-management skills, such as the ability to set personal goals, monitor progress, or reward progress toward such goals

- Lack encouragement, support, or companionship from family and friends

- Do not have parks, sidewalks, bicycle trails, or safe and pleasant walking paths convenient to their homes or offices

Source: "Overcoming Barriers To Physical Activity," Department of Health and Human Services, Centers for Disease Control and Prevention (CDC), May 2005.

Making Activity Easy

Our understanding of fitness has evolved since the fitness craze first took hold. Scientific evidence now clearly indicates that regular moderate-intensity physical activity offers many of the health benefits traditionally associated with more intense exercise. Moderate-intensity activity includes many of the things you may already be doing during a day. For many people, being more active may simply mean taking advantage of or creating opportunities for activity.

For example, walking to school can help you accumulate active time. So can foregoing the elevator for the stairs, gardening or mowing the lawn with a push mower, or doing other things that can give you a workout. The point is not to make physical activity an unwelcome chore, but to seize the opportunities you have and make the most of them.

There's really no mystery to fitness. And though there may be barriers, there are also solutions. Once you commit yourself, the barriers to fitness will be easily surmountable, and the rewards of better living will be yours.

✔ **Quick Tip**

If boredom is your activity barrier, try these tips.

Vary your activities so you don't tire of one.

Enlist a friend or family member as an exercise partner.

Use different jogging, walking, or biking paths for scenic variety.

Choose activities you really enjoy, that are fun and offer a reward, such as hiking for a great view or walking to a friends house.

Make activities into social occasions such as tennis tournaments among friends.

Earn one or more Presidential Sports Awards.

Source: "The Nolan Ryan Fitness Guide," President's Council on Physical Fitness and Sports, October 2004.

Take The First Step Toward Fitness

Most of us need to take a simpler approach—do something. The first step is just being more active even if it's only a little. Start by walking. It can always be worked into your day. Anyone can do it any time, in almost any place, without any special equipment. The opportunities are plentiful. Go for a walk after dinner instead of watching television, walk to school, walk to the store rather than driving, or take the dog for a long walk. A moderately brisk pace is preferable, but build up to it gradually.

Of course, there are lots of other activities besides walking that will give you the benefits of an aerobic workout, and you should pursue as many as you can and want to. Choose the ones you enjoy most, and have a great time while you get in shape.

Sports Injuries: How To Stay In The Game

Nothing is more frustrating than finally getting involved in an activity you enjoy, only to hurt yourself and be forced into a prolonged rehabilitation period. Although some injuries may be unavoidable, proper conditioning and attention to the details of warm-ups, cool-downs, and stretching will help keep you off the disabled list.

An Ounce Of Prevention...

Preventing injuries requires both common sense and careful preparation. By following a few basic principles, you can help ensure that your activity won't put you out of commission.

Warm Up: This is the number one tenet of injury prevention and should consist of three to five minutes of low-level activity followed by a few minutes of stretching.

Stay Flexible: Stretching during the warm-up and cool-down phases will help prevent muscle pulls and strains as well as the general aches and pains that can occur after exercising.

Build Gradually: Start out slowly and build up gradually in intensity and duration of activity. Weekend athletes are famous for trying to do too much, too soon. Don't fall into this trap.

Be Prepared: Use the right equipment for your sport whether its a good pair of running shoes or knee pads for inline skating. Be sure the equipment is in good condition and appropriate for your skill level (for example, skis for beginners versus experts).

✔ Quick Tip
Don't Know Where To Start?

- Start by making the most of the activities you do already and increase their frequency, duration, or intensity.

- Ask a friend or someone who has the experience and is willing to help you.

- Go to health fairs, sports expositions, and clinics to learn from the variety of offerings presented.

- If you've been inactive for a long time, start off slowly. Walk for 10 minutes or just around the block.

- Match your activity to your fitness level.

- Don't concern yourself with fancy equipment or health club memberships.

- Just activate!

Source: "The Nolan Ryan Fitness Guide," President's Council on Physical Fitness and Sports, October 2004.

Rehydrate: Water is the best sports drink and you should drink plenty of it before, during, and after exercise especially in warm weather. Keep drinking it throughout the day.

Avoid Extremes: Try not to exercise outdoors in extreme hot or cold weather, but if you do, be sure to dress properly. Use caution against heat exhaustion or, at the other extreme, frostbite.

Cool Down: Gradually decrease the intensity of your activity to restore a normal heart rate. Post exercise stretching should not be overlooked.

Hitting A Grand Slam

Now that you know just how easy being more physically active can be, the only thing left is to do it. Just think about all the great things being physically fit will do for your health and well being, and activate yourself. Involve your family and your friends—anyone and everyone that you can. Start incorporating more active pursuits into your lifestyle, and before you know it, activity will be the most natural and enjoyable part of your day. Every single day you do something physically active—even if its just walking home from school—is one day closer to realizing the mental and physical benefits of fitness. And that can make you feel like you hit a grand slam in the World Series.

Chapter 37

Don't Let Health Issues Keep You On The Sidelines

Meeting The Challenge: Don't Let Asthma Keep You Out Of The Game

Who Has Asthma?

Asthma, which makes it hard to breathe—and causes coughing and wheezing—affects about five million American kids and teens. That's almost one in 10.

Famous people like rapper Coolio have asthma, although he's better known for his hit songs like "Gangsta's Paradise" than for his fight against the illness. Olympians like Misty Hyman and Amy VanDyken, Tom Dolan and Karen Furneaux, and Kurt Grote also have asthma.

Physical Activity And Asthma

Things like cold or dry air, dust, pollen, pollution, cigarette smoke, or stress can trigger asthma. This can make your body pump out chemicals

About This Chapter: This chapter includes information from "Meeting The Challenge: Don't Let Asthma Keep You Out Of The Game," 2001; and "Expert's Opinion On Diabetes," 2005, Centers for Disease Control and Prevention (CDC). Additional text from the American College of Sports Medicine and American Heart Association is cited separately within the chapter.

that close off your airways, making it hard for air to get into to your lungs, and cause an asthma attack.

Physical activity can trigger asthma attacks too. Experts don't know for sure why physical activity sometimes brings one on, but they suspect that fast breathing through the mouth (like when you get winded) can irritate the airways. In addition, because air pollution levels rise later in the day, physical activity is harder on the lungs than morning activity.

Get Fit

So, should you get a doctor's note and skip gym class? No. Doctors want their asthma patients to get active, especially in asthma-friendly activities like these: swimming, bicycling, golf, inline skating, and weightlifting.

Why are these good choices if you want to be physically active?

• They let you control how hard and fast you breathe

• They let you breathe through your nose at all times

• They don't dry out your airways

• They mix short, intense activities with long endurance workouts

---

♣ It's A Fact!!

Today, more than ever, asthma is not a barrier to physical activity. In fact, if you keep your asthma under control, you can do it all. Need proof?

• At the 1984 summer Olympics, 67 of the 597 American athletes had asthma. Among them, they won 41 medals.

• Twenty percent of the athletes at the 1996 summer Olympics had asthma brought on by physical activity.

• Almost 30 percent of the American swimmers on the 2000 summer Olympic team had asthma and used inhalers.

Asthma didn't hold them back, and it shouldn't hold you back, either.

Source: From "Meeting the Challenge: Don't Let Asthma Keep You Out of the Game," Centers for Disease Control and Prevention (CDC), 2001.

- You can do them in a controlled environment (for example, a gym with air that's not too cold or dry)

- Usually you do them with other people, who can help you if an attack comes on

Getting regular physical activity can improve your breathing and lead to fewer asthma attacks. Just remember to follow these tips—in fact, this is good advice for everyone, not just those with asthma.

- **Ease into exercise.** Start your workout with a warm-up, and don't overdo it by running five miles on your first day, if you get winded walking around the block. Finish up with a cool down.

- **Take a buddy.** It's more fun and a friend can help if you get into trouble.

- **Respect your body.** Stay away from the things that trigger your asthma. Help out your airways by breathing through your nose instead of your mouth, take it easy on days when your asthma symptoms are really bugging you, and stick to the medicine routine that your doctor has set up.

- **Take breaks.** Treat yourself to rest and drink plenty of water.

- **Mix it up.** For example, try going inline skating one day and taking a long walk the next.

Feel Good

To feel your best, do the right stuff to control your asthma, and listen to your doctors because they're on your team.

According to Dr. Stephen Redd, an asthma expert at the Centers for Disease Control and Prevention (CDC), people with asthma "should expect to live a life that really isn't affected by asthma, except for having to follow the directions." He also says to speak up if you are having symptoms, and remember to "keep a good attitude and keep working to control the disease."

So, get out there and get moving. With good habits and today's medicines, you can go for the gold or just join your friends on the basketball court.

Exercise-Induced Asthma

"Exercise-Induced Asthma," reprinted with permission of the American College of Sports Medicine. Copyright © 2005 American College of Sports Medicine. This information is a product of ACSM's Consumer Products Committee.

"Out Of Shape?" Maybe Not...

Many people incorrectly believe that they are "out of shape," when in fact they may have exercise-induced asthma (EIA). Because the symptoms of EIA are similar to poor fitness—shortness of breath and a tight feeling in the chest—it is difficult to tell the difference between them. Increased training does not stop the problem, and for some, the symptoms of EIA may deter them from exercising. Exercise-induced asthma may not be life threatening, but it is uncomfortable. EIA affects more people than was originally believed. Clinicians estimate that up to 15 percent of the general population may suffer from this easily over-looked condition. Approximately 11 percent of the 1984 United States Olympic Team had symptoms of exercise-induced asthma. The good news is that EIA is controllable.

What Is Exercise-Induced Asthma?

Exercise-induced asthma is a reaction of the passages of the lunges that is caused by exercise. The bronchial tubes become irritated during exercise and begin to constrict. The bronchial muscles around the tube go into spasm, thus the term "broncho spasm." Mucus builds up in the tubes, and the cells that line the airways also start to swell, closing the airways even more. Thus, you have problems getting air in and out of your lungs.

Probable Cause

What triggers an EIA attack is not yet completely known. Your airway warms and moistens incoming air, which is usually cooler and drier. In the process the airways can cool down and dry out, which can irritate sensitive tissues. The amount of air moved in and out of the lungs increases during exercise, thus increasing the amount of cooling and drying. The bronchial tubes react to this process with EIA. Although chronic asthma sufferers are more likely to have EIA, the presence of EIA does not lead to chronic asthma.

Symptoms Of Exercise-Induced Asthma

The symptoms of EIA include: shortness of breath during or after exercise, chest tightness or pain, coughing, and wheezing. These symptoms start a few minutes into exercise and may last for 30-60 minutes. In contrast, if the problem is poor fitness, the symptoms will usually disappear a few minutes after stopping exercise.

What To Do

You should speak with your doctor if you think you have exercise-induced asthma. Only a doctor can decide whether you have EIA. An exercise test can be used to determine EIA. However, this test will not be positive for everyone with EIA. Many doctors will base their diagnosis on your history and symptoms, and may have you use a trial of bronchodilator therapy prior to exercise. Although chest pain is a symptom of EIA, it is important for your doctor to rule out cardiovascular disease.

You can take several simple steps to reduce the chance of having an EIA attack. Breathing through your nose will help warm and moisten the air before it reaches the bronchial tubes, though it's not very easy during anything but a mild workout. Staying out of cold, dry air may be the best course of action, but if you do exercise outdoors, wear a facemask or scarf, which enriches inhaled air with heat and moisture from your skin. If you exercise inside, such as on an indoor track, on a treadmill, or in the warm, moist air of an indoor swimming pool, you are less likely to have an EIA episode. Lower intensity sports, such as golf, baseball, or weight lifting, are less likely to stimulate EIA (though they provide less cardiovascular benefits). And no matter what your activity, if high amounts of airborne irritants, like pollen, increase your chance of an attack, it makes good sense to exercise indoors on days when those pollutants are high.

Most importantly you should continue to exercise. Exercise training will improve fitness so that a lower level of breathing is needed at a given exercise level. Good cardiovascular fitness will enable you to exercise at a higher intensity before causing an EIA attack.

Tips To Train By

- Exercise indoors

- Cover mouth and nose when outdoors

- Warm-up 45–60 minutes before training

- Use interval training

Additional Workout Strategies

Nature has created an EIA loophole called the refractory period. The refractory period lasts up to two hours after an exercise-induced asthma attack. During this time your lungs are less likely to react as strongly. If you warm up 45 minutes to an hour before your workout you may be able to exercise without too many symptoms. In addition, EIA usually starts several minutes into a workout. Some athletes have found they can exercise easier by using alternating work and rest periods (interval training).

Medicines For EIA

Though some people can keep their exercise-induced asthma under control with simple workout strategies, you may need medication. There are two broad types of medications that your physician might prescribe.

Bronchodilators work to keep the airways relaxed and open, and are used before, or during exercise. A relatively new class of drugs called leukotriene inhibitors blocks the chemical the body uses to constrict the bronchial muscles. The other main categories of medicines are the anti-inflammatories. These include inhaled corticosteroids, which reduce the sensitivity to airways.

While most available medications are inhaled, some are taken in pill form. No one medicine works best for everyone and you may need a combination for best control. The accompanying table (Table 37.1) lists the generic medicines, indicate how they work, and for how long. Side effects, in cases where they exist, are possible tremors, nausea, or heart palpitations. If you are an athlete, it is important to check that the medication suggested for you is legal, as several of these have been on the list of banned medications for different sports.

Table 37.1. Medicines For Exercise-Induced Asthma

Medication	How Long Before Exercise?	Lasts How Long?
Short-acting beta agonists (B)	15–30 min.	2 hrs.
Salmeterol (B)	30–60 min.	12 hrs.
Cromolyn sodium or nedocromil sodium (A)	10–20 min.	2 hrs.
Inhaled corticosteroids (A)	Ongoing therapy	Ongoing therapy
Ipratropium bromide (B)	1 hr.	2–3 hrs.
Oral theophylline (B)	Ongoing therapy	Ongoing therapy
Leukotriene inhibitors (B)	Ongoing therapy	Ongoing therapy
A = Anti-inflammatory	B = Bronchodilator	

Source: American College of Sports Medicine Copyright © 2005

Physical Activity And Exercise: Information For People With Heart Defects

"Physical Activity And Exercise," reprinted with permission from www .americanheart.org. © 2008 American Heart Association, Inc.

One of the most common questions people with heart defects ask is, "Do I have to limit my physical activity?" Activities like walking, jogging, and swimming help keep the cardiovascular system fit. They're good for almost everyone, including most people with heart defects. But some people with heart defects do need to limit their activities. Usually this means forgoing intense competitive sports and certain exercises including isometric exercises and weightlifting, rope climbing, sit-ups, chin-ups, and push-ups. In some (rare) instances even more restrictions may be needed.

Exercise And Your Heart

Your heart's workload can be increased in two ways: (1) by increasing the amount of blood the heart pumps, and (2) by pumping at a higher blood pressure. Physical activity makes your heart work more in both these ways. The amount of extra work for the heart varies a lot from one activity to another, however.

Low-intensity sports like golf, baseball, and doubles tennis—and activities like dancing, casual swimming, cycling, and power walking—don't put much strain on the heart. They're fine for almost anyone with congenital heart defects. Household activities such as digging in a garden, raking leaves, mowing the grass, and vacuuming are also fine. Shoveling snow isn't a good idea.

People with some heart defects may be asked to avoid high-intensity sports like basketball, competitive swimming, rowing, competitive cycling, jogging, and wrestling.

✔ **Quick Tip**

Expert's Opinion On Diabetes

Want the straight scoop on talking to a friend who has diabetes? Well, it's just like talking to anyone else. Someone with diabetes is just as likely to like the same books, movies, and activities you do, but they do have some special things they need to think about every day.

It can be hard to have a serious disease, and your friend may feel strange about bringing up all the new things he or she has to do. They may worry that you think it's gross when they stick their finger to test blood sugar or if they have to give themselves a shot. One of the best things you can do is give them a chance to talk to you about how they feel and what they worry about. Another thing that can help is learning more about their disease and how you can help them manage it—including warning signs that their blood sugar may be too low. It may be a big relief for them to know that someone else is helping to look out for them.

And here's the inside scoop. There are two big things that every person with diabetes needs to think of every day.

First, they need to think about food. While everyone should try and eat mostly healthy meals and snacks, it's really important for someone with diabetes. Since some carbohydrates can affect blood sugar really quickly, people with diabetes

Finally, certain sports like diving, football, and ice hockey have a significant risk of bodily injury. People with certain problems (for example, a pacemaker or Marfan syndrome) should avoid these sports.

Finding The Right Activity Regimen

Every person with congenital heart disease, whether or not they've had their defect repaired, is different when it comes to participating in sports. Only your cardiologist can tell you for sure which activities are right for you. Sometimes tests to evaluate your heart, like an echocardiogram, Holter monitor, or exercise test may help your doctor determine what level of activity is safest. If you have chest pain, palpitations, shortness of breath, or faintness, stop exercising immediately! Contact your doctor as soon as you can—even if your symptoms go away.

---

need to make sure they eat mostly complex carbohydrates like whole grain bread and pasta, fruits and vegetables, and low-fat dairy products. These are broken down more slowly by the body and help keep blood sugar stable. Carbohydrates like white bread, juice, soda, or candy can send blood sugar soaring—just what people with diabetes need to avoid. Eating small meals every few hours also helps keep blood sugar levels from going up and down too much.

So, if a friend turns down cake at your birthday, don't take it personally or try to make him eat it anyway. And, it's even better if you can plan ahead to make sure that you have plenty of stuff they can eat there, too. There are even special cake recipes that use artificial sweetener that people with diabetes (and everyone else) can eat.

Next, they need to make sure they are physically active. It's important that people with diabetes get plenty of activity because it helps them to keep their blood sugar down.

Being active can also help prevent diabetes. Keeping your weight at the level that's right for you is one way to reduce the chance of getting type 2 diabetes yourself.

Source: Reprinted from "Expert's Opinion on Diabetes," Centers for Disease Control and Prevention (CDC), 2005.

Job Restrictions

Most people with heart defects can work in virtually any occupation. Some may be asked to avoid intense physical activities like heavy lifting. If your heart condition has a high risk of causing fainting or dizziness, you may need to avoid jobs where fainting could be dangerous to you or others. If you have concerns about how your occupation might affect your health, ask your cardiologist.

Chapter 38

Cold Weather, Hot Weather, And Cardiovascular Disease

Cold Weather And Cardiovascular Disease

How does cold weather affect the heart?

Many people aren't conditioned to the physical stress of outdoor activities and don't know the dangers of being outdoors in cold weather. Winter sports enthusiasts who don't take certain precautions can suffer accidental hypothermia (hi-po-ther-me-ah).

Hypothermia means the body temperature has fallen below normal. It occurs when your body can't produce enough energy to keep the internal body temperature warm enough. It can kill you. Heart failure causes most deaths in hypothermia.

Symptoms include lack of coordination, mental confusion, slowed reactions, shivering, and sleepiness.

Children, the elderly, and those with heart disease are at special risk. As people age, their ability to maintain a normal internal body temperature often

About This Chapter: This chapter includes information from "Cold Weather And Cardiovascular Disease" and "Hot Weather And Cardiovascular Disease," reprinted with permission from www.americanheart.org. © 2008 American Heart Association, Inc.

decreases. Because elderly people seem to be relatively insensitive to moderately cold conditions, they can suffer hypothermia without knowing they're in danger.

People with coronary heart disease often suffer chest pain or discomfort called angina pectoris (an-jih-nah or an-jih-nah pek-tor-is) when they're in cold weather. Some studies suggest that harsh winter weather may increase a person's risk of heart attack due to overexertion.

Besides cold temperatures, high winds, snow, and rain also can steal body heat. Wind is especially dangerous, because it removes the layer of heated air from around your body. At 30 degrees Fahrenheit in a 20-mile-per-hour wind, the cooling effect is equal to calm air at four degrees. Similarly, dampness causes the body to lose heat faster than it would at the same temperature in drier conditions.

To keep warm, wear layers of clothing. This traps air between layers, forming a protective insulation. Also, wear a hat or headscarf. Much of your body's heat can be lost through your head. And ears are especially prone to frostbite. Keep your hands and feet warm, too, as they tend to lose heat rapidly.

Don't drink alcoholic beverages before going outdoors or when outside. Alcohol gives an initial feeling of warmth because blood vessels in the skin expand. Heat is then drawn away from the body's vital organs.

♣ It's A Fact!!
American Heart Association Recommendation

People who are outdoors in cold weather should avoid sudden exertion like lifting a heavy shovel full of snow. Even walking through heavy, wet snow or snowdrifts can strain a person's heart.

Source: "Cold Weather And Cardiovascular Disease," AHA, © 2007.

Hot Weather And Cardiovascular Disease

How does hot weather affect the heart?

Extremely hot weather causes dehydration, heat exhaustion, and heat stroke. These risks increase when the humidity is above 70 percent and the temperature is above 70 degrees Fahrenheit. Heat and humidity interfere with the body's natural cooling process.

Exercising outside in hot and humid conditions can be hard on your heart. This is true even for athletes who haven't yet adapted to the heat. The problem is made worse because the heart is trying to deliver blood and oxygen to your working muscles while your body is trying to cool off by sweating. If you sweat too much, you lose fluid. This decreases your total blood volume. That means your heart has to pump even harder to get the smaller volume of blood to your working muscles, skin, and the other body parts. When you lose too much fluid, your body temperature rises and your nervous system doesn't work properly. Extreme fluid loss can lead to brain and heart damage.

A good way to monitor your body fluid level is to weigh every morning after using the bathroom. If you weigh two pounds less than normal in the morning, you're probably dehydrated and need to drink more water before doing any vigorous physical activity. (You may have lost weight as water but not as fat.)

If you plan to exercise outside in hot and humid weather, wear very light, comfortable clothing and work out in the early morning or late evening, if possible. Know the symptoms of heat exhaustion and heat stroke. If any symptoms appear, stop exercising and cool down immediately by dousing yourself with cold water. You may need to get medical attention. Heat exhaustion can progress quickly to heat stroke, which can kill you.

What are the symptoms of heat exhaustion?

- Heavy sweating
- Cold, clammy skin
- Dizziness or fainting (syncope)
- A weak and rapid pulse
- Muscle cramps

- Fast, shallow breathing

- Nausea, vomiting, or both

What are the symptoms of heat stroke?

- Warm, dry skin with no sweating

- Strong and rapid pulse

- Confusion and/or unconsciousness

- High fever

- Throbbing headaches

- Nausea, vomiting, or both

Chapter 39

Dealing With Sports Injuries

Worried about sports injuries? Don't sweat it. Think of avoiding injury as just another part of playing by the rules—only this rulebook is the one that keeps you from getting hurt. That's because the best way to deal with sports injuries is to prevent them. Prevention includes knowing the rules of the game you're playing, using the proper equipment, and playing it safe.

But you've practiced with your team, played it safe on the field, and still sustained an injury. Don't worry, it's not the end of the world—just the beginning of a healing process. Read on to find out what this process is and how you can deal with a sports injury.

What Are Sports Injuries?

Sports injuries are injuries that typically occur while participating in organized sports, competitions, training sessions, or organized fitness activities. These injuries may occur in teens for a variety of reasons, including improper training, lack appropriate footwear or safety equipment, and rapid growth during puberty.

About This Chapter: This chapter includes information from "Dealing With Sports Injuries," June 2007, reprinted with permission from www.kidshealth.org. Copyright © 2006 The Nemours Foundation. This information was provided by KidsHealth, one of the largest resources online for medically reviewed health information written for parents, kids, and teens. For more articles like this one, visit www.KidsHealth.org or www.TeensHealth.org.

There are two general types. The first type is called an acute traumatic injury. Acute traumatic injuries usually involve a single blow from a single application of force—like getting a cross-body block in football. Acute traumatic injuries include the following:

- **A Fracture:** Crack, break, or shattering of a bone

- **A Bruise (Known Medically As A Contusion):** Caused by a direct blow, which may cause swelling and bleeding in muscles and other body tissues

- **A Strain:** A stretch or tear of a muscle or tendon the tough and narrow end of a muscle that connects it to a bone

- **A Sprain:** Stretch or tear of a ligament, the tissue that supports and strengthens joints by connecting bones and cartilage

- **An Abrasion:** A scrape

- **A Laceration:** A cut in the skin that is usually deep enough to require stitches

The second type of sports injury is called an overuse or chronic injury. Chronic injuries are those that happen over a period of time. Chronic injuries are usually the result of repetitive training, such as running, overhand throwing, or serving a ball tennis. These include:

- **Stress Fractures:** Tiny cracks in the bone's surface often caused by repetitive overloading (such as in the feet of a basketball player who is continuously jumping on the court)

- **Tendinitis:** Inflammation of the tendon caused by repetitive stretching

- **Epiphysitis Or Apophysitis:** Growth plate overload injuries such as Osgood-Schlatter disease

Often overuse injuries seem less important than acute injuries. You may be tempted to ignore that aching in your wrist or that soreness in your knees, but always remember that just because an injury isn't dramatic doesn't mean it's unimportant or will go away on its own. If left untreated, a chronic injury will probably get worse over time.

Head And Neck Injuries

Head injuries include concussions, contusions, fractures, and hematomas. A concussion is a violent jarring or shock to the head that causes a temporary jolt to the brain. If severe enough, or recurrent, concussions can cause brain damage but fortunately this is not common in teens. A hematoma is a bleeding or pooling of blood between the tissue layers covering the brain or inside the brain. All of these injuries can be caused by impact to the head from a fall, forceful shaking of the head, a blow to the head, or whiplash. Whiplash is an injury to the neck caused by an abrupt jerking motion of the head.

Always wear helmets for contact sports and when doing activities like biking and in-line skating to prevent head injuries.

Neck injuries are among the most dangerous. You can hurt your neck through a sudden traumatic injury in sports like mountain climbing, skydiving, horseback riding, gymnastics, diving, rugby, judo, or boxing.

Neck injuries include strains, fractures, contusions, and sprains. Another very common sports-related neck injury is a stinger or burner from stretched nerves in the neck. Most neck injuries are caused by impact to the head or neck sustained during a fall or a blow. Your neck can also be injured a little at a time. Too much strain on your neck can cause increasing pain, sometimes only on one side of your neck. Sometimes you may feel only a slight pain when you move a certain way.

If the injury is severe and there is a chance that the neck might be injured, it's very important to keep the injured person still with the head held straight while someone calls for emergency medical help. If the person is lying on the ground, do not try to move him or her. Never try to move someone who may have a neck injury—a mishandled neck fracture could lead to permanent paralysis or even death.

How do these injuries happen? Serious head and neck injuries occur most often in athletes who participate in contact sports (like football or rugby) or sports with the potential for falling accidents, such as horseback riding.

♣ It's A Fact!!
Common Knee Injuries And Problems

- **Chondromalacia:** Refers to softening of the articular cartilage of the kneecap. This disorder occurs most often in young adults and can be caused by injury, overuse, misalignment of the patella, or muscle weakness. Instead of gliding smoothly across the lower end of the thighbone, the kneecap rubs against it, thereby roughening the cartilage underneath the kneecap. The most frequent symptom is a dull pain around or under the kneecap that worsens when walking down stairs or hills.

- **Cruciate Ligament Injuries:** Sometimes referred to as sprains, these injuries don't necessarily cause pain, but they are disabling. The anterior cruciate ligament is most often stretched or torn (or both) by a sudden twisting motion (for example, when the feet are planted one way and the knees are turned another). The posterior cruciate ligament is most often injured by a direct impact, such as in an automobile accident or football tackle. You may hear a popping sound, and the leg may buckle when you try to stand on it.

- **Tendinitis:** Knee tendon injuries range from tendinitis (inflammation of a tendon) to a ruptured (torn) tendon. If a person overuses a tendon during certain activities such as dancing, cycling, or running, the tendon stretches and becomes inflamed. Tendinitis of the patellar tendon is sometimes called jumper's knee because in sports that require jumping, such as basketball, the muscle contraction and force of hitting the ground after a jump strain the tendon. After repeated stress, the tendon may become inflamed or tear. People with tendinitis often have tenderness at the point where the patellar tendon meets the bone. In addition, they may feel pain during running, hurried walking, or jumping.

- **Osgood-Schlatter Disease:** A condition caused by repetitive stress or tension on part of the growth area of the upper tibia. It is characterized by inflammation of the patellar tendon and surrounding soft tissues at the point where the tendon attaches to the tibia. The disease may also be associated with an injury in which the tendon is stretched so much that it tears away from the tibia and takes a fragment of bone with it. The disease most commonly affects active young people, particularly boys between the ages of 10 and 15, who play games or sports that include frequent running and jumping. People with this disease experience pain just below the knee joint that usually worsens with activity and is relieved by rest. A bony bump that is particularly painful when pressed may appear on the upper edge of the tibia (below the kneecap). Usually, the motion of the knee is not affected. Pain may last a few months and may recur until the child's growth is completed.

- **Iliotibial Band Syndrome:** An inflammatory condition caused when a band of tissue rubs over the outer bone (lateral condyle) of the knee. Although iliotibial band syndrome may be caused by direct injury to the knee, it is most often caused by the stress of long-term overuse, such as sometimes occurs in sports training and, particularly, in running. A person with this syndrome feels an ache or burning sensation at the side of the knee during activity. Pain may be localized at the side of the knee or radiate up the side of the thigh. A person may also feel a snap when the knee is bent and then straightened. Swelling is usually absent and knee motion is normal.

- **Osteochondritis Dissecans:** Results from a loss of the blood supply to an area of bone underneath a joint surface. It usually involves the knee. The affected bone and its covering of cartilage gradually loosen and cause pain. This problem usually arises spontaneously in an active adolescent or young adult. It may be due to a slight blockage of a small artery or to an unrecognized injury or tiny fracture that damages the overlying cartilage. A person with this condition may eventually develop osteoarthritis. Lack of a blood supply can cause bone to break down.

- **Plica Syndrome:** Occurs when plicae (bands of synovial tissue) are irritated by overuse or injury. Synovial plicae are the remains of tissue pouches found in the early stages of fetal development. As the fetus develops, these pouches normally combine to form one large synovial cavity. If this process is incomplete, plicae remain as four folds or bands of synovial tissue within the knee. Injury, chronic overuse, or inflammatory conditions are associated with this syndrome. Symptoms of plica syndrome include pain and swelling, a clicking sensation, and locking and weakness of the knee.

Source: "Knee Problems," National Institute of Arthritis and Musculoskeletal and Skin Diseases (NIAMS), National Institutes of Health, Department of Health and Human Services, May 2006.

Back Injuries

Back injuries include sprains, fractures, contusions, stress fractures, and strains and are caused by twists or overexertion of back muscles during bending or lifting movements. These injuries can occur in contact sports like football and ice hockey or in weight lifting, figure skating, gymnastics, dancing, baseball, and basketball.

Sex Organs

When it comes to injuries to the sex organs, guys usually suffer more trauma than girls because the penis and testicles are outside the body and lack natural protection during contact sports. Guys should always wear athletic supporters, or in some sports a cup, protect the genitals from serious injury.

Injuries to the uterus or ovaries are rare, but breast injuries are common complaints among teen girls. As the breasts develop, they can often be sore, and a blow from a softball or a jab from an elbow, for example, can be painful. Girls should wear supportive sports bras while playing sports or exercising.

♣ **It's A Fact!!**
Sports Injuries On Your Body

You may think of your back or your arms and legs as the only places where you could get hurt while playing, but you can get a sports injury anywhere on your body, including your face, neck, head, back, sex organs, hands, and feet.

Source: "Dealing With Sports Injuries," June 2007, reprinted with permission from www.kidshealth.org. Copyright © 2006 The Nemours Foundation.

Hand And Wrist Injuries

Hand, finger, and wrist injuries include fractures, dislocations, and sprains and often occur in contact sports such as football, lacrosse, and hockey. Hand injuries can result from a fall that forces the hand or fingers backward, a forceful impact to the hands, or a direct blow.

Foot Injuries

Foot injuries can include ligament strains, stress fractures, heel bruises, and swollen growth plates. Because your feet support all of your weight and must absorb a lot of force over and over again, they can be particularly susceptible to injury. Another reason some teens may suffer foot injuries is because of differences in their feet. For example, some people have flat feet or high arches. These differences don't mean that sports should be avoided, but it does mean that precautions, such as a special shoe insert, may be needed.

Taking Care Of Sports Injuries

If your pain progressively increases with activity (what sports medicine doctors call an "upward crescendo") and causes swelling, limping, or loss of range of motion, you need to see a doctor soon as possible.

What kinds of pain should you be on the lookout for? Any injury that results in swelling, numbness, intense pain or tenderness, stiffness, or loss of flexibility should be taken seriously.

You should also know the difference between soreness and chronic pain. Soreness is temporary, but chronic pain continues over a greater length of time. For example, it's not always necessary to see a doctor right away if your shoulder is sore, but you should schedule an appointment if the pain is worsening at any time or if it persists for a week or more. You should also see a doctor if your pain progresses from happening only after playing to happening during sports or if you notice it when you wake up or are doing daily activities.

The most important thing to do when you suspect you are injured is to stop doing whatever sport has caused the injury right away and go see a doctor.

For more severe or complicated injuries, it may be best to see a doctor who specializes in sports medicine.

The doctor will examine your injury and use diagnostic tools such as x-rays and magnetic resonance imaging (MRI) to determine the extent of your injury. MRI allows doctors to see soft tissues more clearly than x-rays or CT (computed tomography) scans do.

Once the doctor knows the full extent of your injury, he or she usually will start with conservative treatment techniques such as rest and ice to help decrease swelling. Pain relief and anti-inflammatory medicines such as ibuprofen (like Advil or Motrin) may be prescribed. Splints, casts, and surgery also may be needed, depending on the injury.

One of three things will happen next. Your doctor may recommend that you not play while you heal, that you play and use a protective device (a knee brace or wrist guard, for example), or that you undergo rehabilitation (physical therapy). Sports medicine doctors won't let you play if you are at risk for getting another injury or aggravating an injury you are recovering from.

When Can You Play Again?

If your doctor has asked you to stop playing, your number one question is probably "When can I play sports again?" This depends on your specific injury, so make sure you discuss this with your doctor. There are things you can do while injured to stay fit without making your injury worse—but make sure you check with your doctor first. These activities are known as cross training, and they include using stationary cycles, swimming, water therapy, and rowing machines.

Your rehabilitation program will also help you stay fit as you recover. Rehabilitation, or rehab, is the process that gets you back in shape and ready for action again. Rehab may be part of your treatment program and can include exercise, manual therapy from a physical therapist (a specialist who is trained to help you recover from a sports injury), and technology such as ultrasound. Ultrasound equipment is used to heat the injured area. This heat relieves pain, promotes healing, and increases your range of motion.

Playing Safe

What can you do to protect yourself from getting hurt again? Use protective gear—such as helmets for contact sports like football—that is appropriate to the specific sport.

When you return to play, you might need some new protective gear, including modified shoes (such as those with inserts or arch supports or those designed for use in a particular sport), tapings (tape used to wrap a knee, for example, to provide extra support), knee and elbow braces, and mouth guards. These devices help support and protect your body part from strains, direct blows, and possible reinjury.

To help prevent reinjury, be sure to warm up adequately before practice and games. Remember to take it slow when you first get back into your sport and gradually build back up to your preinjury level.

Also, know your limits. If the previously injured part (or any body part) begins to hurt, stop immediately and rest. Don't delay in seeking medical attention if the pain persists. It's your body's way of telling you something is not right.

So, play, but play safe. Try to learn from your experience and do the things that can help you avoid getting hurt again.

Chapter 40

Drugs In Sports

General Information On Drugs In Sports

What is the background of drug use in sports?

During the past 30 years, the use of performance enhancing substances in athletics increased at every level of competition. Athletes have used different supplements including vitamins and minerals, amino acid supplements, anabolic steroids, and other anabolic substances, stimulants, painkillers, and a variety of illegal street drugs. Husch (1995) and Wagner (1991) suggested that student athletes use substances due to complex social, psychological, physiological, economic, and political factors.

What are some reasons why student athletes take different kinds of drugs?

Student athletes have used drugs:

• to cope with academic and athletic stress;

• to speed up increases in strength and physical size;

• to socialize and relax after competition.

About This Chapter: This chapter includes information excerpted from "Drugs In Sports," © 2002 National Center for Drug Free Sport, Inc. (www.drugfreesport.com). Reprinted with permission. The complete report can be viewed at http://www.drugfreesport.com/choices/drugs/index.html.

Human Growth Hormone (HGH)

What are the sources of HGH?

HGH is a naturally occurring polypeptide hormone produced by the anterior pituitary gland and secreted into the general circulation. HGH is released from the somatotroph cells of the anterior pituitary, which is under the control of the hypothalamic hormones.

What are the actions/effects of HGH?

HGH is one of the major hormones influencing growth and development in humans. A major function of HGH is the maintenance of normal linear growth from birth to adulthood. The metabolic action of HGH is also important in the regulation of energy production and storage.

Why would some student athletes want to use HGH?

Some individuals use HGH because they perceive that it is as effective as anabolic steroids with fewer side effects and is not detectable in a drug test. Therefore, they may also choose to use HGH as a steroid substitute to prevent loss of muscle after discontinuing the use of steroids.

♣ It's A Fact!!
Drug Use In Sports

In general, findings from different surveys indicate that:

- decisions not to use drugs and alcohol are personal ones and were not based on coaches' rules or laws;

- since 1989, fewer athletes feel there is a problem of illegal drug use by college athletes;

- some student athletes perceive institutionally-based and the National Collegiate Athletic Association (NCAA) drug testing to be "easy to beat" and report that either they or a teammate have "beaten" a drug test in the past;

- student athletes are more aware of the drug education efforts of their schools and generally rate their school's drug education and counseling services to be either "good" or "excellent;"

- additional research is needed relative to the alcohol and drug use habits of college student-athletes.

What are the effects of HGH on performance?

According to some controlled scientific studies, HGH does not increase muscle strength. Most reports on HGH efficacies are either anecdotal or based on animal studies.

What are the side effects of HGH use?

The side effects of using HGH may lead to life threatening health conditions, especially since some estimates report that athletes who use HGH to enhance performance are taking 10 times the therapeutic dosage.

♣ It's A Fact!!
Reported Side Effects Of Human Growth Hormone (HGH)

- Developing irreversible acromegaly (abnormal growth of bones of the hands and feet and face)
- High blood pressure
- Heart damage
- Premature aging and death
- Soft tissue swelling
- Thickening of the skin, abnormal hair growth

- Colonic polyps
- Liver damage and glucose intolerance
- Muscle weakness
- Enlargement of the internal organs
- Arthritis
- Impotence

Adrenocorticotropic Hormone (ACTH)

Why would a student athlete be interested in using ACTH?

A student athlete might perceive that this substance would enhance muscular development.

What are some of the adverse reactions associated with the use of ACTH?

ACTH may mask signs of infection. Diabetics may have increased requirements for insulin or oral hypoglycemics. ACTH can also cause fluid and electrolyte disturbances, muscle weakness and loss of muscle mass, ulcerative esophagitis and peptic ulcer, impaired wound healing, headache and vertigo, increased intracranial pressure, menstrual irregularities, suppression of growth in children, ophthalmic, metabolic, and allergic reactions.

Erythropoietin (EPO)

What are the actions/effects of erythropoietin (EPO)?

EPO is a glycoprotein that stimulates red blood cell production.

What are the therapeutic uses of EPO?

The Food and Drug Administration (FDA), for treatment of anemia, approves EPO.

Why would some student athletes want to use EPO?

The use of EPO is believed to increase oxygen absorption, reduce fatigue and improve endurance by increasing the rate of red cell production. Promoters of EPO claim that this drug increases the metabolism and the healing process of muscles because the extra red cells carry more oxygen and nutrients.

What are the adverse effects associated with using EPO?

EPO causes an increase in the total number of circulating red bloods cells. This can lead to increased thickening (blood viscosity) of the blood. Added to the dehydration that frequently occurs in endurance sports, excess thickening of the blood takes place.

The risk for coronary and cerebral artery blockages increases when the hematocrit (percentage of red blood cells in the blood) level exceeds 55%.

✔ **Quick Tip**

What are some of the most important recent findings from the National Collegiate Athletic Association (NCAA) National Study of the Substance Abuse Habits of Student Athletes?

Find out the current information related to this topic directly from the NCAA website at www.ncaa.org/wps/portal.

Diuretics

What are the therapeutic uses of diuretics?

Diuretics are drugs that increase urination. These drugs are used medically used to control hypertension, or high blood pressure, reduce edema, and to treat congestive heart failure.

Why would some student athletes want to use diuretics?

Diuretics have been used by athletes to achieve rapid weight loss, to reduce the concentration of drugs in the urine through rapid diuresis, and to reduce the likelihood of detection of banned drugs in a urine test. Athletes involved in weight-category sports have used a combination of heat exposure, exercise, food and water restriction, self-induced vomiting, laxatives, and diuretics to lose weight. Diuretics have also been used by female athletes in conjugation with strict dieting which could lead to anorexia. Diuretics have also been used to manage premenstrual fluid retention.

What are some potential adverse effects associated with using diuretics?

Some individuals may experience dehydration, muscle cramps, dizziness, high potassium levels, high calcium levels, low blood sugar levels, headache, nausea, vomiting, and drowsiness.

Central Nervous System Stimulants (CNS)

What are central nervous system (CNS) stimulants?

CNS stimulants increase brain activity. Many CNS stimulants have direct effects on cardiovascular functions and on the sympathetic nervous system.

How do CNS stimulants work in the body?

Stimulants pass easily into the brain tissue. Once the stimulant in the brain it can increase the release of neurotransmitters onto receptor sites, directly stimulate the postsynaptic receptors, or inhibit neurotransmitter reuptake. Two major examples of CNS stimulants are amphetamines and epinephrine/norepinephrine.

A variety of compounds contain amphetamine substances such as dextroamphetamine (Dexedrine), methamphetamine (Desoxyn). Other similar drugs are phenmetrazine (Preludin), methylphenidate (Ritalin).

What are the general effects of amphetamines?

Amphetamine limits appetite, increases plasma free fatty acid levels and body temperature, and has sympathetic effects on the cardiovascular and respiratory functions. Amphetamines increase alertness and arousal; however, an extended level of arousal may change to anxiety or panic.

♣ It's A Fact!! Illegal Forms Of Amphetamine

Illegal forms of amphetamine appears as crystals, chunks, and fine to coarse powders, off-white to yellow in color, and supplied loose (in plastic or foil bags) or in capsules or tablets of various sizes, and colors. The drug may be sniffed, smoked, injected, or taken orally in tablet or capsule form.

Common street names for amphetamines include: crystal, speed, meth, bennies, dexies, uppers, pep pills, diet pills, jolly bean, copilots, hearts, footballs, crosstops, and ice.

Why would student athletes want to use amphetamines?

Student athletes have taken amphetamines to improve mood states, improve confidence, increase alertness and concentration, and increase endurance.

What are some of the unwanted side effects of amphetamines on athletic performance?

Amphetamine causes blood to flow away from the skin and increase the risk of heat stroke.

What are some of the main effects of amphetamines on the body?

Amphetamines increase heart rate and blood pressure, decrease appetite and increase weight loss, increased respiration, increase inability to sleep, increase dry mouth, headache and dizziness, heat intolerance, increase kidney damage, increase the risk for cerebral hemorrhage and seizures. Regular amphetamine use may lead to dependency, irritability, fearfulness (in some cases, paranoia) and apprehension, hallucination, and even psychosis. Heavy

users of amphetamines may be prone to sudden, violent, and irrational acts
self-centeredness, distortions of perception, and paranoid delusions.

Alcohol

What are the physiological and psychological effects of alcohol use?

Alcohol acts on the central nervous system as a depressant. Users of moderate amounts of alcohol experience relief from anxiety and disinhibition.
The effects of alcohol on individuals vary and are often unpredictable. One
person can become euphoric, friendly and talkative, while others become
aggressive and hostile.

Alcohol interferes with motor activity, reflexes and coordination. In moderate quantities alcohol increases heart rate, and dilated peripheral blood
vessels. Alcohol is diffused in the blood stream after ingestion by passing
through the gastrointestinal walls. Once alcohol is in the small intestine its
absorption is not affected by food. The effect of alcohol on the body depends
on the amount of alcohol in the blood (commonly referred to as BAC or
blood alcohol level).

☞ Remember!!

Heavy drinking over a long period of time can
result in serious mental disorders and permanent brain
damage. Liver disorders are most common causes of death
among alcoholics. Prolonged use of alcohol may cause ulcers,
hiatal hernia, and cancers throughout the digestive track. The pan-
creas is also damaged by heavy alcohol use.

Other serious consequences of chronic alcohol abuse includes heart
disease, malnutrition and vitamin deficiencies, sexual malfunction-
ing, atrophy of testicles and lowered sperm count. Females
experience menstrual delays, ovarian abnormalities, and
infertility. Alcohol abuse also can cause severe kidney damage, urinary tract infections, mental disorders, and brain damage.

What are the uses of alcohol?

A student athlete may drink alcohol because they wish to relax, socialize, reduce inhibitions, and cope with everyday stress.

What are the effects of alcohol use on performance?

Although alcohol has been used by student athletes to cope with anxiety and stress related to competition and academics, and to enhance mental status before competition, the use of alcohol decreases reaction time and fine muscle coordination, balance, speech, vision and hearing. The feeling of disinhibition and reduced anxiety is accompanied by loss of motor coordination, decreased reaction time, lack of balance and coordination and judgment. Alcohol also lowers muscle glycogen.

Cocaine

What is the pharmacology of cocaine?

Cocaine has two main pharmacological actions. This drug is a strong central nervous system (CNS) stimulant and an effective vasoconstrictor when used as a local anesthetic. The effects described by Sigmund Freud included: euphoria, a perceived increase in self control, greater work capacity, perceived long-lasting mental or physical work without fatigue, perceived ability to forego food and sleep; these effects have also been referred to as the "perfect illusion." Cocaine affects the brain by stimulating the release of dopamine and norepinephrine, while also blocking their reuptake.

What are the adverse effects associated with the use of cocaine?

Cocaine is a highly addictive drug. Individuals who use cocaine experience psychotic symptoms and euphoria, paranoid psychosis delirium and confusion, seizures, and strokes caused by rupture cerebral vascular vessels.

What are the side effects of cocaine use specific to student athletes and the general population?

Cocaine related deaths from heart failure of Len Bias and Don Rogers in 1986 increased public attention to the harmful effects of cocaine use and abuse among athletes and the general population. Cardiovascular side effects such as ventricular arrhythmia, angina pectoris, myocardial infarction, cerebrovascular complications (such as cerebral infarction), and cerebral hemorrhage can result from use. Individuals differ in their ability to metabolize cocaine, and some experience seizures, headaches, optic neuropathy, insomnia, delirium, confusion, paranoia, hallucinations, psychosis, anorexia, sexual dysfunction, liver toxicity, and loss of smell.

Caffeine And Other Xanthines

What is the chemistry of caffeine and other xanthines?

Caffeine is one member of the group called xanthines. The other xanthines are theophylline and theobromine. Caffeine is found in 63 species of plants.

How are caffeine and other xanthines processed in the body?

Caffeine is absorbed in the body almost 100%. After oral administration caffeine appears in the blood in about five minutes after ingestion. Caffeine is absorbed more slowly from soft drinks than from tea or coffee. Caffeine is rapidly distributed to the tissues from plasma into the brain by simple diffusion. Caffeine is broken down by the liver and eliminated in the urine. Moderate exercise seems to increase peak plasma concentrations of caffeine.

What are the effects of caffeine and other xanthines on the central nervous system?

Xanthines stimulate the central nervous system. Caffeine effects the central nervous system in doses ranging from 85 to 250 mg; the amount contained in one to three cups of coffee. Many individuals use caffeine to reduce drowsiness and fatigue, improve mood, alertness and productivity. Caffeine increases capacity for sustained intellectual effort with clearer flow of thought. Doses above 250-mg produce nervousness, insomnia, restlessness, and tremors.

What are the adverse effects associated with the use of caffeine and other xanthines?

Student athletes who use large amounts of caffeine may experience nervousness, irritability, insomnia, increased heart beat, hypertension, gastric distress, peptic ulcer, delirium, seizures, coma, and increased serum cholesterol.

What are the effects of caffeine on athletic performance?

Some studies have reported that long term endurance exercise has been shown to be positively enhanced by caffeine. Caffeine has been found to have no significant effect on high intensity, short-term work. Reports on caffeine's effect on maximal oxygen consumption (VO2 max) are inconsistent. The delay in the onset of fatigue is attributed to the sparing of muscle glycogen and to caffeine's lipolytic effect, or ability of the body to release more fat for energy. Coordination and other fine motor skills are not enhanced or diminished following caffeine ingestion.

Tobacco

What are the patterns of tobacco use in the United States?

Every day 3000 young people become regular smokers. Every day 6000 teens under 18 smoke their first cigarette. Every day more than 1000 adults die prematurely as a result of an adolescent decision.

What are the physiological effects of nicotine?

Briefly, nicotine can stimulate the brain at all levels, significantly increase breathing, lower HDL (the good fats) levels, increase blood pressure, and constrict peripheral blood vessels. Some individuals experience nausea and vomiting, decreased urinary flow, and increased free fatty acids. Nicotine increases the oxygen requirements of the heart muscle, but lowers oxygen supply, and this effect may lead to heart attacks. Nicotine initially stimulates the salivary and bronchial secretions and then inhibits them. Cigarette smoke causes the excessive saliva associated with smoking. Nicotine inhibits hunger and also causes a slight increase in blood sugar, and deadens the taste buds. Smokers often report weight gain and appetite increase after quitting smoking.

What are the psychological effects of nicotine?

Nicotine is a highly addictive drug. More than 24 billion packages of cigarettes are purchased annually in the United States and approximately 400,000 deaths are attributed to cigarette smoking. Nicotine is so addictive that approximately 70% of smokers who want to quit smoking cannot and about 83% of smokers smoke every day. Smokers report that cigarettes help them to relax. Nicotine is a cholinergic agonist and stimulates the brain. Smokers experience withdrawal symptoms when trying to quit smoking.

What are the effects of nicotine on athletic performance?

Athletes participating in an National Collegiate Athletic Association (NCAA) survey (2001) reported using spit tobacco for recreational or social purposes, to deal with the stresses of college athletics and to feel good. About 53% of the athletes who use spit tobacco reported using it 1–5 times daily. The use of nicotine in high doses is toxic and can cause nicotine poisoning.

Signs of nicotine poisoning are vomiting, sweating, mental confusion, diminished pulse rate, headache, breathing difficulty, respiratory failure caused by muscle paralysis, and death. Impaired oxygen transport secondary to increases in carboxyhemoglobin. In many cases smoking will increase breathing rate during submaximal exercise, and this will reduce athletic performance.

Marijuana

What is the chemistry of marijuana?

Marijuana is derived from the plant *Cannabis sativa* that grows in many parts of the world. Most researchers agree that there is only one species (sativa) and all the variants belong to that species. Others believe that the variants are three distinct species.

Cannabis consists of a male and female plant. After releasing its pollen, the male plant usually dies and the male plant is removed once the female plant has been pollinated.

There are more than 400 different chemicals in the cannabis plant. Delta-9-tetrahydrocannabinol or THC is the primary psychoactive agent in marijuana. THC is mostly concentrated in the flowering tops and upper leaves of the female plant.

What are the behavioral effects of marijuana use?

A general analysis of the pharmacology of marijuana is difficult due to the variations in dosage, presence of contaminants, and the many additives and adulterants (such as PCP) added to marijuana products.

Marijuana produces both central nervous system excitation and depression. These effects are expressed both behaviorally and neurophysiologically. In most individuals low to moderate doses of marijuana produce euphoria and relaxation. After a few minutes of holding the smoke in the lungs most people experience the "high." During this state, the individual experiences a dry mouth, increased heart rate, loss of coordination and balance and slower reaction times; however, the state of euphoria is usually short lived.

What are the physiological effects of marijuana use?

Marijuana affects the central nervous system. The effects of marijuana on the CNS can vary depending on the route of administration, the dosage, the setting, and previous use. Marijuana users report a sense of altered perceptions associated with hunger. High doses can cause hallucinations, delusions, and paranoia and anxiety. Long-term users show a decreased interest in goals, decreased concentration, and making appropriate decisions and memory loss. Marijuana use can also cause serious damage to the lungs and impair respiratory function. Cannabis produces more tar than an equivalent weight of tobacco. Blood vessels of the eyes expand due to vasodilation causing a reddening of the eye. Some users experience high blood pressure.

What are the effects of marijuana use on athletic performance?

Marijuana use can cause changes in personality, induce hallucinations, delusions, and symptoms of psychosis. The primary effects of marijuana produced on the CNS can impair short-term memory and perception.

Narcotic Analgesics (Pain Killers)

What are narcotic analgesics (pain killers)?

The most common use of narcotic analgesics is to relieve pain. Narcotic analgesics or painkillers are categorized as agonists, mixed agonist antagonists, or partial agonists by their activity at opioid receptors.

What are some therapeutic uses of narcotic analgesics?

Narcotic analgesics are use to treat coughs and are effective antitussive agents. For example codeine is used in cough medication. The drugs are also used to relieve diarrhea.

What are some adverse effects of narcotic analgesics on athletic performance?

Athletes who use narcotic analgesics or painkillers can experience feelings of euphoria or psychological stimulation and false feelings of invincibility. Narcotic analgesics increase the pain threshold and as a result an athlete may fail to recognize injury and suffer more serious injury. Athletes may also use painkilling drugs to mask injury in order to continue to participate in their sports. As a result athletes who use painkillers might place themselves at greater risk for injury.

What are the major adverse effects associated with narcotic analgesics?

One of the most common side effects of the opioid narcotics is constipation. Other side effects include drowsiness, mental clouding, itching, inability to urinate, and low blood pressure. Narcotic analgesics produce physical and psychological dependence. Most of these drugs have major side effects, including dose-related respiratory depression, apnea circulatory depression, respiratory arrest, coma, shock, and cardiac arrest. Most frequent adverse effects are lightheadedness, dizziness, sedation, nausea, and vomiting.

Nonsteroidal Anti-Inflammatory Drugs (NSAIDs)

What are nonsteroidal anti-inflammatory drugs (NSAIDs)?

Medications known as non-steroidal anti-inflammatory drugs (NSAIDs), have analgesic (pain killing) and anti-inflammatory actions and are used to alleviate problems associated with pain and swelling of injuries. NSAIDs that have been used for the treatment of sports injuries include diclofenac (Voltaren), ibuprofen (Advil, Aleve, Motrin), ketoprofen (Orudis), naproxen (Anaprox), etc. and compounds such as Indomethacin (Indocin) and sulindac (Clinoril), and Celebrex.

What are the common side effects of NSAIDs?

Some student athletes who use NSAIDs may experience common gastrointestinal side effects such as nausea, vomiting, diarrhea, constipation, abdominal distress, cramps and pain, dyspepsia, flatulence, anorexia, and stomatitis. Other adverse side effects include dizziness, headache, vertigo, drowsiness, tremor, psychic disturbances, mental confusion, congestive heart failure, hypotension, hypertension and renal, hematologic, dermatologic, and respiratory problems.

What are the symptoms of overdosing NSAIDs?

Sometimes users of NSAIDs may experience drowsiness, dizziness, mental confusion, disorientation, lethargy, vomiting, numbness, ringing in the ears, sweating, convulsions, coma, blurred vision, seizures, diminished urinary flow, low blood pressure, and kidney failure.

🖙 Remember!!

Student athletes should be aware that treatment with NSAIDs might effectively reduce pain, swelling, and inflammation; however, when painkillers are used to reduce pain the injury may still be present. Therefore, it is important to proceed with caution when exercising the injured area (that is now pain-free) to prevent further damage.

Chapter 41

Are Steroids Worth The Risk?

Dominic has baseball on the brain. Just being good isn't enough—he wants to be the best. He dreams of playing in the majors someday, but worries about the intense competition for a position on a major league team. His girlfriend, Deborah, is also a highly competitive athlete whose appearance and performance are very important to her. She wants to stand out—both physically and athletically.

Because of the pressure they each feel to excel, Dominic and Deborah wonder whether steroids would help them. They've heard rumors about the bad side effects of steroids, but they don't have many facts. Here's the scoop on steroids.

What Are Steroids?

Steroids, sometimes referred to as roids, juice, hype, weight trainers, gym candy, arnolds, stackers, or pumpers, are the same as, or similar to, certain hormones in the body. The body produces steroids naturally to support such functions as fighting stress and promoting growth and development. But some people use steroid pills, gels, creams, or injections because they think steroids can improve their sports performance or the way they look.

About This Chapter: This chapter includes information from "Are Steroids Worth The Risk?," September 2006, reprinted with permission from www.kidshealth.org. Copyright © 2006 The Nemours Foundation. This information was provided by KidsHealth, one of the largest resources online for medically reviewed health information written for parents, kids, and teens. For more articles like this one, visit www.KidsHealth.org or www.TeensHealth.org.

Anabolic steroids are artificially produced hormones that are the same as, or similar to, androgens, the male-type sex hormones in the body. There are more than 100 variations of anabolic steroids. The most powerful androgen is testosterone (pronounced: tess-toss-tuh-rone). Although testosterone is mainly a mature male hormone, girls' bodies produce smaller amounts. Testosterone promotes the masculine traits that guys develop during puberty, such as deepening of the voice and growth of body hair. Testosterone levels can also affect how aggressive a person is.

Athletes sometimes take anabolic steroids because of their testosterone-like effects.

Another group of steroids, sometimes called steroidal supplements, contains dehydroepiandrosterone (DHEA) and/or androstenedione (also known as andro). For the most part, steroidal supplements, which used to be found at health food stores or gyms, are now illegal and require a prescription. DHEA is one of the few exceptions and can still be bought over the counter.

Steroid supplements are weaker forms of androgen. Their effects aren't well known, but it's thought that, when taken in large doses, they cause effects similar to other androgens like testosterone. Here's what is known about steroidal supplements: Companies that manufacture them often use false claims and very little is known about the long-term effects some of these substances have on the body. That's one reason why the government took action to citizens by passing laws controlling steroid distribution.

♣ It's A Fact!!
Steroids–Just What
The Doctor Ordered...Sometimes

The term "steroids" is also used to describe some types of non-anabolic steroids, such as cortisone, that have medical uses and are available by prescription to treat problems like asthma or arthritis. These steroid medications do not have the male hormone effects of androgens.

How Do Anabolic Steroids Work?

Anabolic steroids stimulate muscle tissue to grow and "bulk up" in response to training by mimicking the effect of naturally produced testosterone on the body. Anabolic steroids can remain in the body anywhere from a couple of days to about a year. Steroids have become popular because they may improve endurance, strength, and muscle mass. However, research has not shown that steroids improve skill, agility, or athletic performance.

Dangers Of Steroids

Anabolic steroids cause many different types of problems. Some of the more serious or long-lasting side effects are:

- Premature balding or hair loss;

- Dizziness;

- Mood swings, including anger, aggression, and depression;

- Seeing or hearing things that aren't there (hallucinations);

- Extreme feelings of mistrust or fear (paranoia);

- Problems sleeping;

- Nausea and vomiting;

- Trembling;

- High blood pressure that can damage the heart or blood vessels over time;

- Aching joints;

- Greater chance of injuring muscles and tendons;

- Jaundice or yellowing of the skin; liver damage;

- Urinary problems;

- Shortening of final adult height;

- Increased risk of developing heart disease, stroke, and some types of cancer.

Specific risks for girls associated with anabolic steroids include:

- Increased facial hair growth;

- Development of masculine traits, such as deepening of the voice, and loss of feminine body; characteristics, such as shrinking of the breasts;

- Enlargement of the clitoris;

- Menstrual cycle changes.

Specific risks for guys include:

- Testicular shrinkage;

- Pain when urinating;

- Breast development;

- Impotence (inability to get an erection);

- Sterility (inability to have children).

> **♣ It's A Fact!!**
> **Buff But Rough**
>
> One of the major reasons why people decide to take steroids is because they think steroids will improve their appearance. But actually, they can do the reverse. Some less serious side effects of steroid use include acne, oily hair, purple or red spots on the body, swollen legs and feet, and persistent bad breath.

Steroids can also have serious psychological side effects. Some users become aggressive or combative, developing "roid rage"—extreme, uncontrolled bouts of anger caused by long-term steroid use.

Steroid users who inject the drugs with a needle are at risk for infection with HIV (human immunodeficiency virus), the virus that causes AIDS, if they share needles with other users. People who dirty needles are also at greater risk for contracting hepatitis, a disease of the liver, or bacterial endocarditis, an infection of the inner lining of the heart.

Steroids: Stacking And Addiction

Some people combine or "stack" anabolic steroids with other drugs. Other steroid users may "pyramid" or "cycle" their steroid doses, starting with a low dose of stacked drugs and then periodically increasing and decreasing the dosage of the steroid, which users believe helps their bodies recuperate from the drugs.

Remember!!

Some of the long-term effects of steroids may not show up for many years. People who use steroids also appear to be at higher risk for using other drugs, such as alcohol or cocaine.

Because even scientists don't understand exactly how steroids interact with each other or possibly cause reactions to other medications, it's possible that a person who stacks or cycles steroids can take a deadly combination. Emergency departments have reported cases of vomiting, tremors, dizziness, and even coma (unconsciousness) when patients were admitted after taking combinations of steroids.

A lot of people tell themselves they'll only use steroids for a season or a school year. Unfortunately, steroids can be addictive, making it hard to stop taking them.

Steroid users can spend lots of time and money trying to get the drugs. And once users stop taking steroids, they're at risk of developing irritability, paranoia, and severe depression, which may lead to suicidal thoughts or attempted suicide.

What Is Human Growth Hormone?

You may have heard of something called Human Growth Hormone, or hGH, in relation to sports supplements and maybe even related to steroids. Like steroids, hGH is only legal when prescribed by a doctor for a medical condition. Doctors prescribe hGH for people whose bodies don't naturally make enough growth hormone, a condition known as growth hormone deficiency. However, recent trends show an increase in growth hormone being abused as an athletic supplement. A lot of myths surround hGH and its effects on athletes. As with steroids, there is absolutely no evidence that growth hormone helps to improve athletic performance. Here are some risks you should be aware of:

- Any type of hGH that is not obtained by prescription is not regulated by the government and could be almost anything.

- If you buy what may be called "growth hormone," "growth stimulators," or "growth factors" online, it's likely they're not really hGH. Many websites claim to be selling growth hormone, but they're really selling amino acids that don't significantly increase growth hormone levels in your body.

- If the false claims of performance benefits from hGH don't bother you, the price probably will—$5,000 for a month's prescription, meaning that the street value for just a month could run anywhere from $5,000–$10,000.

- Because growth hormone can only be injected, like some steroids, there's a risk of contracting HIV or other diseases (like hepatitis) if people share needles.

Strong Alternatives To Steroids

Anabolic steroids are controversial in the sports world because of the health risks associated with them and their unproven performance benefits. Most are illegal and are banned by professional sports organizations and medical associations. As seen in the high-profile cases, if an athlete is caught using steroids, his or her career can be destroyed.

When it comes right down to it, harming your body or getting disqualified aren't smart ways to try to improve your athletic performance. Being a star athlete means training the healthy way: eating the right foods, practicing, and strength training without the use of drugs.

Chapter 42

Compulsive Exercise

Rachel and her cheerleading team practice three to five times a week. Rachel feels a lot of pressure to keep her weight down—as head cheerleader, she wants to set an example to the team. So she adds extra daily workouts to her regimen. But lately, Rachel has been feeling worn out, and she has a hard time just making it through a regular team practice.

You may think you can't get too much of a good thing, but in the case of exercise, a healthy activity can sometimes turn into an unhealthy compulsion. Rachel is a good example of how an overemphasis on physical fitness or weight control can become unhealthy. Read on to find out more about compulsive exercise and its effects.

Too Much Of A Good Thing?

We all know the benefits of exercise, and it seems that everywhere we turn, we hear that we should exercise more. The right kind of exercise does many great things for your body and soul: It can strengthen your heart and muscles, lower your body fat, and reduce your risk of many diseases.

About This Chapter: This chapter includes information from "Compulsive Exercise," October 2007, reprinted with permission from www.kidshealth.org. Copyright © 2006 The Nemours Foundation. This information was provided by KidsHealth, one of the largest resources online for medically reviewed health information written for parents, kids, and teens. For more articles like this one, visit www.KidsHealth.org or www.TeensHealth.org. Additional information is cited within the chapter.

Many teens who play sports have higher self-esteem than their less active pals, and exercise can even help keep the blues at bay because of the endorphin rush it can cause. Endorphins are chemicals that naturally relieve pain and lift mood. These chemicals are released in your body during and after a workout and they go a long way in helping to control stress.

So how can something with so many benefits have the potential to cause harm?

Lots of people start working out because it's fun or it makes them feel good, but exercise can become a compulsive habit when it is done for the wrong reasons.

Some people start exercising with weight loss as their main goal. Although exercise is part of a safe and healthy way to control weight, many people may have unrealistic expectations. We are bombarded with images from advertisers of the ideal body: young and thin for women, strong and muscular for men. To try to reach these unreasonable ideals, people may turn to diets, and for some, this may develop into eating disorders such as anorexia and bulimia. And some people who grow frustrated with the results from diets alone may overexercise to speed up weight loss.

Some athletes may also think that repeated exercise will help them to win an important game. Like Rachel, they add extra workouts to those regularly scheduled with their teams without consulting their coaches or trainers. The pressure to succeed may also lead these people to exercise more than is healthy. The body needs activity but it also needs rest. Overexercising can lead to injuries like fractures and muscle strains.

Are You A Healthy Exerciser?

Fitness experts recommend that teens do at least 60 minutes of moderate to vigorous physical activity every day. Most young people exercise much less than this recommended amount (which can be a problem for different reasons), but some—such as athletes—do more.

Experts say that repeatedly exercising beyond the requirements for good health is an indicator of compulsive behavior. Some people need more than

✔ **Quick Tip**

If you are concerned about your own exercise habits or a friend's, ask yourself the following questions.

- Do you force yourself to exercise, even if you don't feel well?

- Do you prefer to exercise rather than being with friends?

- Do you become very upset if you miss a workout?

- Do you base the amount you exercise on how much you eat?

- Do you have trouble sitting still because you think you're not burning calories?

- Do you worry that you'll gain weight if you skip exercising for a day?

If the answer to any of these questions is yes, you or your friend may have a problem. What should you do? See "How To Get Help" in this chapter.

the average amount of exercise, of course—such as athletes in training for a big event. But several workouts a day, every day, when a person is not in training is a sign that the person is probably overdoing it.

People who are exercise dependent also go to extremes to fit activity into their lives. If you put workouts ahead of friends, homework, and other responsibilities, you may be developing a dependence on exercise.

How To Get Help

The first thing you should do if you suspect that you are a compulsive exerciser is get help. Talk to your parents, doctor, a teacher or counselor, a coach, or another trusted adult. Compulsive exercise, especially when it is combined with an eating disorder, can cause serious and permanent health problems, and in extreme cases, death.

Because compulsive exercise is closely related to eating disorders, help can be found at community agencies specifically set up to deal with anorexia, bulimia, and other eating problems. Your school's health or physical education department may also have support programs and nutrition advice available. Ask your teacher, coach, or counselor to recommend local organizations that may be able to help.

You should also schedule a checkup with a doctor. Because our bodies go through so many important developments during the teen years, guys and girls who have compulsive exercise problems need to see a doctor to make sure they are developing normally. This is especially true if the person also has an eating disorder. Female athlete triad, a condition that affects girls who overexercise and restrict their eating because of their sports, can cause a girl to stop having her period. Medical help is necessary to resolve the physical problems associated with overexercising before they cause long-term damage to the body.

👉 Remember!!
Make A Positive Change

Changes in activity of any kind—eating or sleeping, for example—can often be a sign that something else is wrong in your life. Girls and guys who exercise compulsively may have a distorted body image and low self-esteem. They may see themselves as overweight or out of shape even when they are actually a healthy weight.

Compulsive exercisers need to get professional help for the reasons described above. But there are also some things that you can do to help you take charge again:

- **Work on changing your daily self-talk.** When you look in the mirror, make sure you find at least one good thing to say about yourself. Be more aware of your positive attributes.

- **When you exercise, focus on the positive, mood-boosting qualities.**

- **Give yourself a break.** Listen to your body and give yourself a day of rest after a hard workout.

- **Control your weight by exercising and eating moderate portions of healthy foods.** Don't try to change your body into an unrealistically lean shape. Talk with your doctor, dietitian, coach, athletic trainer, or other adult about what a healthy body weight is for you and how to develop healthy eating and exercise habits.

Exercise and sports are supposed to be fun and keep you healthy. Working out in moderation will do both.

Chapter 43

The Female Athlete Triad

With dreams of college scholarships in her mind, Hannah joined the track team her freshman year and trained hard to become a lean, strong sprinter. When her coach told her losing a few pounds would improve her performance, she immediately started counting calories and increased the duration of her workouts. She was too busy with practices and meets to notice that her period had stopped—she was more worried about the stress fracture in her ankle slowing her down.

Although Hannah thinks her intense training and disciplined diet are helping her performance, they may actually be hurting her—and her health.

What Is Female Athlete Triad?

Sports and exercise are part of a balanced, healthy lifestyle. Girls who play sports are healthier; get better grades; are less likely to experience depression; and use alcohol, cigarettes, and drugs less frequently than girls who aren't athletes. But for some girls, not balancing the needs of their bodies and their sports can have major consequences.

About This Chapter: This chapter includes information from "The Female Athlete Triad," October 2006, reprinted with permission from www.kidshealth.org. Copyright © 2006 The Nemours Foundation. This information was provided by KidsHealth, one of the largest resources online for medically reviewed health information written for parents, kids, and teens. For more articles like this one, visit www.KidsHealth.org or www.TeensHealth.org.

Some girls who play sports or exercise intensely are at risk for a problem called female athlete triad. Female athlete triad is a combination of three conditions: disordered eating, amenorrhea, and osteoporosis. A female athlete can have one, two, or all three parts of the triad.

Triad Factor #1: Disordered Eating

Most girls with female athlete triad try to lose weight primarily to improve their athletic performance. The disordered eating that accompanies female athlete triad can range from avoiding certain types of food the athlete thinks are "bad" (such as foods containing fat) to serious eating disorders like anorexia nervosa or bulimia nervosa.

Triad Factor #2: Amenorrhea

Because a girl with female athlete triad is simultaneously exercising intensely and not eating enough calories, when her weight falls too low, she may experience decreases in estrogen, the hormone that helps to regulate the menstrual cycle. As a result, a girl's periods may become irregular or stop altogether. Of course, it is normal for teen girls to occasionally miss periods, especially in their first year of having periods. A missed period does not automatically mean a girl has female athlete triad. A missed period could mean something else is going on, like pregnancy or a medical condition. If you have missed a period and you are sexually active, talk to your doctor.

Some girls who participate intensively in sports may never even get their first period because they've been training so hard. Other girls may have had periods, but once they increase their training and change their eating habits, their periods may stop.

Triad Factor #3: Osteoporosis

Low estrogen levels and poor nutrition, especially low calcium intake, can lead to osteoporosis, the third aspect of the triad. Osteoporosis is a weakening of the bones due to the loss of bone density and improper bone formation. This condition can ruin a female athlete's career because it may lead to stress fractures and other injuries.

Usually, the teen years are a time when girls should be building up their bone mass to their highest levels—called peak bone mass. Not getting enough calcium during the teen years can also have a lasting effect on how strong a girl's bones are later in life.

Who Gets Female Athlete Triad?

Most girls have concerns about the size and shape of their bodies, but girls who develop female athlete triad have certain risk factors that set them apart. Being a highly competitive athlete and participating in a sport that requires you to train extra hard is a risk factor.

Girls with female athlete triad often care so much about their sports that they would do almost anything to improve their performance. Martial arts and rowing are examples of sports that classify athletes by weight class, so focusing on weight becomes an important part of the training program and can put a girl at risk for disordered eating.

Participation in sports where a thin appearance is valued can also put a girl at risk for female athlete triad. Sports such as gymnastics, figure skating, diving, and ballet are examples of sports that value a thin, lean body shape. Some girls may even be told by coaches or judges that losing weight would improve their scores.

Even in sports where body size and shape aren't as important, such as distance running and cross-country skiing, girls may be pressured by teammates, parents, partners, and coaches who mistakenly believe that "losing just a few pounds" could improve their performance.

The truth is, though, that losing those few pounds generally doesn't improve performance at all. People who are fit and active enough to compete in sports generally have more muscle than fat, so it's the muscle that gets starved when a girl cuts back on food. Plus, if a girl loses weight when she doesn't need to, it interferes with healthy body processes such as menstruation and bone development.

In addition, for some competitive female athletes, problems such as low self-esteem, a tendency toward perfectionism, and family stress place them at risk for disordered eating.

How Doctors Help

An extensive physical examination is a crucial part of diagnosing female athlete triad. A doctor who thinks a girl has female athlete triad will probably ask questions about her periods, her nutrition and exercise habits, any medications she takes, and her feelings about her body. This is called the medical history.

Poor nutrition can also affect the body in many ways, so a doctor might order blood tests to check for anemia and other problems associated with the triad. The doctor also will check for medical reasons why a girl may be losing weight and missing her periods. Because osteoporosis can put a girl at higher risk for bone fractures, the doctor may also request tests to measure bone density.

Doctors don't work alone to help a girl with female athlete triad. Coaches, parents, physical therapists, pediatricians and adolescent medicine specialists, nutritionists and dietitians, and mental health specialists can all work together to treat the physical and emotional problems that a girl with female athlete triad faces.

♣ It's A Fact!!

What Are The Signs And Symptoms Of Female Athlete Triad?

If a girl has risk factors for female athlete triad, she may already be experiencing some symptoms and signs of the disorder, such as:

- Weight loss;
- No periods or irregular periods;
- Fatigue and decreased ability to concentrate;
- Stress fractures (fractures that occur even if a person hasn't had a significant injury);
- Muscle injuries.

Girls with female athlete triad often have signs and symptoms of eating disorders, such as:

- Continued dieting in spite of weight loss;
- Preoccupation with food and weight;
- Frequent trips to the bathroom during and after meals;
- Using laxatives;
- Brittle hair or nails;
- Dental cavities because in girls with bulimia tooth enamel is worn away by frequent vomiting;
- Sensitivity to cold;
- Low heart rate and blood pressure;
- Heart irregularities and chest pain.

✔ **Quick Tip**

Tips For Female Athletes

Here are a few tips to help teen athletes stay on top of their physical condition:

- **Keep track of your periods.** It's easy to forget when you had your last visit from Aunt Flo, so keep a calendar in your gym bag and mark down when your period starts and stops and if the bleeding is particularly heavy or light. That way, if you start missing periods, you'll know right away and you'll have accurate information to give to your doctor.

- **Don't skip meals or snacks.** Girls who are constantly on the go between school, practice, and competitions may be tempted to skip meals and snacks to save time. But eating now will improve performance later, so stock your locker or bag with quick and easy favorites such as bagels, string cheese, unsalted nuts and seeds, raw vegetables, granola bars, and fruit.

- **Visit a dietitian or nutritionist who works with teen athletes.** He or she can help you get your dietary game plan into gear and determine if you're getting enough key nutrients such as iron, calcium, and protein. And if you need supplements, a nutritionist can recommend the best choices.

- **Do it for you.** Pressure from teammates, parents, or coaches can turn a fun activity into a nightmare. If you're not enjoying your sport, make a change. Remember: It's your body and your life. You—not your coach or teammates—will have to live with any damage you do to your body now.

It might be tempting for a girl with female athlete triad to shrug off several months of missed periods, but getting help right away is important. In the short term, she may have muscle weakness, stress fractures, and reduced physical performance. Over the long term, she may suffer from bone weakness, long-term effects on her reproductive system, and heart problems.

A girl who is recovering from female athlete triad may work with a dietitian to help get to and maintain a healthy weight and ensure she's eating enough calories and nutrients for health and good athletic performance. Depending on how much the girl is exercising, she may have to reduce the length of her workouts. Talking to a psychologist or therapist can help a girl deal with depression, pressure from coaches or family members, or low self-esteem and can help her find ways to deal with her problems other than restricting her food intake or exercising excessively.

Some girls with female athlete triad may need to take hormones to supply their bodies with estrogen so they can get their periods started again. In such cases, birth control pills are often used to regulate the menstrual cycle. Calcium and vitamin D supplementation is also common for a girl who has suffered bone loss as the result of female athlete triad.

What If I Think Someone I Know Has It?

A girl with female athlete triad may try to hide it, but she can't just ignore the disorder and hope it goes away. She needs to get help from a doctor and other health professionals. If a friend, sister, or teammate has signs and symptoms of female athlete triad, discuss your concerns with her and encourage her to seek treatment. If she refuses to seek treatment, you may need to mention your concern to a parent, coach, teacher, or school nurse.

You may worry about being nosy when you ask questions about a friend's health, but you're not: Your concern is a sign that you're a caring friend. Lending an ear may be just what your friend needs.

Part Six

If You Need More Information

Chapter 44

The President's Challenge

In Fitness We Trust

The President's Council on Physical Fitness and Sports (PCPFS) strives to make the health and fitness of all Americans a top national priority.

The history of the Council dates back to 1956, when President Eisenhower initiated the first national testing program. Ever since, the Council has included some of America's most distinguished citizens as members. They hail from all walks of life: athletes, civic leaders, educators, businesspeople, and health experts. Together they serve as a shining example, inspiring millions to live more active lives.

The mission of the PCPFS is to promote the benefits of fitness everywhere it can—from local communities all the way to the highest levels of government. That involves partnering with organizations across the country—including schools, boys and girls clubs, corporations, and more.

The Challenge

What began as a national youth fitness test has grown up—in a big way. Today, the President's Challenge takes staying active beyond the school gym, and into everyday life.

The President's Challenge includes a whole series of programs designed to help improve anyone's activity level—young or old. It's about choosing to live healthier—and finding things you really like to do.

No matter how active you are right now, you'll find a program that's right for you.

Taking Part In The Active Lifestyle Program

If you're active less than 30 minutes a day, five days a week (or 60 minutes a day for youths under 18), this program is for you.

> ✔ **Quick Tip**
> ## Contact Information For The President's Challenge
>
> If you have questions about the President's Challenge, here's how you can get in touch with them.
>
> - **Address:** The President's Challenge, 501 N. Morton, Suite 203, Bloomington, IN 47404
>
> - **Phone:** 1-800-258-8146, Monday to Friday, 8 a.m. to 5 p.m. (Eastern Time)
>
> - **Fax:** 1-812-855-8999
>
> - **E-mail:** preschal@indiana.edu

The Active Lifestyle program shows you how to make a commitment to staying active and how to stick to it. The program helps you set realistic goals to encourage fitness for a lifetime. The rules are simple. You can choose from all kinds of activities, and you can get a personal activity log to guide you every step of the way.

Because your hard work shouldn't go unrecognized, you can also earn awards. You can earn the Presidential Active Lifestyle Award (PALA) by performing regular activity beyond your daily activity goal of (30 minutes a day for adults/60 minutes a day for youths under 18) at least five days per week, for a total of six weeks. As an alternative you can count your daily activity steps using a pedometer.

That means if you stick with the program, you can earn an award in a little over a month. So what are you waiting for?

The Rules For The Active Lifestyle Program

- **Choose an activity.** Just about any physical activity where you're using large muscle groups and burning energy counts. Taking a long walk.

Playing basketball or tennis. Taking an aerobics class. Even doing chores around the house if you do these activities in addition to what you normally do. There is a wealth of scientific evidence showing that as little as 30 minutes of moderate-intensity physical activity (equal in intensity to brisk walking) done on most, if not all, days of the week has substantial health benefits for adults. Sixty minutes has been recommended as a minimum amount of regular activity for youth.

- **Get active.** Your goal is to meet your daily activity goal (30 minutes a day for adults/60 minutes a day for children under 18) at least five days a week, for a total of six weeks. You can take up to eight weeks to complete the program.

- **Track your activity.** A personal activity log makes it easy for you to track the time you spend on activities. You can log your time as often as you want, in amounts as short as five minutes. Accumulating your activities in periods of 10 minutes or more is even better. Although you can't log time for activities you haven't done yet, you can go back a maximum of 14 days to enter past activities. Track of your progress online at www.presidentschallenge.org once you've registered for the President's Challenge.

✔ Quick Tip
What Activities Count?

The President's Challenge lets you choose from almost 100 different activities, so you're sure to find at least one you like. Here are some of the activities. Go to www.presidentschallenge.org for a complete list.

- **Gym activities:** Aerobics, calisthenics, weight lifting, yoga, stretching, plus many others
- **Sports:** Baseball, basketball, hockey, tennis, soccer, squash, badminton, as well as other fun sport activities
- **Outdoor activities:** Canoeing, inline skating, sledding, snorkeling, snowboarding, scuba diving, etc.
- **Other activities:** Household tasks, dancing, cheerleading, children's games, gardening, fishing, and a lot of other everyday activities

- **Order your award.** When you reach your goal, your activity log will remind you that you've earned an award. You can order it right online or by mail. Then you can continue earning awards in the Active Lifestyle program or move on to the next challenge: the Presidential Champions program.

> **✔ Quick Tip**
> Both the Active Lifestyle and the Presidential Champions programs offer a personal activity log to track your progress online (at www.presidentschallenge.org)—along with awards for reaching your goals. You can even join with others to take the Challenge as a group.

Can You Use A Pedometer?

Absolutely. If you like to walk, run, or play games like basketball or tennis, you can use a pedometer—a small device that automatically counts the number of steps you take. Then just record the amount in your activity log. Different people will have different daily step goals:

- Girls 6 to 17 should log at least 11,000 steps a day
- Boys 6 to 17 should log at least 13,000 steps a day

If you want to log minutes one day and pedometer steps the next, that's okay. As long as your meet you daily activity goal of minutes or steps.

Taking Part In The Presidential Champions Program

If you're already active and want a new challenge, this program is for you.

The Presidential Champions program challenges you to see just how high you can raise your activity level. The guidelines are simple. You can choose from a variety of activities. You can also get a personal activity log to help track your progress along the way. There's even a special option for performance athletes and others who train at more advanced levels.

Your goal is to see how many points you can earn by being active. You'll earn points for every activity you log. Points are based on the amount of energy each activity burns. So the more active you are, the more points you'll get.

The first goal to aim for is a Bronze award. Then you can keep going for a Silver or Gold.

So what are you waiting for?

Join A Group And Meet The Challenge Together

Maybe you have a friend you like to walk with. Or your family goes out for a bike ride together every weekend. If you want to stay active with someone else, you can take the President's Challenge as part of a group.

Staying active with others can be a lot of fun. They'll help keep you motivated—even when you don't really feel like it. Groups are a great way to meet new people. There are even programs for people at different activity levels: the Active Lifestyle program aimed at beginners and the Presidential Champions program for those who are already active.

Signing up for a group is simple. There's no limit to how many you can belong to. You can join or leave at any time. You can even create a group of your own. All you have to do is log into our group admin at http://www .presidentschallenge.org/group_admin/index.aspx. There you'll find everything you need to get started.

Chapter 45

Fitness And Health Organizations

General Sports And Fitness Organizations

Aerobics and Fitness Association of America
15250 Ventura Blvd., Suite 200
Sherman Oaks, CA 91403
Toll-Free: 877-YOURBODY;
(877-968-7263)
Phone: 818-905-0040
Fax: 818-990-5468
Website: http://www.afaa.com
E-mail: contactAFAA@afaa.com

Amateur Athletic Union
National Headquarters
1910 Hotel Plaza Blvd.
P.O. Box 22409
Lake Buena Vista, FL 32830
Toll-Free: 800-AAU-4USA
Phone: 407-934-7200
Fax: 407-934-7242
Website: http://www.aausports.org

American Council on Exercise
4851 Paramount Drive
San Diego, CA 92123
Toll-Free: 800-825-3636
Phone: 858-279-8227
Fax: 858-279-8064
Website: http://www.acefitness.org
E-mail: support@acefitness.org

BAM! (Body and Mind)
Centers for Disease Control and Prevention (CDC)
1600 Clifton Road, MD C-04
Atlanta, GA 30333
Toll-Free: 800-311-3435
Phone: 404-498-1515
Website: http://www.bam.gov
E-mail: bam@cdc.gov

About This Chapter: The list of organizations in this chapter was compiled from many sources deemed accurate. Inclusion does not constitute endorsement. All contact information was verified in May, 2008.

Idea, Inc.
10455 Pacific Center Court
San Diego, CA 92121-4339
Toll-Free: 800-999-4332
Phone: 858-535-8979
Fax: 858-535-8234
Website: http://www.ideafit.com

iEmily.com
136 West Street, Suite 201
Northampton, MA 01060
Phone: 413-587-0244
Website: http://www.iemily.com
E-mail:
iemily@healthcommunities.com

National Association for Fitness Certification
Bodybasics Fitness Training
Siera Vista, AZ 85635
Toll-Free: 800-324-8315
Phone: 520-452-8712
Website: http://www.body-basics.com
E-mail:
bodybasics@body-basics.com

National Center for Drug Free Sport, Inc.
2537 Madison Ave.
Kansas City, MO, 64108
Phone: 816-474-8655
Fax: 816-502-9287
Website: http://
www.drugfreesport.com
E-mail: info@drugfreesport.com

National Collegiate Athletic Association (NCAA)
P.O. Box 6222
Indianapolis, IN 46206-6222
Phone: 317-917-6222
Fax: 317-917-6888
Website: http://www.ncaa.org

National High School Athletic Coaches Association
P.O. Box 4342
Hamden, CT 06514
Fax: 203-288-8224
Website: http://www.hscoaches.org
E-mail: office@hscoaches.org

National Women's Health Information Center (NWHIC)
Office on Women's Health
Dept. of Health and Human Services
200 Independence Ave., SW Rm. 712E
Washington, DC 20201
Toll-Free: 800-994-9662
Phone: 202-690-7650
Fax: 202-205-2631
Website: http://www.4women.gov

President's Challenge
501 N. Morton, Suite 104
Bloomington, IN 47404
Toll-Free: 800-258-8146
Fax: 812-855-8999
Website: http://
www.presidentschallenge.org
E-mail: preschal@indiana.edu

President's Council on Physical Fitness and Sports
200 Independence Ave. SW, Rm. 738-H
Washington, DC 20201-0004
Phone: 202-690-9000
Fax: 202-690-5211
Website: http://www.fitness.gov

Shape Up America!
c/o WebFront Solutions Corporation
15009 Native Dancer Road
N. Potomac, MD 20787
Fax: 240-632-1075
Website: http://www.shapeup.org
E-mail: customer-care@shapeup.org

Special Olympics
1133 19th Street, N.W.
Washington, DC 20036
Phone: 202-628-3630
Fax: 202-824-0200
Website: http://
www.specialolympics.org
E-mail: info@specialolympics.org

Women's Sports Foundation
1899 Hempstead Turnpike, Suite 400
East Meadow, NY 11554
Toll-Free: 800-227-3988
Phone: 516-542-4700
Fax: 516-542-4716
Website: http://
www.womenssportsfoundation.org
E-mail: wosport@aol.com

Fitness Organizations For The Disabled

Disabled Sports USA
451 Hungerford Drive, Suite 100
Rockville, MD 20850
Phone: 301-217-0960
Fax: 301-217-0968
Website: http://www.dsusa.org
E-mail: information@dsusa.org

United States Olympic Committee
U.S. Paralympics Division
One Olympic Plaza
Colorado Springs, CO 80909
Phone: 719-866-2030
Fax: 719-866-2029
Website: http://
www.usolympicteam.com/paralympics
E-mail: paralympicinfo@usoc.org

Medical Organizations

American College of Sports Medicine (ACSM)
401 West Michigan Street
Indianapolis, IN 46202-3233
P.O. Box 1440
Indianapolis, IN 46206-1440
Phone: (317) 637-9200 National
Center; (317) 637-9200, ext. 138
Regional Chapter Resource Center
Fax: (317) 634-7817
Website: http://www.acsm.org

American Alliance for Health, Physical Education, Recreation, and Dance
1900 Association Dr.
Reston, VA 20191-1598
Toll-Free: 800-213-7193
Phone: 703-476-3400
Website: http://www.aahperd.org

American Academy of Family Physicians (AAFP)
11400 Tomahawk Creek Pkwy.
Leawood, KS 66211-2672
Toll-Free: 800-274-2237
Phone: 913-906-6000
Website: http://www.aafp.org
E-mail: contactcenter@aafp.org

American Academy of Orthopaedic Surgeons (AAOS)
6300 North River Road
Rosemont, IL 60018-4262
Phone: 847-823-7186
Fax: 847-823-8125
Website: http://www.aaos.org
E-mail: pemr@aaos.org

American Dietetic Association
120 S. Riverside Plaza, Suite 2000
Chicago, IL 60606-6995
Toll-Free: 800-877-1600
Website: http://www.eatright.org

American Heart Association
National Center
7272 Greenville Avenue
Dallas, TX 75231
Toll-Free: 800-AHA-USA-1;
800-242-8721
Website: http://www.americanheart.org

American Orthopaedic Foot and Ankle Society
6300 N. River Road, Suite 510
Rosemont, IL 60018
Toll-Free: 800-235-4855
Phone: 847-698-4654
Fax: 847-692-3315
Website: www.aofas.org
E-mail: aofasinfo@aofas.org

National Sleep Foundation
1522 K Street, NW, Suite 500
Washington, DC 20005
Phone: 202-347-3471
Fax: 202-347-3472
Website: http://www.sleepfoundation.org
E-mail: nsf@sleepfoundation.org

National Institute of Child Health and Development (NICHD)
P.O. Box 3006
Rockville, MD 20847
Toll-Free: 800-370-2943
Fax: 301-984-1473
Website: http://www.nichd.nih.gov
E-mail:
NICHDINformationResourceCenter
@mail.nih.gov

National Institute of Arthritis and Musculoskeletal and Skin Diseases (NIAMS)
Information Clearinghouse
National Institutes of Health
1 AMS Circle
Bethesda, MD 20892-3675
Toll-Free: 877-22-NIAMS (226-4267)
Phone: 301-495-4484
Fax: 301-718-6366
Website: http://www.niams.nih.gov
E-mail: NIAMSinfo@mail.nih.gov

Nutritional Information

Iowa State University Extension Service
Website: http://
www.extension.iastate.edu/
healthnutrition

International Food Information Council Foundation
1100 Connecticut Ave. NW,
Suite 430
Washington, DC 20036
Phone: 202-296-6540
Fax: 202-296-6547
Website: http://www.ific.org
E-mail: foodinfo@ific.org

National Eating Disorders Association
603 Stewart St., Suite 803
Seattle, WA 98101
Toll-Free: 800-931-2237
Phone: 206-382-3587
Website: http://
www.nationaleatingdisorders.org
E-mail:
info@nationaleatingdisorders.org

Weight-Control Information Network
1 Win Way
Bethesda, MD 20892-3665
Toll-Free: 877-946-4627
Phone: 202-828-1025
Fax: 202-828-1028
Website: http://www.niddk.nih.gov/
health/nutrit/win.htm
E-mail: win@info.niddk.nih.gov

Sports-Specific Organizations

Baseball And Softball

Amateur Softball Association of America
2801 NE 50th Street
Oklahoma City, OK 73111
Toll-Free: 800-654-8337
Phone: 405-424-5266
Website: http://www.asasoftbal.com

Little League Baseball International
P.O. Box 3485
Williamsport, PA 17701
Phone: 570-326-1921
Fax: 570-322-2376
Website: http://www.littleleague.org

National Softball Association (NSA)
P.O. Box 7
Nicholasville, KY 40340
Phone: 859-887-4114
Fax: 859-887-4874
Website: http://www.playnsa.com
E-mail: nsahdqtrs@aol.com

PONY Baseball and Softball
International Headquarters
P.O. Box 225
Washington, PA 15301-0225
Phone: 724-225-1060
Fax: 724-225-9852
Website: http://www.pony.org
E-mail: pony@pony.org

USA Baseball Headquarters
P.O. Box 1131
Durham, NC 27702
Phone: 919-474-8721
Fax: 919-474-8822
Website: http://www.usabaseball.com
E-mail: info@usabaseball.com

Basketball

Jr. NBA and Jr. WNBA
P.O. Box 8066
Wasau, WI 54402
Phone: 715-261-9390
Fax: 715-261-9560
Website: http://www.nba.com/jrnba
E-mail: fanrelations@NBA.com

Mid-America Youth Basketball
2309 South Kansas
P.O. Box 348
Newton, KS 67114
Phone: 316-284-0354
Fax: 316-284-0294
Website: http://www.mayb.com
E-mail: mayb@mayb.com

National Junior Basketball
1500 Anaheim Blvd., Suite 200
Anaheim, CA 92805
Phone: 714-541-4450
Fax: 714-541-5145
Website: http://www.njbl.org
E-mail: info@njbl.org

Youth Basketball of America
10325 Orangewood Blvd.
Orlando, FL 32821
Phone: 407-363-9262
Fax: 407-363-0599
Website: http://www.yboa.org

Boating And Watercraft

American Canoe Association
1340 Central Park Blvd., Suite 210
Fredericksburg, VA 22401
Phone: 540-907-4460
Fax: 703-636-0296
Website: http://www.acanet.org
E-mail: aca@americancanoe.org

National Safe Boating Council
P.O. Box 509
Bristow, VA 20136
Phone: 703-361-4294
Fax: 703-361-5294
Website: http://
www.safeboatingcouncil.org
E-mail:
NSBCdirect@safeboatingcouncil.org

USA Canoe/Kayak
301 South Tryon St., Suite 1750
Charlotte, NC 28282
Phone: 704-348-4330
Fax: 704-348-4418
Website: http://www.usacanoekayak.org
E-mail: info@usack.org

Bicycling

Bicycle Helmet Safety Institute
4611 Seventh Street South
Arlington, VA 22204-1419
Phone/Fax: 703-486-0100
Website: http://www.bhsi.org
E-mail: info@helmets.org

USA Cycling
1 Olympic Plaza
Colorado Springs, CO 80909
Phone: 719-866-4581
Fax: 719-866-4628
Website: http://www.usacycling.org
E-mail: membership@usacycling.org

Cheerleading

American Cheerleading
Lifestyle Media, Inc.
110 William Street, 23rd Floor
New York, NY 10038
Phone: 646-459-4800
Fax: 646-459-4900
Website: http://
www.americancheerleader.com
E-mail:
acmail@americancheerleader.com

Pop Warner Little Scholars, Inc.
586 Middletown Blvd., Suite C-100
Langhorne, PA 19047
Phone: 215-752-2691
Fax: 215-752-2879
Website: http://www.popwarner.com

Varsity.com
6745 Lenox Center Court
Memphis, TN 38115
Toll-Free: 800-238-0286
Phone: 901-387-4306
Fax: 901-387-4357
Website: http://www.varsity.com

Football

NFL for Kids
280 Park Avenue
New York, NY 10017
Website: http://www.playfootball.com

Pop Warner Little Scholars, Inc.
586 Middletown Blvd., Suite C-100
Langhorne, PA 19047
Phone: 215-752-2691
Fax: 215-752-2879
Website: http://www.popwarner.com

Golf

Hook a Kid On Golf
2050 Vista Parkway
West Palm Beach, FL 33411
Toll-Free: 800-729-2057
Fax: 561-712-9887
Website: http://
www.hookakidongolf.org
E-mail: info@hookakidongolf.org

Junior Links
United States Golf Association
Copper Building
1631 Mesa Ave.
Colorado Springs, CO 80906
Phone: 719-471-4810
Website: http://www.juniorlinks.com
E-mail: juniorlinks@usga.org

U.S. Kids Golf
3040 Northwoods Parkway
Norcross, GA 30071
Toll-Free: 1-888-3-US KIDS
(1-888-387-5437)
Phone: 770-441-3077
Fax: 770-448-3069
Website: http://www.uskidsgolf.com
E-mail:
customerservice@uskidsgolf.com

Gymnastics

International GYMNAST Magazine
P.O. Box 72120
Norman, OK 73070
Phone: 405-447-9988
Fax: 405-447-5810
Website: http://www.intlgymnast.com
E-mail:
customerservice@intlgymnast.com

USA Gymnastics
Pan Am Plaza, Suite 300
201 S. Capitol Avenue
Indianapolis, IN 46225
Toll-Free: 800-345-4719
Phone: 317-2375050
Fax: 317-237-5069
Website:
http://www.usa-gymnastics.org

Hockey

USA Hockey, Inc.
1775 Bob Johnson Drive
Colorado Springs, CO 80906-4090
Phone: 719-576-USAH (8724)
Fax: 719-538-1160
Website: http://www.usahockey.com
E-mail: usah@usahockey.org

United States Field Hockey
1 Olympic Plaza
Colorado Springs, CO 80909-5773
Phone: 719-866-4567
Fax: 719-632-0979
Website: http://
www.usfieldhockey.com
E-mail: usfha@usfieldhockey.com

Martial Arts And Kickboxing

American Athletic Union
AAU National Headquarters
Phone: 407-828-3459; 407-235-8063
Fax: 407-934-7242
Website: http://aautaekwondo.org
E-mail: dan@aausports.org

FightingArts.com
Phone: 718-549-2151
Website: http://www.fightingarts.com

International Kickboxing Federation
P.O. Box 1205
Newcastle, CA 95658
Phone: 916-663-2467
Fax: 916-663-4510
Website: http://
www.ikfkickboxing.com
E-mail: main@ikfkickboxing.com

Racquet Sports

College and Junior Tennis
100 Harbor Road
Port Washington, NY 11050
Phone: 516-883-6601
Fax: 516-883-5241
Website: http://
www.clgandjrtennis.com
E-mail:
info@collegeandjuniortennis.com

U.S. Racquetball Association
1685 West Uintah
Colorado Springs, CO 80904-2906
Phone: 719-635-5396
Fax: 719-635-0685
Website: http://usra.org

U.S. Tennis Association
70 West Red Oak Lane
White Plains, NY 10604
Phone: 914-696-7223
Website: http://www.usta.com
E-mail: foundation@usta.com

Skating And Skateboarding

Aggressive Skaters Association
ASA Entertainment, LLC
5855 Green Valley Circle, Suite 308
Culver City, CA 90230
Phone: 310-410-3020
Website: http://www.asaskate.com

International Association of Skateboard Companies (IASC)
22431 Antonio Pkwy. Suite B160-412
Rancho Santa Margarita, CA 92688
Phone: 949-455-1112
Fax: 949-455-1712
Website: http://
www.skateboardiasc.org

International Inline Skating Association
7210 Trailmark Dr.
Wilmington, NC 28405
Website: http://www.iisa.org
E-mail:info@iisa.org

U.S. Figure Skating
20 First Street
Colorado Springs, CO 80906
Phone: 719-635-5200
Fax: 719-635-9548
Website: http://
www.usfigureskating.org
E-mail: info@usfigureskating.org

Soccer

American Youth Soccer Organization
12501 South Isis Ave.
Hawthorne, CA 90250
Toll-Free: 800-872-2976
Fax: 310-643-5310
Website: http://soccer.org

CC United
P.O. Box 62
Cedar Park, TX 78630
Phone: 512-535-1177
Website: http://www.ccunited.com
E-mail: admin@ccunited.com

Major League Soccer
420 5th Ave., 7th floor
New York, NY 10018
Phone: 212-450-1200
Fax: 212-450-1300
Website: http://web.mlsnet.com

US Youth Soccer
9220 World Cup Way
Frisco, TX 75034
Toll-Free: 800-4SOCCER
(476-2237)
Fax: 972-334-9960
Website: http://www.usyouthsoccer.org
E-mail:
nationaloffice@usyouthsoccer.org

Swimming And Other Water Sports

Aquatic Exercise Association
P.O. Box 1609
Nokomis, FL 34274
Toll-Free: 888-232-9283
Phone: 941-486-8600
Website: http://www.aeawave.com
E-mail: info@aeawave.com

National Scholastic Surfing Association (NSSA)
P.O. Box 495
Huntington Beach, CA 92648
Phone: 714-378-0899
Fax: 714-964-5232
Website: http://www.nssa.org
E-mail: jaragon@nssa.org

Surfing America, Inc.
33157-B Camino Capistrano
San Juan Capistrano, CA 92675
Phone: 949-276-4660
Fax: 949-496-9190
Website: http://
www.surfingamerica.org

Surfrider Foundation USA
P.O. Box 6010
San Clemente, CA 92674-6010
Phone: 949-492-8170
Fax: 949-492-8142
Website: http://surfrider.org
E-mail: info@surfrider.org

USA Diving
201 S. Capitol Ave.,
Suite 430
Indianapolis, IN 46225
Phone: 317-237-5252
Fax: 317-237-5257
Website: http://www.usadiving.org
E-mail: usadiving@usadiving.org

USA Swimming
1 Olympic Plaza
Colorado Springs, CO 80909
Phone: 719-866-4578
Fax: 719-866-4669
Website: http://www.usaswimming.org

United States Synchronized Swimming
201 S. Capitol Avenue, Suite 901
Indianapolis, IN 46225
Phone: 317-237-5700
Fax: 317-237-5705
Website: http://www.usasynchro.org

USA Water Polo, Inc.
2124 Main Street, Suite 210
Huntington Beach, CA 92648
Phone: 714-500-5445
Fax: 714-960-2431
Website: http://www.usawaterpolo.org

USA Water Ski
1251 Holy Cow Road
Polk City, FL 33868
Phone: 863-324-4341
Fax: 863-325-8259
Website: http://www.usawaterski.org
E-mail: usawaterski@usawaterski.org

Volleyball

Starlings Volleyball Clubs, USA
P.O. Box 61
Imperial Beach, CA 91933-0061
Website: http://www.starlings.org
E-mail: info@Starlings.org

United States Youth Volleyball League
22710 Plaza Del Amo, Suite 808
Torrance, CA 90503
Toll-Free: 888-988-7985
Phone: 310-212-7008
Fax: 310-643-8396
Website: http://volleyball.org/usyvl
E-mail: volleyballorg@hotmail.com

USA Volleyball
715 South Circle Drive
Colorado Springs, CO 80910
Phone: 719-228-6800
Fax: 719-228-6899
Website: http://www.usavolleyball.org
E-mail: postmaster@usav.org

Walking, Running, Jumping, And Climbing

American Double-Dutch League
P.O. Box 567
Cherry Hill, NJ 08003-0567
Phone: 800-982-ADDL (2335)
Website: http://www.usaddl.org
E-mail: ADDLNYC@msn.com

American Hiking Society
1422 Fenwick Lane
Silver Spring, MD 20910
Toll-Free: 800-972-8608
Phone: 301-565-6704
Fax: 301-565-6714
Website: http://www.americanhiking.org
E-mail: info@americanhiking.org

American Running Association
4405 East-West Highway, Suite 405
Bethesda, MD 20814
Toll-Free: 800-776-2732
Phone: 301-913-9517
Website: http://www.americanrunning.org
E-mail: run@americanrunning.org

North American Race Walking Foundation

358 W. California Blvd., #110
Pasadena, CA 91105-2926
Website: http://www.philsport.com/narf
E-mail: narwf@sbcglobal.net

The American Alpine Club

710 Tenth Street,
Suite 100
Golden, CO 80401
Phone: 303-384-0110
Fax: 303-384-0111
Website: http://www.americanalpineclub.org

USA Climbing

P.O. Box 3405
Boulder, CO 80307
Toll-Free: 888-944-4244
Fax: 561-423-0715
Website: www.usaclimbing.net
E-mail: info@usaclimbing.org

Weight Training

National Gym Association, Inc.

P.O. Box 970579
Coconut Creek, FL 33097-0579
Phone: 954-344-8410
Fax: 954-344-8412
Website: http://www.nationalgym.com
E-mail: info@nationalgym.com

National Strength and Conditioning Association (NSCA)

1885 Bob Johnson Drive
Colorado Springs, CO 80906
Toll-Free: 800-815-6826
Phone: 719-632-6722
Fax: 719-632-6367
Website: http://www.nsca-lift.org
E-mail: nsca@nsca-lift.org

Winter Sports

U.S. Ski and Snowboard Association

P.O. Box 100
1500 Kearns Blvd. Building F-100
Park City, UT 84060
Phone: 435-649-9090
Fax: 435-649-3613
Website: http://www.ussa.org
E-mail:webmaster@ussa.org

U.S. Ski Team

P.O. Box 100
Park City, UT 84060
Washington, DC 2007-7684
Toll-Free: 800-809-SNOW (7669)
Website: http://www.usskiteam.com

Chapter 46

Suggested Additional Reading

Books

Bicycling Magazine's New Cyclist Handbook
By Ben Hewitt, Published by Rodale Books, 2005; ISBN: 1594863008

Breathe: Yoga for Teens
By Mary Kay Chryssicas, Published by DK CHILDREN, 2007; ISBN: 0756626617

Fueling the Teen Machine
By Ellen Shanley, Colleen Thompson, Published by Bull Publishing Company, 2001; ISBN: 0923521577

Fitness
By Joanna Watson, Joanna Kedge, Published by Raintree Publishers, 2005; ISBN: 1844431525

Fitness Made Simple
By John Basedow, Published by McGraw-Hill; 1 edition, 2007; ISBN: 0071497080

About This Chapter: The books, articles, webpages, magazines, and newsletters in this chapter were selected from a wide variety of sources deemed accurate. Inclusion does not constitute endorsement. To make topics readily apparent, they are listed alphabetically by title within each category.

Get Rolling, the Beginner's Guide to In-line Skating, Third Edition
By Liz Miller, Published by Get Rolling Books, 2003; ISBN: 0963219634

I Love Yoga: A Source Book for Teens
By Ellen Schwartz, Published by Tundra Books, 2003; ISBN: 088776598X

"I'm, Like, SO Fat!": Helping Your Teen Make Healthy Choices about Eating and Exercise in a Weight-Obsessed World
By Dianne Neumark-Sztainer, Published by The Guilford Press, 2005; ISBN: 1572309806

Rock Climbing: Mastering Basic Skills
By Craig Luebben, Published by Mountaineers Books, 2004; ISBN: 0898867436

RopeSport: The Ultimate Jump Rope Workout
By Martin Winkler, Published by Wiley, 2007; ISBN: 0470036311

Runner's World Complete Book of Women's Running: The Best Advice to Get Started, Stay Motivated, Lose Weight, Run Injury-Free, Be Safe, and Train for Any Distance
By Dagny Scott Barrios, Published by Rodale Books, 2007; ISBN: 1594867585

Street Skateboarding: Endless Grinds and Slides: An Instructional Look at Curb Tricks
By Evan Goodfellow, Doug Werner, Published by Tracks Publishing, 2005; ISBN: 1884654231

Teen Fit For Guys: Your Complete Guide to Fun, Fitness and Self-Esteem
By Gerard Thorne, Published by Robert Kennedy Publishing, 2006; ISBN: 1552100308

The Art of Snowboarding
By Jim Smith, Published by International Marine/Ragged Mountain Press, 2006; ISBN: 0071456880

The Beginning Runner's Handbook: The Proven 13-Week Walk-Run Program
By The Sports Medicine Council, British Columbia, Published by Greystone Books, 2005; ISBN: 1553650875

The Best You Can Be: A Teen's Guide To Fitness And Nutrition
By Christopher Hovius, Published by Mason Crest Publishers, 2005; ISBN: 1590848489

The Performance Zone: Your Nutrition Action Plan for Greater Endurance & Sports Performance
By John Ivy, Robert Portman, Published by Basic Health Publications, 2004; ISBN: 1591201489

Toning for Teens: The 20-Minute Workout that Makes You Look Good and Feel Great!
By Joyce L. Vedral, Published by Grand Central Publishing, 2002; ISBN: 0446678155

Weight Loss Confidential: How Teens Lose Weight and Keep It Off—and What They Wish Parents Knew
By Anne M. Fletcher, Published by Houghton Mifflin, 2007; ISBN: 061843366X

Weight Loss Confidential Journal: Week-by-Week Success Strategies for Teens from Teens
By Anne Fletcher, Published by Houghton Mifflin, 2008; ISBN: 0618433724

Articles

"3 Critical Stretching Exercises," by Dionne McClain, *Volleyball*, vol. 18, no. 1 (January 2007), p. 46-8.

"5 Exercises to Improve Court Movement," by Sarah Walls, *Volleyball*, vol. 19, no. 1 (January 2008), p. 48-51.

412 Fitness Information For Teens, Second Edition

"7 Ways To Make A Heart Rate Monitor Work for You," by Michelle Lovitt, *Volleyball*, vol. 18, no. 4 (April 2007), p. 38-41.

"An Asthma Update," by Joy Bennett Kinnon, *Ebony*, vol. 60, no. 9 (July 2005), p. 84-5.

"Being Disabled Yet Personally Fit," by Jerry Levinson, *The Exceptional Parent*, vol. 36, no. 3 (March 2006), p. 100.

"Cardio Kickboxing: An Effective Way to Spice Up Your Winter Workout," by Lynette Holloway, *Ebony*, vol. 63, no. 2 (December 2007), p. 186, 188, 190.

"Don't Let Excuses Stop You From Getting Fit," *Jet*, vol. 109, no. 15 (April 17 2006), p. 22, 49.

"Eat Breakfast, Drink Milk, Play Xbox," by Charlene O'Hanlon, *T.H.E. Journal*, vol. 34, no. 4 (April 2007), p. 34-6, 38-9.

"Fitting in Fitness," by Jen Chapman, *Current Health 2*, vol. 31, no. 8 (April/May 2005), p. 23-5.

"Gym Quiz," by Jen Chapman, *Current Health 2*, vol. 31, no. 5 (January 2005), p. 21-2.

"Hard-Core [fitness]," by Sabrina McLaughlin, *Current Health 2*, vol. 32, no. 2 (October 2005), p. 14-15.

"Overexercising: Just Don't Do It!" *Ebony*, vol. 63, no. 5 (March 2008), p. 48.

"Rolling, Rolling, Rolling: Get and Stay Fit with Skating," by Stephanie Johnson, *Ebony*, vol. 61, no. 12 (October 2006), p. 90, 92, 94.

"Spice Up Your Workout Routine With Martial Arts," *Ebony*, vol. 62, no. 1 (November 2006), p. 96, 98, 100.

"Test Your Fitness IQ," by Jeff Ives, *Current Health 2*, vol. 34, no. 5 (January 2008), p. 16-18.

"The Importance Of A Balanced Workout," by Asha Taylor, *Ebony*, vol. 61, no. 1 (November 2005), p. 190, 192-3.

"Total-Body Water Workout," by Dina Roth Port, *Prevention* (Emmaus, Pa.), vol. 57, no. 8 (August 2005), p. 109-12, 114.

"Walk It!" by Marianne McGinnis, Merritt Watts, and Natalie Gingerich, *Prevention* (Emmaus, Pa.), vol. 60, no. 1 (January 2008), p. 116.

"Walk the Weight Off—Anywhere," by Kessie Knadler, *Prevention* (Emmaus, Pa.), vol. 59, no. 1 (January 2007), p. 99-102.

Internet Pages, Magazines, And Newsletters

American Cheerleader Magazine
http://www.americancheerleader.com

American Medical Association: Adolescent Health Information
http://www.ama-assn.org/ama/pub/category/1947.html

Bicycling Magazine
http://www.bicycling.com

Black Belt Magazine
http://www.blackbeltmag.com

Climbing Magazine
http://www.climbing.com

Eat Smart Play Hard
http://www.fns.usda.gov/eatsmartplayhard

Fitness For Youth
http://www.fitnessforyouth.umich.edu

GirlPower!
http://www.girlpower.gov

HealthierUS
http://www.healthierus.gov

Healthy People 2010
http://www.healthypeople.gov

Inline Fitness Magazine
http://www.inlinefitnessmag.com

Nutrition.gov
http://www.nutrition.gov

PaddleNews (Kayaking And Canoeing)
http://www.paddling.net

Runner's World
http://www.runnersworld.com

Sports Illustrated for Kids
http://www.sikids.com

Swimming World
http://www.swimmingworldmagazine.com

TeensHealth
http://teenshealth.org

Tennis Magazine
http://www.tennis.com

Transworld Snowboarding Magazine
http://www.transworldsnowboarding.com

USA Junior Hockey Magazine
http://www.usajuniorhockey.com

VERB
http://www.verbnow.com

Water Ski Magazine
http://www.waterskimag.com

Index

Index

Page numbers that appear in *Italics* refer to illustrations. Page numbers that have a small 'n' after the page number refer to information shown as Notes at the beginning of each chapter. Page numbers that appear in **Bold** refer to information contained in boxes on that page (except Notes information at the beginning of each chapter).